Phenomenology for Therapists

Phenomenology for Therapists

Researching the Lived World

By Linda Finlay

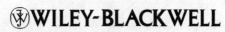

WILEY-BLACKWELL

A John Wiley & Sons, Ltd., Publication

Wiley-Blackwell is an imprint of John Wiley & Sons, formed by the merger of Wiley's global
Scientific, Technical and Medical business with Blackwell Publishing.

Registered Office
John Wiley & Sons Ltd, The Atrium, Southern Gate, Chichester, West Sussex, PO19 8SQ, United
Kingdom

Editorial Offices
350 Main Street, Malden, MA 02148-5020, USA
9600 Garsington Road, Oxford, OX4 2DQ, UK
The Atrium, Southern Gate, Chichester, West Sussex, PO19 8SQ, UK

For details of our global editorial offices, for customer services, and for information about how to
apply for permission to reuse the copyright material in this book please see our website at
www.wiley.com/wiley-blackwell.

Library of Congress Cataloging-in-Publication Data

Finlay, Linda, 1957–
  Phenomenology for therapists : researching the lived world / Linda Finlay.
      p. cm.
  Includes bibliographical references and index.
  ISBN 978-0-470-66646-3 (cloth) – ISBN 978-0-470-66645-6 (pbk.)
  1. Psychotherapy–Methodology.   2. Phenomenology.   3. Spiritual care (Medical care)
4. Psychotherapists.   5. Allied health personnel.   I. Title.
  RC437.5.F56 2011
  616.89′14–dc22

                                                        2011006422

A catalogue record for this book is available from the British Library.

This book is published in the following electronic formats: ePDFs 9781119975113; Wiley Online
Library 9781119975144; ePub 9781119975120

Set in 10.5/13pt Minion by Aptara Inc., New Delhi, India
Printed in Malaysia by Ho Printing (M) Sdn Bhd
1   2011

Contents

About the Author

Linda Finlay is an integrative psychotherapist, occupational therapist and freelance consultant who offers training and mentorship on how to apply qualitative research in health care. In addition to her psychotherapy practice, she teaches psychology and writes with the Open University. Her books include *Groupwork in Occupational Therapy* (1993), *The Practice of Psychosocial Occupational Therapy* (3rd edition, Nelson Thornes, 2004), *Qualitative Research for Allied Health Professionals: Challenging Choices* (co-edited with C. Ballinger, John Wiley & Sons, 2006) and *Relational-centred Research for Psychotherapists* (with K. Evans, Wiley-Blackwell, 2009).

Preface

A personal reflection: As I sit down to write this book, hesitation takes hold of me. It's as if a fog has descended, a wary presence whispering words of caution. I take a moment to dwell with the sensation – I feel warned off. In all probability it springs from my own experience of negotiating the muddy mire of phenomenological theory, of knowing there is not one phenomenology but many . . . I want to navigate a simple path that will guide my readers sure-footedly through this shifting, boggy landscape with its myriad contested ideas and experiences. My shame-voice asks, 'Am I up to the task?' . . . All too easily your own hesitancy and reluctance are summoned: why, after all, should you follow? Then I remember the unexpected and perplexing delights that lie ahead, the strange and irresistible beauty of the phenomenological universe. I want so much to share them with you. The mist of hesitancy lifts a little . . .

Therapists (allied health professionals and psychotherapists alike) are increasingly called upon to do research. Many are drawn to phenomenology; its holistic appreciation of everyday human experience resonates for them. Yet, as novice researcher-practitioners engage the field they are frequently brought up short, baffled by the language and sheer depth of ideas in this strange new world. Soon the novice is faced with bewildering choices. What version of phenomenology should they employ? *Descriptive or hermeneutic? Idiographic or normative? Realist or relativist?* When I engaged my own PhD, I was similarly bamboozled. Just what was phenomenology? And more urgently, how was I supposed to use it for my research?

Phenomenology studies taken-for-granted, everyday examples of the lived world, making explicit the meanings we attach to our human experience. In this book – *Phenomenology for Therapists* – I have tried to show how phenomenology approaches this study and to map the territory (the names, ideas and methods). Rather than being a 'how to' book, I offer a glimpse of the extraordinarily rich and varied terrain of phenomenology, aiming to help budding researchers find their preferred path. Rather than honing in on one particular approach or methodology to the exclusion others, I want to honour the wealth of choices to access and evoke lived experience. I give pointers and examples of how to handle data collection and analysis but I do not spell out the mechanics of the process. I want to show, as Merleau-Ponty expresses it, that phenomenology is 'a problem to be solved and a hope to be realized' (1945/1962, p. viii).

In my writing I have drawn heavily on many *practical examples* of phenomenological research – attempting to show phenomenology in action rather than just talking about it. I invite you to dwell with these examples and feel the register, style and sheer poetry of what is possible. At the end of each chapter I offer some *personal reflections* where I invite you to 'dialogue' with me about the issues and debates at stake.

I belong to three professional communities: occupational therapy, psychology and psychotherapy, but it is in the world of phenomenology that I feel at 'home'. Here I am able to bring my professional identities together, for example, through my research on the life world of the therapist and on the lived experience of disability. And so it is that the process of writing this book has been an integrative and healing project for me. The exercise of explicating phenomenology as a whole has also helped me better understand, and to feel easier about, the apparently divergent voices which have risked sundering the phenomenological world. Phenomenology is not either–or. It is not either 'descriptive' or 'interpretive'; it is both. It enjoys both structure and texture. It is concerned with individuals' experience and with more general phenomenon.

Many people have helped with the evolution of this book. I want first to acknowledge my husband Mel Wilder whose loyal encouragement and judicious editing has helped me to find my 'voice'. Extra special thanks needs to go to David Seamon, Les Todres, Ken Evans and Steen Halling who have so generously given me their time and support, and whose work so inspires. I also would not have been able to write this book without the nourishing conversations over many years with my friends and colleagues in the human science community, particularly: Chris Aanstoos, Rosemary Anderson, Peter Ashworth, Scott Churchill, Karin Dahlberg, Virge Eatough, Kate Galvin, Andy Giorgi, Kevin Krycka, George Kunz, Darren Langdridge, Ilja Maso, Bep Mook, Jim Morley, Eva Simms, Jonathan Smith, Fred Wertz, Peter Willis and Aki Yoshida. The misunderstandings, omissions and all inelegancy within the book are, of course, mine alone. Finally, my thanks needs to be extended to Sue Ram for her invaluable editing and to Andrew Peart (commissioning editor), Karen Shield (project editor), Suchitra Srinivasan (production editor) and the rest of the publishing team for seeing the manuscript through to publication.

Linda Finlay
October 2010

Part I

The Phenomenological Project: Concepts, Theory and Philosophy

Introduction to Part I

Phenomenology invites us to slow down, focus on, and dwell with the 'phenomenon' – the specific qualities of the **lived world** being investigated. 'Our world is our home, a realization of subjectivity' (1972, p. 340), says the philosopher van den Berg. To understand another person, phenomenologists do not inquire about some inner, subjective realm. Instead, understanding comes from asking how the person's *world* is lived and experienced.

Unlike other research approaches, phenomenology does not categorize or explain behaviour nor does it generate theory. It seeks solely to do justice to everyday experience, to evoke what it is to be human. In his celebrated rallying cry, '*Zu den Sachen selbst!*' ('Back to the things themselves!'), Husserl exhorted phenomenologists to go all out to capture the richness and ambiguity of the 'thing'. The process he laid down was one of reflecting on the visceral texture of experience, the sensuous perceiving of life, as it is 'given' to the experiencer, pregnant with layers of implicit meanings.

The introductory chapters which follow seek to present the key concepts as well as the philosophical base of phenomenology. *Chapter 1* invites you into the world of qualitative phenomenological research, which I see as offering a bridge across the **chasm between practice and research**. From my own experience I know that while therapists are exhorted to carry out research and draw on evidence-based practice, many find the lofty world of research far removed from their work at the 'coalface.' Phenomenology, I argue, offers the opportunity to draw these two worlds together.

Phenomenology for Therapists: Researching the Lived World, First Edition. Linda Finlay.
© 2011 Linda Finlay. Published 2011 by John Wiley & Sons, Ltd.

Chapter 2 lays out the **basic principles** of phenomenology, helped by illustrations from actual research projects. I define and explore what I see as the six essential features that make phenomenological research specifically *phenomenological.*

In *Chapter 3*, examples from everyday life, therapy, philosophy and re-search are used to explore the idea (central to phenomenology) that **body and world are intimately intertwined.**

The **philosophical foundations** of phenomenology are laid out in *Chapter 4*. I try to map the key names and main ideas relevant to research in order to give a feel of the richness and complexity of the field. Although the language is frequently dense and obscure, I hope your soul, like mine, will be stirred by what the philosophers in the phenomenological tradition have revealed.

The fifth and final chapter of Part I explores '**the phenomenological attitude**': the special stance – open and non-judgemental – that researchers endeavour to adopt and maintain. In adopting this stance, researchers seek to put aside pre-existing ideas and assumptions (Husserl's 'reduction') and ready themselves to be filled with curiosity and wonder as they engage in what I describe as the 'reductive-reflexive dance'.

Chapter 1

Phenomenology: Bridging the Practice–Research Divide?[i]

We need an imaginative, even outlandish, science to envision the potential of human experience . . . not just tidy reports. (Braud & Anderson, 1998, p. xxvii)

Therapists of all modalities are increasingly exhorted to undertake research. We are pushed to be accountable, to provide evidence of our effectiveness and to draw on 'evidence-based practice' to improve the quality of our services. We may even be threatened with funding cuts and the withdrawal of our services if we fail to use and produce research.

But research can seem remote from, even irrelevant to our practice. Dry language and impenetrable jargon can make academic journal articles confusing, even boring. Much research around seems to be carried out by postgraduate researchers far removed from everyday experiences of work with patients and clients. Clinicians are often short of time, research experience, support and confidence; and this makes the very thought of undertaking research a daunting prospect.

How can the chasm that lies between clinical practice and academic research be bridged? How can research be made relevant to practice so that clinicians actively rejoice in the integration of research findings into their practice? How can research benefit from the insight and understanding of experienced clinicians?

These are wide-ranging questions and only partial or provisional answers can be offered here. There is not the space to address the politics involved to

Phenomenology for Therapists: Researching the Lived World, First Edition. Linda Finlay.
© 2011 Linda Finlay. Published 2011 by John Wiley & Sons, Ltd.

do with money and power (such as the way that policy-driven research may be more about cost cutting and ideologically driven research may be more to do with defining one group as more deserving than another).[ii] Instead, this chapter seeks to demonstrate how phenomenology might build helpful bridges between practice and research.

I start by considering some general **links between practice and research**. The 'chasm' may be smaller than it sometimes feels. The following two sections discuss the implications of using **qualitative research** and **phenomenology** to bridge the divide. Phenomenology, I argue, focuses on issues of concern to therapists and therefore offers valuable knowledge to the profession. Also it nests easily with the skills and professional values of our practice. A research example is offered to demonstrate the potential of phenomenology as a research methodology for therapists.

Research For and In Practice: Linking Therapy and Research

I had a client recently who was challenged by chronic fatigue and struggling to cope with her life. In my effort to better understand her needs and experience, I investigated what current research was saying about the condition, with its profound interlacing of physical and emotional factors. My client was also seeing a complementary therapist and I wanted to learn more about how we could work together. I began by conducting a *literature search*, with the aim of finding out more about chronic fatigue.

My client had explained the impact of her condition on her daily life activities. She told her story and I listened – both to what she was saying and to her *underlying meanings*, to the things she was not saying. I checked out my own evolving understandings with her, and sought to help her describe the experience in richer detail.

In short, I engaged a process of **reflective enquiry**. Together we were 'doing therapy' but there was also a sense in which it was 're-search', or *searching again*. McGuire (1999) well captures these twin dimensions:

> Every counsellor is a researcher: for every time we form an understanding of what is going on for a client, and work with that, we are testing out a hypothesis, and altering our activity in the light of evidence (1999, p. 1).

Here McGuire is referring specifically to counselling but in my view the words apply to every therapy field. Every time we seek to know and understand more about our service users, we are doing research. Every time we reflect upon and evaluate our therapy practice, we are doing research. Every time we take part in auditing our service, we are doing research.

These therapy skills and qualities are directly transferable to the research domain – and vice versa. Both therapy and phenomenological research involve a journey of evolving self–other understanding and growth. They involve similar skills, values and interests, like interviewing skills; critical, reflexive intuitive interpretation; inferential thinking; bodily awareness; and a capacity for warmth, openness and empathy: these are all qualities needed in both therapy practice and qualitative research (Finlay & Evans, 2009). The spirit of the holistic goals we strive for, such as enabling people through rehabilitation to re-enter their 'real world' away from hospital or clinic, and our focus on an individuals' everyday ways of being, doing and functioning are entirely phenomenological in spirit.

The reverse applies too. Some research approaches offer techniques and concepts that can be usefully imported back into therapy. For example, Moustakas (1990) sees his heuristic phenomenological research method, utilizing techniques of self-searching and self-dialogue, as being directly applicable to practice in the form of '*heuristic psychotherapy*'. Gendlin's concept of '*felt-sense*' has a direct application in both therapy and research. Narrative-phenomenological methods have been applied as a form of enquiry in therapy (e.g. Angus & McLeod, 2003) and have influenced the evolution of occupational therapists' *clinical reasoning* (Mattingly, 1998; Mattingly & Fleming, 1994). Also, practice in narrative research has morphed into the practice of *narrative therapy*[iii] (White & Epston, 1990).

Therapists like us, therefore, have distinct advantages over other professionals when it comes to learning about and doing research. With the valuable professional competencies we bring to qualitative or phenomenological research (Finlay & Evans, 2009) we are indeed wanted and needed in research. Further, research stands to be enhanced considerably by our contribution.

If you have been hesitating to cross the bridge between therapy practice and research, I urge you to stride forth. But be warned, you need to choose your route through research territory with care. As for any journey, you need to plan and perhaps get some advice before starting off as there are challenging choices to make (Finlay & Ballinger, 2006). Thinking through the following questions should help you plan your route: What kind of evidence would best show the value of the work you do? What type of evidence should service users and funders rely on to make their choices? Perhaps most importantly, what kind of research are you drawn to and do you want to do?

Choosing the Qualitative Route

The prevailing view of the *evidence-based practice movement*[iv] is that evidence should be 'scientific' and that the best – indeed the only – way to achieve this is through rigorous measurement of (observable) behaviour and the use of standardized protocols and quantification.

This view is erroneous; in fact there are other choices that can be made. While quantitative outcome studies have much to recommend them, they are not the *only* ways to evaluate our practice and explore the value of therapy. As therapists, we know instinctively that some things cannot be sensibly measured or quantified. Measured outcomes do not necessarily reflect the value of our work or inform our practice. Our interests go beyond simplistic behavioural evaluations and qualitative research provides a possible answer.

Qualitative research illuminates the less tangible meanings and intricacies of our social world. Applied to the therapy field it offers the possibility of hearing the perceptions and experience of service users. How do service users experience their health and well-being? What does their illness or disability mean to them? How do they understand and experience therapy? What factors do they see are beneficial? How can in-depth understanding of one patient's experience be presented so as to give insight that informs future practice? And, what do therapists think and feel? What is their experience? How do they understand the processes involved in therapy?

In order to better understand the value of qualitative research we need to begin by considering the ways in which it differs from research based on quantitative methods and approaches – see Table 1.1.

Qualitative research **aims** to be inductive and exploratory, typically asking 'what' and 'how', and posing questions related to description and understanding. Quantitative research, in contrast, seeks to explain and 'prove'. Hypothesis-testing is used with the aim of proving or disproving:

Table 1.1 Contrasting qualitative with quantitative research.

	Qualitative	*Quantitative*
Aims	Inductive and exploratory aiming to describe or explain experience and meanings of the social world	Investigates causal relationships and tests hypothesis aiming to prove or disprove scientifically
Method	*Human* science: interviews, participant observations, creative media, groupwork, etc.	*Natural* science: primarily experiments and surveys
Researcher's role	Research is more subjective: relationship between researcher, participants and the social world acknowledged	Researcher is objective, neutral and detached
Findings	Uses words and creative arts	Uses numbers

it asks, for example, 'why' or 'whether' one treatment is more effective than another.[v]

In **method,** too, there are important differences. Qualitative research is a *human science* rather than a natural science. It explores the textured meanings and subjective interpretations of a fluid, uncertain world. It uses interviews, participant observation, focus groups, creative/projective techniques, reflection and first person writing or diary studies. Quantitative research, in contrast, strives for objectivity. The methods employed are more straightforward and usually involve either experiments (for instance, comparing the results of treatment group A with control group B) or attitude surveys and questionnaires.

The **researcher's role** differs too. In qualitative research the relationship between participants, researchers and their wider social world is actively acknowledged. The researcher recognizes his or her central role in a co-construction of tentative data and is required to explore these dynamics reflexively. Quantitative researchers, on the other hand, assume themselves objective outsiders looking in and obtaining hard data to analyse. The researcher strives for objectivity, detachment and neutrality. In short, qualitative approaches celebrate researcher subjectivity and quantitative ones see subjectivity as 'bias' and claim to eliminate it.

Unsurprisingly, these different aims and methods generate different kinds of **findings.** Qualitative research findings tend to be complex, rich, messy and ambiguous. They are usually expressed through words or through creative arts. Quantitative research favours specific, numerated outcomes with emphasis on scientific rigour (which can sometimes prove reductionist) (Finlay, 2006a).

To help illustrate the special qualities of qualitative research, consider the research of Qualls (1998) into the phenomenon of 'being with suffering'. Nine individuals who had travelled to Eastern Europe to work as volunteers with children in a Romanian orphanage wrote descriptions of their own internal worlds. This was followed by a 'walk-through interview' where they were able work through their accounts with the researcher. On analysing the data phenomenologically, the researcher found that the experience of seeing children being inhumanely treated had drained the participants' personal reserves and challenged their sense of the world and their faith in God. The participants experienced powerful and ambivalent emotions, including simultaneous feelings of love, fear and disgust. Strong supportive bonds with colleagues and a sense of community helped them cope, both during the experience and for years afterwards. This research revealed with clarity and poignancy the struggles and long-term trauma of volunteers in challenging situations. Finding that volunteers required debriefing and long-term support also brought clear policy implications.

The research undertaken by Gilbert (2006) into the impact of the death of a child on social services staff reveals the ability of qualitative research to tap into powerful emotions. As Gilbert recalls the experience:

> I was aware of carrying the feelings of shame, that we should not be talking about C's death and that in raising the issue I was breaking a taboo... co-researchers may not have been aware of its presence, projecting it outwards so I carried the feelings for them. (2006, p. 6)

By drawing on her subjectivity, Gilbert was able to offer valuable 'evidence' to better inform practice and policy regarding the staff support.

To explore other relevant studies see the lists on these useful websites:

http://www.artfulsoftware.com/humanscienceresearch.html and
http://www.phenomenologyonline.com/articles/articles.html.

Choosing Phenomenology as the Qualitative Method of Choice

I hope these examples have reinforced your inclination to consider the qualitative research route. If you have chosen to read this book, you are probably interested in qualitative research already. But what has phenomenology to do with all this? What exactly does it involve, and what does it offer therapists?

The aim of phenomenology is *to describe the lived world of everyday experience*. Lived experience can be general, such as what being a therapist is like, or else specific, such as being pregnant, dying of cancer, or having a sense of 'losing one's footing' after a trauma. Phenomenological research into individual experiences gives insight into, and understanding of, the human condition. Sometimes it languages things we already know tacitly but have not articulated in depth. At other times quite surprising insights reveal themselves. Phenomenology also deepens our understanding of therapy practice and processes helping us in both our personal and professional development.

Phenomenological research is potentially **transformative** for both researcher and participant. It offers individuals the opportunity to be **witnessed** in their experience and allows them to '**give voice**' to what they are going through. It also open new possibilities for both researcher and researched to **make sense of** the experience in focus.

In order to demonstrate the special value of phenomenology, I offer an extended quotation from a published study – see Example 1.1. I conducted this research collaboratively with my co-researcher, Pat, to explore her lived experience of her rehabilitation following a cochlear implant. Drawing on data from participant observation, interview and email correspondence over the course of several months, the resulting analysis focused on Pat's dramatically evolving sensory experience as she learned what sound is and how to hear it.

Example 1.1   A phenomenological study of a changing lifeworld following a cochlear implant[vi]

All her energy was poured into coping with the hyper-noise. As Pat put it, "Everything is so noisy! Putting on a coat, trousers, writing on paper. It is so noisy! Sometimes I can't bear it".

On good days she relished her explorations of the new world unfolding before her . . . She felt a thrill each time she was able to distinguish a sound and hear it for the first time in 50 years . . .

On *bad* days, the surreal quality of all these strange crackling sensations in her head, together with her altered perceptions, made her feel "distracted" and "confused, out of control". It was all so big and overwhelming. With her previous habitual way of being-in-the-world now under constant challenge, her self-confidence took a battering. She struggled to put her deafness in context, experiencing her existence as what she called a "messy limbo":

> "... How many mistakes have I made in my work and interactions that are based in the wrong interpretation of information? I cringe when I think about it ..."

As Pat learned to map an expanding range of sounds, she also had to confront the fact that her relationships with people were changing. People somehow *felt* different, but Pat recognised that she was in fact the one who was changing . . . "Everything has been affected", Pat said, "... my body, my thinking". . . Pat found herself wanting to withdraw from social contact, to hide from the gaze of others. She craved solace from the tensions of her deafness which continue to be revealed to her in her disrupted interactions . . .

> "I don't want to face deafness, disability, implants anymore. I don't like deafness as other people see it . . . I cannot follow things like others do even with the implant."

. . . The full extent of her profound level of deafness, which she felt she had kept hidden [from her self and others], is now uncovered. She feels that she's been caught out and left unprotected in the eyes of the public. She feels this shame both in relation to her present disability and to what she now understands as her past deep-going hearing disablement . . .

She is struggling to accept herself (both her hearing self and her deaf self) while simultaneously seeking to hide from herself. (This extract has been reproduced from Finlay, L. and Molano-Fisher, P. (2008) 'Transforming' self and world: A phenomenological study of a changing lifeworld following a cochlear implant. *Medicine, Health Care and Philosophy*, 11, 255–267, with the kind permission of Springer Publications.)

This research had a major impact on both Pat and myself. For Pat, the process of being witnessed was a powerful and beneficial experience. She valued the opportunity to talk through, and make sense of, the surgery and rehabilitation she felt had derailed her life for a time. On several occasions we recognized a 'therapeutic' element to our research – an unlooked for outcome. For my part, I gained from a deepening friendship with Pat and a new perception of the world.

On a more professional level, the research had an influential 'spreading the word' effect. People considering the option of cochlear surgery have expressed their gratitude to us and the research has affirmed their experience. Doctors and audiologists from different parts of the world have been in touch to thank us for providing a glimpse into their patients' experience. In one case, a somewhat surprised doctor unfamiliar with qualitative research told us 'I have found this very illuminating and I will now give this information to my patients considering the surgery.' Could there be a better validation of the use of qualitative, phenomenological methods?

Reflections

In this chapter I have suggested that qualitative research in general, and phenomenological approaches specifically, offer a bridge across the gulf that separates research from clinical practice within the field of therapy. In addition, I would also argue for small-scale, 'practitioner research' (McLeod, 1999) and **practice-based evidence** to study the value, processes and challenges of therapy. While such practitioner research does not rule out the use of quantitative approaches, I am a strong advocate of qualitative research that explores what health or illness means to individuals and the ways in which they experience therapy. Qualitative research also enables us to hear about practitioners' own views, theories, approaches to, and intuitive hunches about practice allowing us to draw on their experience.

As I see it, phenomenology has a special role in all of this. I want to do and hear about research that teaches me something new and, ideally, moves me in some way. I want research with the potential to contribute something to my practice, to help me to better understand the therapeutic process and my clients' needs. I seek research that enables them to make sense of their own experiences and have this witnessed. I also want to spread the word to others. All this, I argue, can be made possible through recourse to phenomenology, with its enriching and transformative possibilities.

For me, phenomenology has become more than a research methodology. It is a *way of being*.

Between 1977 and 1991, I practised as an occupational therapist (and/or was in the therapeutic field) and then returned to clinical practice in 2008. I spent the intervening years studying phenomenology, getting my PhD and then retraining as an integrative psychotherapist. As I began seeing clients again, I was curious about how 'rusty' my skills would be. Somewhat to my surprise, I realized that I had become a vastly better therapist, more aware of myself, more 'present' with my clients, and far better attuned to their experience. Becoming a phenomenologist has transformed my being and doing.[vii] My capacity to *be-with* an Other has grown. I can sustain an approach to the Other that is open, respectful, non-instrumental and relationally oriented. I can dwell with them as they seek to describe their journey in all its richness and complexity.

Phenomenology has given me these *gifts*. She is a generous friend. You, too, will be richly rewarded if you come with me and cross the bridge.

Notes

[i] Some of the material in this chapter has been drawn from Chapter 4 of Finlay, L. and Evans, K. (2009) *Relational-centred Research for Psychotherapists: Exploring Meanings and Experience,* and has been reproduced here with kind permission of the publisher, Wiley-Blackwell.

[ii] A key politically orientated question to ask about any research is '*In who's interests is this?*' There is a danger that therapy knowledge as published in books/research becomes ever more dominated by academic and policy-driven (and ideologically driven) research. This can only open up the divide between practice and research even more. It also means that practitioners at the coalface who are less engaged in the research world may be silenced, marginalized and undervalued (McLeod, 1999).

[iii] The recognition that humans use narrative structure as a way to organize the events of their lives and to provide a scheme for their own self-identity is of importance for the practice of psychotherapy . . . The telling of the story in itself is held to have therapeutic value, and sharing one's own narrative with others helps bring cohesion to the support group (Polkinghorne, 1988, p. 178).

[iv] I prefer the concept of **practice-based evidence** instead of 'evidence-based practice'. This approach enables relatively small-scale research in natural, everyday clinical settings. It places staff and service users' experiences of therapy at the core of research (Finlay & Evans, 2009; Mellor-Clark & Barkham, 2003). Practice-based evidence can draw on both quantitative and qualitative research approaches. In practice-based research, clinicians are usually the main researchers (perhaps in collaboration with academics) and the research is usually integrated within a therapy programme (or the research is, itself, therapeutic). In such research, practitioners might offer detailed descriptions of some aspect of their clinical case work, perhaps including descriptions of the context and the work with patients/clients. Clinical or narrative **case studies** and/or studies that **audit** particular facets of practice are typical examples of practice-based evidence.

[v] Akihiro Yoshida (2010) offers a detailed explication of the implications of 'why' versus 'what' questions in a teaching context and suggests that both are needed in collaboration.

'Why questions' produce more focused patterned answers providing *explanation* while 'what questions' invite more freeing creative reflections towards understanding.

[vi] This extract has been reproduced from Finlay and Molano-Fisher (2008), 'Transforming' self and world: a phenomenological study of a changing lifeworld following a cochlear implant, in *Medicine, Health Care and Philosophy*, *11*, 255–267, with kind permission of Springer Publications.

[vii] Phenomenology has also impacted on my way of *being-in-the-world* more generally. I think and act phenomenologically: I use my bodily intuitions more readily and I have a greater awareness of the existential issues calling me. I find that when I go to a new place now, I will 'feel myself into' that space. Even the decisions taken in the design of my house were assisted by taking a phenomenological approach!

Chapter 2

The Phenomenological Project

Phenomenology begins in silence . . . Rushing into descriptions before having made sure of the thing to be described may even be called one of the main pitfalls of phenomenology. (Spiegelberg, 1982, p. 693)

Phenomenologists seek to capture **lived experience** – to connect directly and immediately with the world as we experience it. The focus is on our personal or shared meanings, as distinct from the objective physical world explored by science. The aim is to clarify taken-for-granted human situations and events they are known in everyday life but typically unnoticed and unquestioned (Seamon, 2000).

Some phenomenologists talk about lived experience in terms of the nature of 'consciousness' and how experience arises in (or is 'given to') our consciousness. Others favour the concept of 'lifeworld' which is the world that is subjectively lived. However expressed, there is an engagement with, and a faithful commitment to, describing experience in all its richness and layers.

What does this mean in practice? How is lived experience researched? In this chapter I explore and illustrate six facets of what is involved in the phenomenological project. I contend that some measure of each of the following facets needs to be present in every research project if a researcher is really 'doing phenomenology':

1) A focus on lived experience and meanings;
2) The use of rigorous, rich, resonant description;

Phenomenology for Therapists: Researching the Lived World, First Edition. Linda Finlay.
© 2011 Linda Finlay. Published 2011 by John Wiley & Sons, Ltd.

3)   A concern with existential issues;
4)   The assumption that body and world are intertwined;
5)   The application of the 'phenomenological attitude';
6)   A potentially transformative relational approach.

These ideas are introduced here and developed in subsequent chapters. Here, I offer numerous illustrative examples and invite you to dwell with these in order to get a feel for the phenomenological project.

A Focus on Lived Experience and Meanings

Phenomenologists are interested in *embodied* lived experience and the meanings held about that experience. The aim is to describe the phenomenon (i.e. an event, object, situation, process) as it is known through our everyday experience of it.

The phenomena that are open to phenomenological research are many and varied. The sheer range can bemuse novice researchers trying to grapple with what a phenomenon represents. In practice, research can be focused on specific phenomena such as 'the moment of insight in therapy' or 'experiencing the rush of doing a bungee jump' at one end of the spectrum, to broader studies such as those exploring 'the experience of first love' or 'the lifeworld of a therapist'. Often, studies will focus on specific moments of experience and yet from such seeds a whole 'world' can sometimes be discovered. (We see this in psychotherapy when a focus on the *here-and-now* in the therapy encounter also seems to contain a *there-and-then* of the client's wider history and world.)

Phenomenologists vary in the degree to which they focus on the specific as opposed to the general. Mostly phenomenologists attend to specific instances of a phenomenon as part of a larger project to describe its more general qualities. Instances of lived experience get transformed, through in-depth analysis, into textual description of the essences of the phenomenon – a description which hopefully resonates and evokes the experience. In other words, analysis typically moves from individual experience to general insight. The challenge here is to break free of the basic data (e.g. participants' accounts) and **focus on the phenomenon**. A further challenge is to break free of literal meanings of what participants say is their experience and to intuit **implicit meanings**.

The following example shows how individuals' stories of lived experience may be merged into an overarching general description. It comes from my PhD research exploring lifeworld of 12 occupational therapists (Finlay, 1998a). Here I summarize one dimension of the therapists' lifeworld: their sense of professional self. If you are an occupational therapist, as you read, see if this description resonates with your own experience. If you are not an occupational therapist, does any of the experience apply to your work?

> They search for an identity. They struggle to negotiate the boundaries of their ambiguous role – a task made more difficult in a changing health care context. Whilst they embrace their profession's values, they are also ambivalent, to the extent of rejecting certain elements of occupational therapy . . . They struggle to apply their holistic values in a work context which demands more efficient, reductionist practice. Feeling misunderstood and under-valued by others, they internalise others' dismissiveness, and this damages their sense of professional self-esteem.
>
> But the therapists are committed to their mission to help others. They value what occupational therapy can offer and believe that it can make a significant and meaningful contribution in treatment. 'Doing occupational therapy' is experienced as being satisfying, interesting and enjoyable, though often difficult. They enjoy their craft, using themselves as treatment tools and participating in treatment activities. They are challenged by the problem-solving process which draws on both creative inspiration and scientific techniques. Whilst the daily therapy routines can be boring and/or frustrating, they take much pleasure in achievement. The therapists are particularly thrilled when they see any transformation in their patients/clients . . . it raises their professional self-esteem. (Finlay, 1998a, p. 246)

Such descriptions of lived experience often arise out of participants' narratives which the researcher synthesizes and elaborates further, as in the example above. Descriptions may also be based on **personal reflection**. Consider, for example, Milloy's (2005) research on the lived experience of doing research and writing where she offers a description of the process of how words can be generated in the body – what she calls the 'proprioceptive register':

> The whole body is poised in between . . . Paperthin, the page weighs nothing. The words slowly weigh it down, and page by page, the heaviness transfers and shifts, yet I don't become lighter: there is more. More to breathe, more to feel, more to birth, more to penetrate. The words re-invent themselves after the coitus of momentary truth, pass further into more . . . Writing is the moisture I excrete, the air I breathe. (Milloy, 2005, pp. 546–547)

The Use of Rigorous, Rich, Resonant Description[i]

Phenomenological accounts seeks to describe experience systematically in all its density, poignancy, richness and paradox. Full description is prized above any kind of explanation or theorising. *Why* a person might have said something matters less than *what* might be being revealed in the saying/experiencing.

Aanstoos, for instance, obtained vivid concrete written descriptions from 25 students of their own particular experiences of 'feeling left out'. He then synthesized these into a '**composite structural description**' to capture a sense of one's world when feeling left out. Note how he uses language to evoke the experience:

> Experiencing ourselves as left out evokes an intensely disquieting and painful emotional storm. Previously taken for granted meanings of who we are for others, and who they are for us, are sundered from their past familiar anchors . . . The smooth reciprocity of self-other relations gives way, and we are confronted by a disturbing negativity. This negativity expresses itself as a tear in the unfolding tapestry of mutual recognition between ourselves and the others . . . We look, with trepidation, to the other; but our appeal goes unheeded, even unnoticed . . . we discover . . . in horror that we are invisible to others . . . The previous gnawing possibility of isolation proves inescapable; its preceding virtuality now becomes an all-consuming reality. (Aanstoos, 1987, cited in Moustakas, 1994, p. 141)

With phenomenological description, researchers tap into the **ambiguity** and contradictions inherent in experience in order to capture layers of complexity.[ii] For example, research into the lifeworld of patients following flexor tendon injury and surgery (Fitzpatrick & Finlay, 2008) sheds light on the lived experience of the rehabilitation phase following flexor tendon surgery. It reveals how profoundly challenging the experience is at every level: emotional, practical and social. Every hour of every day is a frustrating, painful struggle as individuals seek to cope with the pain and trauma of the injury, the surgery, the rehabilitation exercise programme and the challenge of one-handed living. Participants are immersed in a world of ambivalence; they struggle *and* adapt; retreat *and* do battle; deny *and* accept. They fight against the body while also protecting it and caring for it. They feel overwhelmed with pain while at the same time that they try to hide and deny it. They oscillate between:

> Needing care from others while rejecting it; between enacting a new disabled identity while hanging on to a non-disabled identity; between curtailing involvement in the world while determinedly forging ahead. (Fitzpatrick & Finlay, 2008, p. 150)

Phenomenological descriptions often blur the boundaries between **science and art** (between empirical studies and literary evocations) although individual researchers will have their preferences.[iii] Some phenomenological researchers are more concerned to be rigorous and systematic, taking a science-like approach to offering fine-grained, normative descriptions. Others take imaginative flight using poetic flourishes, images and metaphors.

Rather than seeing phenomenology as either science or art, it might best be considered along a continuum with pure rigorous, scientific description on one end and fluidly poetic interpretation at the other, with most practice falling somewhere in the middle. Todres (2007; Todres & Galvin, 2006), for example, argues for the balanced harmony of a middle ground where both **structure** and **texture** can be attended to. He suggests that scientifically orientated phenomenologies run the risk of offering drier, more distanced accounts while attending excessively to textual dimensions can result in poetic presentations where meanings are left too implicit. Bringing structure and texture together, he describes the process of moving between closeness and distance:

> In exercising 'closeness' I attempted to enter my informants' experiences and bring the 'heart' of these textures to language. In exercising 'distance' I entered a more academic moment and attempted to tease out some of the meanings in a more thematic way (Todres, 2007, p. 58).

A Concern with Existential Issues

Like phenomenologically orientated therapy, phenomenological research is concerned with existential issues (i.e. that which relates to the experience of existence; our human condition). It engages our human concerns relating to life, ageing and death, being and becoming, embodiment and identity, choice and meaningfulness, belonging and needs, sense of time and space, freedom and oppression, and so on.

Continental phenomenological philosophers such as Sartre (1943/1969), Heidegger (1927/1962) and Merleau-Ponty (1945/1962) have outlined key structures of human existence (also called '**lifeworld**'). They argue that we all have an *embodied sense of self* which is always in *relation to others*, while our consciousness is shared with others through *language, discourse, culture and history*. We experience *time* in our recollection of past joys and trauma. We also anticipate what is to come in the future. We are placed into a matrix of *spatial relations* in the world surrounded by things which have *meaning* while we engage with ideas and activities which become our *projects*. We are thrown into the world in order to live: we act, make choices, strive, become. And ultimately we die.

language, discourse how have if cannot hea

Applying these concepts to research, van Manen (1990, p. 101) recommends that we use four fundamental lifeworld themes – he calls them 'existentials' – as helpful guides for reflection on our research: '*lived space* (spatiality), *lived body* (corporeality), *lived time* (temporality), and *lived human relation* (relationality or communality)'. **Lived space** is the way place or space is experienced, for instance, how a dark alley can be threatening or a home can feel cosy. **Lived body** is the way we feel our body such as when we are sluggish, energized or we have a 'bad hair' day. **Lived time** is subjective time rather than clock time such as how a boring meeting can feel endless or an enjoyably dramatic film can flash by in no time. It is also the way meanings of past experience can become superimposed on present and future ones (and vice versa) such as the way a client in a negative transference with a psychotherapist may anticipate persecution or neglect. **Lived relations** is our experience of others such as when we can feel shamed by another's critical gaze or how we can blossom under a loving one.

The next extract is from Carel's (2008) book on her experience of living with illness (specifically the rare disease of lymphangioleiomyomatosis – LAM). She takes a broader existential focus touching on lived space, time and body. Note also her rich descriptions, including her artful use of imagery and metaphor:

> My future held no promise but the promise of decline and a rapidly shrinking world. Because I am exposed to so much uncertainty, I had to find a way not to worry about it too much ... My lungs could collapse at any time, rendering them useless ... In the first days after my diagnosis I was terrified and walked delicately, sensing danger everywhere ... The fragility, but also the preciousness, of the present became a fundamental building-block of my experiences. I learned to dwell in the present and stop the terrain of thoughts about the future, about all the scary painful things that could happen, about needing a lung transplant. Things that seemed surreal became my daily bread. Using oxygen, having a life-threatening illness, suffering severe breathlessness at every twist and turn of my daily routine; these became my breakfast, lunch and dinner. They are with me when I first open my eyes each morning and are the last thought of the day. I struggle not to let them fill every thought in between ... All my energy and happiness are funnelled into the *now*, into today: how nice it feels to be *here*, in the sun, having a massage, listening to beautiful music, laughing until I am dizzy, sitting by a warm fire, experiencing friendship, love, sunshine, the lazy sensation of waking up after a deep sleep, the sharp authority of beauty. (Carel, 2008, pp. 124–125)

Carel's words above are imbued with her embodied, emotional way of being in the world of daily activities. Ratcliffe (2008)[iv] talks about **existential feelings** as background orientations through which experience is structured and which involve our bodily relationship with the world e.g.

'feeling trapped in a situation'; 'feeling fulfilled'; 'feeling safe and secure'; 'feeling distant'; 'feeling of depersonalization'. He considers them to be *more than* emotion in that they are not directed *to* something like 'feeling angry' or 'in love'. Instead they are woven into our perception, bodily being and experience of the world. Existential feelings challenge dualisms of: self versus world, inside versus outside self, affect versus cognition, bodily versus non-bodily, subject versus object. None of these polarized ways of looking at the world apply to the way we find ourselves in it. *Self and world are experientially related*. This is the point made in the next section.

The Assumption that Body, Self and World are Intertwined

Examples like Carel's above remind us how our body becomes absorbed in life activities and mostly drifts into the background as a kind of taken-for-granted horizon (although it can suddenly become figural when we become ill or are made to feel self-conscious). The point is that, *viewed phenomenologically*, body-self-world are intertwined.

Phenomenology champions a holistic, non-dualist approach to life. The dualist distinction between the mental and material world is woven into our Western thinking and language (Ashworth, 2006). Our Western science has taught us to split mind–body, split mental processes from the physical world. Phenomenology wants us to relinquish our conditioning and to bring together the polarities of mind-body, self-other, individual-social, feelings-thoughts, body-soul, nature-nurture, mental-physical, subject-object. The hyphen signifies intertwining rather than separation: the world does not exist 'out there' separate from our perceptions, rather it is part of us and us of it. 'The world is not an object', says Merleau-Ponty, it is the 'field for, all my thoughts and all my explicit perceptions . . . [It is] what I live through . . . I am in communication with it' (1945/1962, p. xvii).

So, for instance, while scientists might talk of perception as arising in the senses and interpreted by the brain, phenomenologists see perception as arising from our bodily engagement with the world. The world's colours, tones and textures proclaim themselves through our senses; space is disclosed through our body movements; a sense of self arises through our relations with others and is revealed to us through our own embodied reaching out. It is only in the world that we can come to know ourselves.

The following extract recognizes the interconnection between body and world. Here, Jager (2010) slowly, painstakingly and evocatively describes a scene in true phenomenological fashion. One day, he happened to be walking in a shopping centre past an improvised children's zoo enclosed within a circular space boundaried by bales of straw. He is delighted to notice the lively interest of children observing animals:

> I noticed a dozen chickens, a few rabbits, a sleeping pig undisturbed by her litter of suckling piglets, a young calf and a most beautiful, fairy-tale white young goat. The zoo had no doubt been arranged to amuse the city children, many of whom had never before seen a rooster stride across a barnyard or heard a piglet squeal . . .
>
> A young girl of perhaps four years old drew my particular attention. The child looked with uncommon concentration at [the] white goat that, as if in response to the girl's curiosity, slowly walked over to where she stood and then stuck her head across the bales of straw in her direction. The animal appeared as curious about the children as the children were about her. It is hard to say what it was that so transfixed the girl's attention on this particular animal.
>
> Perhaps it was the extraordinary shiny whiteness of its coat, or the rosy white snout or perhaps the tiny beard. The girl kept a little distance from the straw encirclement but now, with the animal so close to her she ventured a further step in her direction. She then hesitated for a few more moments before stretching out her arm and gingerly touching the neck of the animal. As she began to stroke the goat stretched her neck, closed her eyes and then stood completely still to receive the child's caress. It was at that moment that I saw the child's face break out in a very broad and triumphant smile . . .
>
> She already understood how to enter into a dialogue with others and to form a bond with an attractive stranger. She did not approach the young goat as a material object contained within a natural universe but as a fellow creature inhabiting a common, cosmic world. The broad smile announced that the goat had consented to be her neighbor and that from that moment on they would no longer fear each other or treat one another as complete strangers . . . This cosmos came into being at the very moment when the child reached out, touched the animal and found it receptive to her touch. A threshold was established at the very spot where the child's hand touched the goat's neck and at the very moment when the goat acknowledged the girl's presence and permitted her to enter her domain. (Jager, 2010, pp. 85–86)

As therapists, we well understand this idea of body-self-world intertwining. In the health care field, we appreciate the infinitely complex interconnections between physical and mental health, between health and social circumstances. In the field of psychotherapy, we use ourselves as tools in the therapy and subtly intertwine with our clients (Finlay, 2010a) exploring their sense of self and lived worldly experience. We accept that the only access we have to the other's unconscious and implicit meanings is through the 'between' – that mysterious intersubjective space where the client and therapist meet and to some extent merge, as empathy and transference overtake us.

Carel's description above of living on the edge of death chronicles this intimate interlacing of body and world. Her illness (and sense of body and self) is encountered in the context of her daily activities within the physical world as well as in the context of her aspirations, history and relationships: the relational and social realms of the lifeworld.

As phenomenologists and researchers, we do not access an 'inner world' so much as an individual's relationship to the world.[v] Person and world are intertwined: 'man [sic] is in the world, and only in the world does he know himself' (Merleau-Ponty, 1945/1962, p. xi). If we could ever get 'inside' a consciousness, Sartre reminds us, we would be seized by a whirlwind and thrown back out into the world(!)

The Application of the 'Phenomenological Attitude'

As the quote at the beginning of the chapter says, 'Phenomenology begins in silence'. At the core of the phenomenological method is a process of intuiting in which the phenomenologist attempts to be open, to meet the phenomenon in as fresh a way as possible. This involves dwelling with the phenomenon and '**bracketing**' (excluding or pushing aside) our habitual ways of perceiving the world. This demanding operation requires deep reflection and critical concentration where the phenomenon is viewed with curiosity and disciplined naiveté (Giorgi, 1985). The aim is to connect directly and immediately with the world as we experience it – as opposed to thinking about it. Here taken-for-granted assumptions, judgements and theories are temporarily suspended (or at least reined in) in order to see the world anew.

All too often the process of bracketing in phenomenology is wrongly understood to be an exercise in objectivity, one undertaken to minimize bias. In fact, rather than striving to be unbiased, distanced or detached, the researcher aims to be fully engaged, involved, interested in and open to what may appear. Researcher subjectivity is prized and intersubjectivity is embraced. Rather than objectivity, the challenge here is to juggle the contradictory stances of being 'scientifically removed from', 'open to' and 'aware of' while simultaneously interlacing with research participants in the midst of their own personal experiencing.

Many contemporary phenomenologists now argue the need for researchers to explicitly and reflexively engage their own subjectivity through both *bracketing* and *reflexivity* (i.e. researcher self-awareness) (Finlay, 2008; Langdridge, 2007; Rennie, 1992; Walsh, 2004). It is seen as inevitable that researchers bring their subjective selves into the research along with preconceptions which both blinker and enable insight. Researchers are an inevitable part of what is being researched. Findings do not emerge by a participant talking to a passive, distant researcher who receives information, but from within a constantly evolving, dynamic and co-created relational process to which both participant and researcher contribute (Finlay & Evans, 2009). There is a dance-like quality to this process, grace essential to skilled application:

> Caught up in the dance, researchers must wage a continuous, iterative struggle to become aware of, and then manage, pre-understandings and habitualities that inevitably linger. Persistence will reward the researcher with special, if fleeting, moments of disclosure in which the phenomenon reveals something of itself in a fresh way. (Finlay, 2008, p. 1)

In the following passage I reflect on my co-researcher's experience of learning to hear following a cochlear implant, having been profoundly deaf for 50 years (see Example 1.1 in *Chapter 1*). Pat had the challenge of learning how to pick up and distinguish sounds through using her 'ears first' rather than relying on the interpretation of visual cues which she had done previously as a lip-reader. She confronted the bewildering babble of a new and noisy world. Over several months following her surgery, Pat and I together set out together to explore, through interview and ongoing emails, her changing perceptions and lived experience. One weekend I witnessed directly how a new world was opening up for her:

> Together we went for a walk in the woods. It was an extraordinary experience. Step by step, I found myself tuning into her world ... I discovered my own perception changing just as Pat's was changing. Previously I would have thought our walk in the woods would have been wonderfully peaceful and quiet. Now, I was seeing/hearing the world differently. What a cacophony: birds, leaves rustling, cars, trains, voices ... Yes, it is an incredibly noisy world! I was reminded of Abram's evocative phrase: "promiscuous creativity of the senses" (Abram, 1996, p. 58). Only now can I appreciate what he was saying. (LF diary entry)

A Potentially Transformative Relational Approach

As the quote above shows, the process of exploring the human condition can throw up unexpected riches that go beyond findings and outcomes. As we engage in research (be it as a participant, researcher or reader), we can be touched and moved. We can be made to cry. In gaining new understandings we are changed.

The relational process of engaging research can itself be transformative – and this applies to both participant and researcher. The research by Padilla (2003) with Clara, a woman who had lived with disability resulting from severe brain injury sustained 21 years earlier in a car accident, offers a good example. He embarked on collaborative in-depth research with Clara, who was prepared to reflect on her experiences. Drawing on data from 11 semi-structured interviews and 72 email exchanges (Clara's preferred mode of communication), Padilla's analysis revealed three key themes:

- *Nostalgia* – Clara was found to constantly and regretfully compare her current and past (prior to the accident) selves.
- *Abandonment* – Clara struggled to retain control over her body and to sustain relationships with significant others. She could be understood to have abandoned both herself and others.
- *Hope* – Through her existential reflections, Clara realized she needed to let go of her past and actively discover meanings and purpose in her present life.

Reflecting on the value of their research, Padilla notes how the phenomenological process enabled Clara's self-exploration, her **search for meaning** and a construction of a new identity. The reflective, collaborative process proved valuable to the researcher, too. He was able to reflect on his own preconceptions and 'able-ist' prejudices, recognizing that they were inherent in occupational therapy practice. He began to question the way therapists may be too quick to focus on restoring function and fail to attend to service users' own experience of disability. His research led him to suggest using collaborative, reflective investigation with clients as a potential tool for therapy as well as for research.

Reading phenomenology can also be transformative. Phenomenology brings us back to our experience – something that we take for granted and 'pass over in silence' (Sartre 1943/1969). Phenomenology grabs our attention and reminds us what it means to be human. Sometimes phenomenological descriptions can prove even more compelling and stirring than the original experience. Phenomenological writing, van Manen notes, can bring 'an otherwise sober-minded person (the reader but also the author) to tears and to a more deeply understood worldly engagement' (van Manen, 1990, p. 129).

Perhaps because we can recognize in others' accounts something our own experience, we are touched and reminded of our human interconnections. But it also has the power to move us into *new* understandings. As therapists we sometimes have to work harder to understand what it is like to, say, have a particular condition which we ourselves have not experienced. Phenomenology has the potential to offer us a window onto new realms.

Reflections

In this chapter I have argued that what makes phenomenological research specifically *phenomenological* is the presence (to a greater or lesser extent) of all six facets discussed above. Through a special open, non-dualist, phenomenological attitude phenomenologists describe, systematically and in rich detail, what it means to be human. Both the process of researching embodied lived experience and the evocative findings that result have the potential to be transformative.

There are many wonderful ethnographical, biographical and grounded theory studies, together with a huge pool of literary works, which successfully disclose aspects of the nature of human existence. However, *not all studies that focus descriptively on lived experience are phenomenological.* Studies that focus on subjective experience (e.g. cognitions or emotions) without attending to the phenomenological attitude and the underpinning non-dualistic philosophical theory are probably best considered to be phenomenologically inspired or orientated rather than phenomenology per se. Similarly, studies that emphasize explanation and analytic interpretation (for instance, categorizing experience using preformed theoretical constructs) also move away from the phenomenological project.

Phenomenology – when it is done well – discloses, transforms and inspires. That is why it excites me, why I am passionate about it. It is not just a research method. It offers a way of both being in *and* of seeing the world, from inside *and* out. It is not just an intellectual project; it is a life practice. It is concerned with the discovery and celebration of our own immersion in body-world experience. The phenomenological project calls the researcher to be reflectively open to connecting with the phenomenon in all its complexity. When I do phenomenological research, I immerse myself in wonder and awe of the other's experience. I want to be caught up inside that experience. Through it, I become enchanted and fascinated with the ambiguity, multiple layers and mysterious paradoxical depths of human existence.

The strength of this method lies in its ability to bring to life the richness of existence through description of what may appear at first sight to be ordinary, mundane living. The magic comes when we focus so deeply on aspects of individuals' ordinary lives we see that what is revealed is, invariably, something special; something *more*. What is revealed is actually quite extra-ordinary.

Notes

[i] The concept of '**description**' as powerful in its own right is central to the phenomenological project. But the term is ambiguous and it is worth considering its different layers.

Description can be contrasted with '**explanation**'. Here we can say that phenomenology aims to describe rather than explain *why* something happens. (A study on the experience of anger would focus on just describing that experience rather than accounting for it.) Description can also be contrasted with '**interpretation**'. While phenomenologists vary about where they sit on the description–interpretation continuum, they all lean to the description side in that they tend – in the first instance anyway – to resist importing external theories and interpretive frameworks, such as bringing in psychoanalytic interpretations.

ii To give a different example, Todres and Galvin (2010) characterize 'existential well-being' in spatial terms as a kind of 'dwelling-mobility' where there is both a feeling of rootedness *and* flowing movement; a being-at-home-with what has been given *and* the adventure of being called into different existential possibilities. Their theory of well-being thus incorporates the value of experiencing a sense of 'not feeling at home' or 'not feeling one's self' (such as when we are ill) which they say can be an energizer. At the same time, there is a sense of safety and contentment in the familiar and habitual.

iii Phenomenology has had a long-standing relationship to the arts in aiming to offer rich description (e.g. Sartre has shown a fascination for the French novelist Flaubert). Descriptions are artful in the way they engage literary forms such as metaphor and poetry. *Chapter 7* expands more fully on this more artful dimension.

iv Ratcliffe is drawing on Heideggerian conceptions of 'mood as atmosphere' related to our ontological disposition ('attunement'). These concepts refer to the way mood is like a pervasive atmosphere or cultural ambience which surrounds us and is already 'there' before being experienced in the body. It is about having a certain attuned relationship toward the world:

> When I am in a mood of sadness, then things address me quite differently or not at all. Here we do not mean feeling in the subjective sense ... Feeling [as existential mood] concerns my whole being-in-the-world ... Attunement ... belongs to being-in-the-world as being addressed by things. (Heidegger, 1987/2001, pp. 202–203)

v Often novice researchers will define phenomenology, not entirely correctly, as being concerned with *inner* realms experience (i.e. what is going on 'within' the person). The focus then becomes an individual's subjective thoughts and feelings. This rather misses the point of what it means to research embodied experience which is lived out in the world. Body and world are intertwined; inside and outside are not polarized. As Merleau-Ponty says, 'To be born is both to be born of the world and to be born in the world' (1945/1962, p. 453).

Chapter 3

The Body in Lived Experience

The body stands before the world and the world upright before it, and between them there is a relation that is one of embrace. (Merleau-Ponty, 1964/1968, p. 271)

It is impossible to separate our bodies from who we are and what we do in the world. Our body is the vehicle for experiencing, doing, being and becoming. We use our bodies before we think about it in everyday life activities. Through our bodies we perceive the world and relate to others, and – in the process – we learn about ourselves. These are, you might say, obvious, common-sense ideas about the body. However, phenomenologists take them further, identifying subtle and profound ways person–body and others–world are intimately *intertwined*.

The mouth that opens when its side is touched . . . orients to and already out-lines the shape of the mother's nipple. The newborn's body molds itself into the mother's arms, fitting along the groove between her arm and abdomen. Newborn eyes can see the perfect distance of twelve inches: the bull's-eye of the breast's aureole and the maternal face. Infants love to gaze at their mothers, a gaze that is one with the rhythm of breathing, sucking, and swallowing, which are reflexive responses as well. Babies are perfectly made for taking in their mother's milk, calling it forth with a gesture or a cry. The skin as the boundary line between two bodies is breached again and again in the evocation and gift of milk . . . Perhaps more than any other substance milk is

Phenomenology for Therapists: Researching the Lived World, First Edition. Linda Finlay.
© 2011 Linda Finlay. Published 2011 by John Wiley & Sons, Ltd.

the visible sign of the invisible, the in-between body, the chiasm, the flesh of mother and infant. Its fluidity refuses to belong to one or the other. (Simms, 2008a, p. 14)

In the above passage Simms reminds us how we begin life not as separate persons but as intertwined beings: the newborn's body and actions merge with that of the (m)other. The primary experience of the newborn involves moving towards a world of others or things while this movement is already prefigured in the child's body. The body is fundamentally implicated in all lived experience.

This chapter explores the phenomenological significance of the body through giving numerous practical examples and quotations. It is worth dwelling with these as a way to understand what phenomenology is striving for.

In the first section I discuss the nature of **embodied lived experience** using different examples, including an extended example of research I conducted with an individual who had multiple sclerosis. In the second section, we turn to phenomenological **philosophy** and examine some of the different ways the body has been theorized. The final section explores how researchers might use their bodies in **research**. I argue the value for researchers to attend *reflexively* to the body – be it the body of participant or researcher.

Embodiment and Lived Experience

The lived body is an *embodied consciousness* which engages with its surrounding world. It is not only directed to things in the world, it is a point of view: it opens up the world as a world of possibilities and potentialities.

In the eyes of phenomenologists, bodily experience and sense of belonging to the world are one and the same. The phenomenological philosopher Sartre picks up this point when he describes when we read with sore, tired eyes, the feeling of the eyes (eyelids) is shown in the reading when words become detached . . . 'they may tremble, quiver; their meaning may be derived only with effort' (1943/1969, p. 332).

Phenomenological researchers aim to tap into the insight that our bodies are in continuous relation with the world by focusing explicitly on the kinaesthetic, sensory, visceral and **'felt sense'** dimensions of bodily lived experience. At the same time, phenomenologists understand that bodies are not removed from our emotional-cognitive, relational and social worlds.

This body-world connection can be shown in: our everyday interactions with the world; in our embodied way of being as therapists; and in terms of what happens to our body-world relations when we are ill.

Everyday body-world interconnections

When we want to watch television, we reach for the remote; when we feel hungry, we check the fridge for food to satisfy our need; when listening to music our foot taps the beat; when someone makes us happy, we smile; when our team scores, we cheer; when greeting a friend, we subtly negotiate whether or not there will be a hug, kiss or more than one kiss; when writing an email to a friend, our fingers fly over a keyboard expressing our thoughts and feelings. Our bodies are the particular point of access to, view of, and way of relating to our worlds.

Mostly we live our body-world interconnection **pre-reflectively**, without thought with the body having its own wisdom and memory. We see this in everyday examples as we act on auto-pilot using our procedural memory. I am struck by this when I travel abroad and drive on the right-hand side of the road. It amazes me how easily my body adapts, yet every so often my left hand still searches fruitlessly for the gear shift. Sometimes, if I have been driving too much, I find that I sit at the dining table and try to put my seat-belt on! When a set of embodied movements are inhabited fully and routinely, they are remembered without consciousness by the fibre of the body.[i]

This phenomenon is exploited by highly skilled performers or sports people when they seek the unconscious **flow**[ii] of their art. In contrast, excessive conscious reflection on skills can cause a breakdown of performance. For example, at the time of writing the British tennis player Andy Murray (currently ranked 4 in the world) has inexplicably lost in the first round of his last four tournaments. Commentators are lining up to talk of performance breakdown ('the yips') caused by over-thinking.

When we are absorbed in life activities, our body drifts into the background becoming a kind of *existential setting* or activity space. It is an ever-present horizon but it can suddenly become figural, for example, when we become ill or injured and can no longer use our bodies in customary ways and/or when consciously reflect on our lived experience (as we ask participants to do in research). Our bodies can also become figural when we suddenly feel watched by another. As we become aware of their regard we begin to exist in a new bodily self-conscious, unnatural way.

> Under the critical gaze the body may turn awkward . . . under the admiring gaze the body surpasses its usual grace . . . the person in love may incarnate his or her erotic mode of being in a subtle glow. (van Manen, 1990, p. 104)

When a gaze is critical and objectifying we can feel embarrassed, even ashamed. More specifically, when our body is seen and experienced as an object somehow separate from our self, it is profoundly objectifying[iii] and thus alienating – not least because we are not in control of what traits are ascribed to us. The following quotation from a study exploring the experience of shame illustrates this point:

> A shamed person feels objectified, put on stage as a thing for others to look at and judge. When a person's devalued or discrediting quality is exposed to the view of others, the subjective reaction against such an exposure is a desire to become invisible, to escape from the situation as soon as possible . . . Individuals experience a "burning in a face"; "My face would be flushed" or "It's like a sting or slap in a face." Avoidance of eye contact is perceived as a common tactic by which persons seek to escape from "facing a world."
> (Ablamowicz, 1992, pp. 41–42)

The body-world of the therapist

Think for a minute about your own body and how you inhabit it when you are working. If you are a psychotherapist you may well use your body consciously and reflexively (i.e. in a self-aware way) as a therapeutic tool. If you are a therapist who does a lot of handling and lifting of patients, you will probably be aware of your body positioning, balance and strength, and using these therapeutically.

The following extract comes from my PhD research on the lifeworld of the occupational therapist. In this study I employed interview, participant observation and personal reflection to explore the lived experience of 12 occupational therapists. Below I summarize my findings of their lived bodily experience showing that, somehow, the body is always involved and subtly implicated in their work, often without conscious thought:

> Through body language therapists present as people to be trusted, people who care. Through touch they express support, comfort, warmth and mutual friendship. They handle, lift, hold and embrace their patients/clients, both physically and mentally, in order to give treatment and keep them safe. In these ways the therapists use their 'trusted-healer body' as a therapeutic tool.
>
> Behind the 'trusted-healer body' is a 'scientist-professional body' which is more clinical, analytical and distant. This body carries keys, wears a white uniform, sits behind a desk. It also observes patients/clients – examines, probes, diagnoses. In these ways therapists display status and power – a remote image they also seek to counteract . . .
>
> They have to be careful about when they use touch and how it will be received. They want to be friendly, trusted and attractive yet deny their sexual body as it contradicts their other bodies. For women therapists, their sexual body is additionally a vulnerable body that can be threatened and invaded. When they come to work, they prefer to leave this more personal body at home.

Finally, the therapists seek to nurture, reassure, enable and care. As patients'/clients' express their needs, so the therapists respond. But . . . their bodies can feel invaded, grabbed at and sucked dry. In this way, the therapists engage a 'mother body' – one that can feel both loving and exhausted. (Finlay, 1998a, pp. 247–248)

The body-world of illness

Now consider the last time you were ill. What changes occurred in your bodily way of being? Phenomenologists highlight how when we are ill there is both an altered experience of one's whole body and an altered experience of the world – and that these are one and the same.

Describing the experience of mental health disorder, van den Berg (1972) talks of how a person's world can 'collapse', how they can feel 'unbalanced' or 'lose their footing'.[iv]

The depressed patient speaks of a world gone gloomy and dark. The flowers have lost their color . . . The patient suffering from mania . . . finds things full of color and beauty . . . The schizophrenic patient sees hears and smell indications of a world disaster . . . The patient is ill; this means that *his world* is ill. (van den Berg, 1972, pp. 45–46)

Kemp (2009) explains the drug addict's existential withdrawal is a withdrawal from the lived body, as well as withdrawal from relations with others and from a meaningful world:

The addict no longer has a lived-body, only a site for instrumental, technological intervention . . . the body cannot be lived any other way. But equally the world is robbed of meaning, now filled with things that are used only to perpetuate the addictive process . . . there is a progressive and painful alienation from self. (Kemp, 2009, p. 130)

To further illustrate the way 'worlds' can collapse and how lived experience is fundamentally embodied, consider the body of a person who develops a physical disability and how changes in motility and mobility can profoundly change their sense of self and world as they are cut adrift from habitual ways of being (Seamon, 2002a, 2002b). If pain makes walking difficult, it becomes a daunting challenge to navigate one's space: distances between points can feel unending while the world shrinks to being one of 'restrictive potentialities' (Merleau-Ponty, 1945/1962, p. 143).

In Example 3.1, I offer a description of an individual's experience of early stage multiple sclerosis which 'Ann' shared with me a few months after she had been diagnosed.

Example 3.1   Ann's experience of early stage multiple sclerosis

In January 2000 – while Ann was recovering from a severe bout of flu – numbness in the finger tips of her right (dominant) hand spread up her arm. After a couple of weeks she lost control over her arm, leaving her unable to write or to use her hand for any fine movements. Although her symptoms were *relatively minor in medical terms*, Ann felt her life had been derailed.

Ann comes to see her right arm as an "it", something *a-part* from herself, something out of control ... She now has to learn to do things in new and different ways, aware that she can no longer take her body for granted. She fatigues easily and certain tasks are no longer easy to do. Describing her difficulty with doing up the buttons on her children's clothes she explains her altered consciousness: "I have to watch, visually do it ... it is much more difficult." Ann notes, with an embarrassed laugh, personal care also presents problems: "I had to learn things like how to clean my 'toilet' with just my other hand." ...

As she seeks to preserve her "mummy role", she also sees it being threatened. Her worst nightmare is having her relationship with her children disrupted. "Initially it was difficult giving the children a proper cuddle which was just so terrible!" She realises with horror that she may permanently lose her ability to touch and feel them ...

With her fatigue and the loss of sensation/co-ordination problems in her arm, the unity between Ann's self-body-world is disrupted. Her on-going engagement with the world – her bodily intentionality – is thwarted, as she can no longer do things she had previously taken for granted. With her arm desensitised and spatially dislocated she has to learn how to carry out everyday living tasks (for herself and children) in new and unfamiliar ways. She must look at her arm, as she does up buttons or reaches into her handbag, to understand what "it" is doing. Certain gestures are no longer within her bodily scope and her possibilities for action shrink. That her arm is out of her control and that she can no longer feel the connection between herself and the world adds to a profound sense of *bodily alienation*.

At the same time, Ann has an acute awareness of *inescapable embodiment*. She cannot, however much she wants to, disassociate herself from her malfunctioning body. She has to cope with her life despite her body feeling fatigued. She cannot separate her arm from herself ... She is forced to negotiate with her arm and gradually learn to incorporate it, in its altered state, back into herself. She learns a new way of Being-in-the-world where her eyes and arm work together engaged in daily living tasks ...

Ann experiences her body ambivalently. Her arm is something both a-part from and a-part of herself and the world ... For Ann, her pre-reflectively lived *subjective body*, is disconnected. The comfortably familiar body . . . which represents her continuing perspective on the world, now contains both an absence and a new, unfamiliar aspect. Her old arm is no longer there and it is as if she has gained a new appendage: an "it", an unseeable, unpredictable attacker, who does things without her volition . . .

Ann scrutinises her body. Her arm is part of her *objective body* – one that she can observe, examine and be disconnected from. Each morning she runs through the different parts of her body, checking they are still there and functioning; evaluating her levels of fatigue and energy. She views her body with a medical gaze. With her professional understandings of multiple sclerosis she 'sees' the myelin sheaths of her peripheral nerves being eroded away. She assesses her own physical functioning as she has assessed others' and as others have assessed her . . .

Yet, even as she 'splits' her body she also seeks to re-connect with her body. Her morning ritual 'check' offers a way of simultaneously embracing both her subjective and objective body. As she runs through her body parts and assesses her functioning level for that day, she is affirming her body identity as a part of herself, apart from herself, as parts of a whole and as part of the world. 'The body, aware of itself in being aware of the world, stands in a relation "of embrace" with the world . . . Each morning I awake to "that blending with the world that recommences for me . . . as soon as I open my eyes". (Merleau-Ponty, 1968, paraphrased by Wider, 1997, p. 138)' (Finlay, 2003a, pp. 162–168).

This extract from the analysis of Ann's story suggests that her sense of self-body-world unity plus her daily life projects and her relationships with others (especially her children) are being threatened. Yet, as her life is derailed by her condition, she is also coming to terms with it and seeking to reclaim it by attempting to connect with her alienated body. Importantly, Ann's illness is encountered in the context of her family and other relationships (i.e. the intersubjective and social realms of her life). Her experience of having/being a body with multiple sclerosis cannot be separated from her world. 'Just as the multiple sclerosis is "in" her, it is "in" her embodied intersubjective relations with others' (Finlay, 2003a, p. 172).

One significant feature of Ann's story is the alien, uncanny, unhomelike[v] quality of her bodily experience where her body is felt as an 'otherness' (Zaner, 1981). The pained or damaged body seems an alien body and no longer *me*. Svenaeus (2001a) describes the experience thus:

Everything that goes on without us paying explicit attention to it when we are healthy – walking, thinking, talking – now offers resistance. The body, our thinking, the world, everything is now 'out of tune', colored by feelings of pain, weakness and helplessness . . . This way of being in the world in illness is best understood as a form of homelessness. (2001, pp. 89–90)

That sense of otherness comes, in part, from the way one's body can be objectified by health professionals, science and technology. Mazis (2001), taking up the theme, argues that medical practice itself can be 'dis-abling':

> The medical objectification of the body with the biotechnological focus of practice exacerbates the same sort of de-contextualizing of the body, the same sort of alienation from the world of the body, with which these disruptive feelings and illness already menace the client. (p. 206)

Philosophizing the Body

In the phenomenological philosophy literature, the body has been theorized in various ways, most notably by Sartre (1943/1969) and Merleau-Ponty (1945/1962), both of whom elaborated Husserl's (1928/1989) original ideas. They pay particular attention to the distinction between **body-subject** (our subjective bodily sense) and **body-object** (our body as a material object); and how body and world are seen to be intertwined (as the example of Ann above shows).

Phenomenologists such as Merleau-Ponty argue that the body is integral to any understanding of the human situation. As he says: 'I perceive in a total way with my whole being; I grasp a unique structure of the thing, a unique way of being, which speaks to all my senses at once.' (1964b, p. 50) We are incarnate; our access to the world is only gained through our bodies, grounded in our corporeal nature. Our body is our openness to the world. But not only am I conscious of the world through the medium of my body, I am also conscious of my body via the world (e.g. through others' views). It is *in the world* (the physical world as well as the world of others, of time and space, of culture), through our bodies, that we can find ourselves.[vi]

With these messages, Merleau-Ponty shows how both our perception of, and our insertion into, the world are embodied. Perception, for Merleau-Ponty, is the way in which we – as embodied beings – are projected into the world. This perception is inherently participatory – an active interplay between the perceiving body and what it perceives, and between the doing body and what it does. There is a mutual relation between the self, body and world.

Abram, mirroring Merleau-Ponty's style of using a poetic metaphorical register, describes the process thus:

> Whenever I quiet the persistent chatter of words within my head, I find this silent or wordless dance always already going on – this improvised duet between my animal body and the fluid, breathing landscape that it inhabits. (Abram, 1996, p. 53)

Human body-world intertwining is based on a key idea of phenomenology that our experience and consciousness are continuously directed towards the world. This is what is meant by the phenomenological term 'intentionality': we are always *conscious of* something in the world.[vii] It is that specific relationship with the world – our intentional relationship – that phenomenologists seek to describe when studying lived experience. And this relationship is fundamentally embodied. For example, consider the lived experience of playing golf and how golfers after hitting the ball will often follow it with their body, leaning right or left as if to pull the ball to move its trajectory. The experience of the golfer then is not within the body as such, nor is it simply about hitting the ball. The golfer *remains with* the ball as it flies. To give a different example, consider my friend who when watching rugby on television, ducks, pushes and grunts unconsciously along with his 'team'. His intentional focus is with the players on the field.

Lingis shows this intentionality in practice in his awareness of how he bodily impacts another through his spoken words. His focus (intentionality) is with the other in a bodily communion:

> With everything I say to him or her, I sense how I affect him, trouble her, question, distress, probe, anger, support, amuse, console him or her. I see it on his or her face, on the quivers and spasms of her skin, on the tightening or recoil of her hands. (Lingis, 2007, p. 5)

Having recognized the centrality of the body and its fundamental intertwining with the world, our task as researchers is to find ways to incorporate these understandings in our research practice.

The Body, Reflexivity and Research

As a therapist you will be very familiar with using yourself and your body as an instrument in therapy. As health professionals, we are trained to observe the way others use their bodies and we rely on their non-verbal cues to tell us what is important, for instance, that they are in pain. In psychotherapy, we draw on our felt-sense and subtle bodily responses to clients to give us insight into their experience. Our bodies act and re-act like a kind of *somatic compass* (Milloy, 2010).

Researchers can focus similarly on embodiment in the research arena. Specifically, I would like to argue for the relevance and importance of researchers attending reflexively to the body of *both* participant *and* researcher. (This is my own approach, however, and not all phenomenologists would agree. Many researchers just focus on participants' embodiment. I invite you to consider this point and to what extent you believe the researcher's body can and should be seen as part of what is being researched.)

Observing others' bodily responses

In my research with Ann (see above), I also attended to her bodily gestures. In the extract below taken from my reflexive diary, I describe the way I used my observations to tune into her lived experience of her struggle with multiple sclerosis – a struggle which I discovered most poignantly impacted her relationships with her children.

> Ann talked quite a bit about how the loss of sensation in her hand interfered with her daily functioning, but it took me a while to tune in. Initially, I fell into the trap of thinking about her experience and her loss of sensation in almost medical terms – I'd been looking at her body as an object. I even found myself thinking, 'well her disability is not that severe – its only partial loss of sensation and she still has some motor function'. Then she did something that yanked me into her life world . . .
>
> She described the sense of almost panic which hit her when she suddenly realised she may not ever again be able reach out to feel the "softness of her babies' skin properly". She gently caressed her own cheek and then reached out to caress the child imagined in front of her. She described this as doing the "mummy thing".
>
> Those fleeting, imaginary, subtle caresses disclosed a profound understanding. Suddenly, I understood that I needed to tune into her bodily experience – specifically her feeling of being unable to connect with – being unable to love – her children. Without sensation, she loses her ability to caress and hold and to express her love to her children. Intimate relations are disrupted as her ability to embody her loving presence is thwarted. A dynamic relation between body-world is revealed when Ann reaches out to touch – and be touched by – her children but discovers she cannot feel them (LF reflexive diary).

This extract shows how, as a researcher, I needed to tune into Ann's embodied presence. I needed to grasp the meaning *to her* of her lived, living body. Through this understanding I could begin to touch her subjectivity. 'It is through his body that the other person's soul is soul in my eyes' (Merleau-Ponty, 1960/1964a, p. 172). Seeing Ann's subtle gesture allowed me to listen and understand better. Because I was I was able to relate to the gesture, I could better understand her experience.

Using our own bodily responses reflexively

Alongside observing our participants' bodily responses we can tune into our own.[viii] The value of attending to the body is similarly celebrated in Gendlin's (1992) psychotherapeutic work, where the body is recognized as having its own special wisdom. Gendlin, who is also a phenomenological philosopher, recommends clients focus on their specific bodily responses, such as having a hollow feeling in the stomach or tightness in the shoulders. This **focusing** technique, he argues, will enable the body of its own accord to bring to the surface the words, images, memories, understandings or new ideas that are needed to solve the problem. When this occurs, the body experiences some easing or release of tension as it registers the rightness of what comes from what Gendlin calls the 'felt sense'. The easing of tension tells the client (and therapist) they have made contact with a deeper level of awareness and are on the right path.

In Example 3.2 I show the way I used my body reflexively and empathetically to better understand my participant's experience. Jenny was a mental health therapist and I was interviewing her about her experience of work and handling violent patients. She described, at some length, her sense of apprehension that one particularly predatory patient, who had a history of being a violent sexual abuser, would eventually 'get her'.

Example 3.2   A bodily experience: Reacting to a predatory patient

Jenny: He's . . . extremely creepy. He will come up, want to touch you . . . He's a bit predatory in that he will follow you down corridors . . . He preyed across the gym . . . crept up behind me . . . "They [colleagues] can't watch all of you all the time . . . I'll get you." . . . He even does things like, there's a large observation window, and even if he can't physically get to you, he'll stand there and rub his groin and drool . . . He'll crawl across the floor to get you.

In my analysis of this interview, I found myself reading and re-reading the transcript with a growing sense of foreboding in the pit of my stomach . . . I started to imagine how I would feel in Jenny's shoes, stalked by this predator:

Suddenly, the world begins to look different. Everything closes round me and somehow grows darker. I can hear the hollow beating of my heart. I think about the unit Jenny works in, seeing it now in terms of the spaces that are safe versus dangerous. She has to walk down public corridors all the time with full awareness she is not 'safe'. I feel her fear, that sense of menace where time is no defence. I experience her loathing, her disgust – my skin creeps in response to his creepiness. I see this same image of a man drooling and clawing at the window to get at me – it won't go away. It feels real, like it has happened to me. It is as if I have become Jenny. . .

This is the moment I wait for in my phenomenological analysis: the moment where I am so immersed in the data and intertwined with my participant I can no longer separate the pieces. Jenny's feeling of being stalked and bodily threatened by this creepy patient is also my feeling. (Finlay, 2003b, pp. 116–117)

In this extract, I demonstrate how an analysis might proceed by tuning empathetically into other and using one's own bodily responses as intuitive cues. The extract also demonstrates how phenomenological analysis involves much *more than* simply paraphrasing participants' words. Instead, researchers reflect intuitively and empathically, aiming to capture meanings and horizons of lived experience.

There are no fixed rules about how such analyses might be done. Researchers vary in how they tune into these implicit horizons (and the extent they try). My research with Jenny shows my own approach where I became so thoroughly immersed in her experience that I momentarily lost sight of my own. This is also illustrated by the work of Churchill (2006) who explores the intersubjective relationship between himself and his 'participants' – in this case, unusually, a bonobo in a zoo. In the following passage, Churchill describes a gestural conversation with one bonobo in which he used a reflexive bodily 'way of knowing':

> When I am engaged in imitating the bonobo … It appears as though he *understands* them *as* responses, this proto-zoologist sitting before me through a looking glass that serves as his entry into my world as much as it serves my entry into his. At this very moment when my awareness now centers on *his* consciousness of the situation, I have magically passed through the glass, transgressed the physical boundary, to the 'other side' where he resides. (Churchill, 2006, p. 18)

Reflections

This chapter has explored how the body is our way of living our experience. It is implicated in who we are and how we relate to others and the world. Phenomenologists agree that the body discloses the world just as the world discloses itself through the body. Yet much phenomenological research focuses on *words* from interview transcripts. The body is strangely absent! Why? I would like to urge you to always return to attending to the body in your research.

I believe that, as therapists (across all modalities), we bring a huge advantage with us when we do phenomenological research because we routinely engage the body in our work. As therapists, we have special understandings of bodily being and we can use our bodies as therapeutic tools. Physiotherapists and other physical therapists have a finely tuned awareness of other people's bodies; psychotherapists gain insight through bodily cues and are trained to consider their own bodily wisdoms.

These skills and understandings can be fruitfully marshalled in phenomenological research. Do you 'agree? Romanyshyn (2007) does when, drawing on Merleau-Ponty's metaphor of 'flesh', he says:

To linger and even loiter in the presence of what is present is to recover the animate flesh. It is the lived body that lingers in an erotic conspiracy with the world ... To begin with the ensouled body and its gestural fields is to acknowledge that between one's flesh and that of the work [research], like the relation in the transference field of therapy between the flesh of the therapist and that of the patient, a secret dialogue has already been in progress, a dialogue that now poses its questions to the researcher. (Romanyshyn, 2007, p. 232)

'The body forms our deepest relational intertwining with the flesh of that world ...' says Aanstoos (1991, p. 95). 'The body-world boundary is a porous one, permitting of unceasing interpenetrability.' It is this complexity that makes the body such a mysteriously elusive yet significant phenomenon.

Notes

[i] David Seamon (1979, 1980) distinguishes between two bodily patterns: *body-routines* (sets of integrated actions and behaviours such as preparing a meal and driving a car); and *time-space routines* (sets of habitual bodily roles and routines such as a 'getting up' routine). He argues that spatial and architectural design – and I would add therapeutic intervention – should pay attention to these bodily routines to ensure a comfortable fit between the lived body and surroundings.

[ii] The concept of **flow** experience has been researched in depth by the American psychologist Csíkszentmihályi (1992). Flow is defined as completely focused, single-minded, energized, joyous motivation – what we colloquially call 'being in the moment' or 'in the zone'. Csíkszentmihályi stresses the importance of absorbing activity and such focusing of attention for psychological well-being.

[iii] The philosopher Levinas (1969) talks, at both a socio-political and personal level, about the concept of 'totalizing' which means reducing something/someone to something non-unique. This totalization is seen as doing violence to the Other – killing their otherness by categorizing and stereotyping them.

[iv] Here van den Berg applies the phenomenological spirit to psychiatry recommending that we should *listen to* our patients and take the reality they are presenting seriously by not imposing our own ideas and not assuming we understand the patient too quickly. Following Heidegger, van den Berg highlights the value of leaving aside 'subjectivist' conceptions in order to focus on how the lived world presents to us (or our patients).

[v] There are many wonderful accounts of the **unhomelike body** in illness. Leder's (1990) account of the searing pain arising from his colon cancer in *The Absent Body* and Toombs' (1993) four-stage model showing the gradual objectification of the body in illness in *The Meaning of Illness* are two particularly good examples.

[vi] This relationship between body-world also relates to our sense of what is 'inside' and 'outside' our bodies. Our habitual tendency in the Western world is to distinguish between our outer physical body which is in contact with the world and our inner body. But, as Morley notes in reference to Pranayama (breath control) yoga, inside-outside are intertwined. 'To breathe is to pull external air into ourselves and rhythmically to release outward something of ourselves' (Morley, 2001, p. 76).

[vii] Developing the theme of a mutual relationship as we inhabit and live our world through our various senses, Merleau-Ponty argues that, in order to act, we need a sense of *proprioceptive bodily awareness* of where we are in space. As we reach out to pick up a cup, we need to understand that we have an arm that can move in that direction. As we see the cup and reach out to drink from it, our bodily intentionality embraces the cup (the world) and (usually occurring below the level of our consciousness) it becomes part of our body.

[viii] Raingruber and Kent (2003) illustrate this in their phenomenological enquiry into clinicians' use of their bodies. They argue that clinicians' bodies can act like a Geiger counter, a detector of meaning that helps them understand and empathize with clients' experiences. For alert professionals, physical sensations such as feeling a 'chill down the spine' or the 'stomach churning' can be crucial cues to attend to certain meanings. 'When clinicians listen to the piercing wisdom and the immediate knowledge of their body', the authors argue, 'they are more likely to make time to reflect and to develop an understanding . . . in personal, professional, and human terms' (p. 466).

Chapter 4

Philosophical Foundations

Husserl's essences are destined to bring back all the living relationships of experience, as the fisherman's net draws up from the depths of the ocean quivering fish and seaweed. (Merleau-Ponty, 1945/1962, p. xv)

At the end of *Chapter 2*, I suggested that research focusing on lived experience could only be considered 'phenomenological' if it embraced underpinning theory and philosophy in some way. In this extended chapter I map some of the key names and ideas (in **bold** type) found in phenomenological philosophy to give you a feel of the richness and diversity of this swampy territory.

The three biggest names in phenomenological philosophy are Husserl, Heidegger and Merleau-Ponty. I start by outlining their contributions and giving their ideas most space. I then touch on the work of other philosophers (in chronological order of their birth) who are most commonly referred to in the therapy world, namely: Buber, Gadamer, Sartre, Levinas, de Beauvoir, Ricoeur and Gendlin.[i]

Of course, writing all this in one chapter does not permit a properly respectful account of these philosophers' ideas. What I offer below is a curtailed summary of my understanding; a few key touchstones which I consider are particularly relevant to therapists embarking on phenomenological research. These are the ideas commonly drawn on when practically applying the philosophy. I try to give a *flavour* of the philosophers' styles,

Phenomenology for Therapists: Researching the Lived World, First Edition. Linda Finlay.
© 2011 Linda Finlay. Published 2011 by John Wiley & Sons, Ltd.

works and concepts but I urge you to read around the subject and, where possible, dip into the writings of the philosophers themselves. Throughout, there are numerous references you might usefully follow up while footnotes (more than usual) expand on social and theoretical points of interest.

For readers new to phenomenological philosophy, can I offer something of a health warning before you read on? This is probably a chapter best dipped into rather than read cover to cover. The material is dense; the ideas difficult. Be prepared to meet radical new concepts as well as strange words.

Husserl: His Search for 'Essences'

Over his lifetime Edmund Husserl, the Austrian-German philosopher[ii] who we might credit as the founder of modern phenomenology, was constantly integrating and reworking his philosophy through numerous dense and extraordinary works such as *Logical Investigations; Ideas I and II; Cartesian Meditations; The Crisis of European Sciences and Transcendental Phenomenology* plus a rich profusion of lectures and working manuscripts (40,000 pages of them!).

Across these works he made important contributions to every area of philosophy, in particular, concerning the nature of thought, logic, science and the problems of both reductionism and positivism. Below I selectively explain the ideas most germane to phenomenological research methodology. (See *Chapter 6* which outlines the descriptive, empirical phenomenological research method based on Husserlian ideas.)

Summary of key ideas

Husserl's project was to forge a new kind of science – one that moved away from the scientific ideal of positivism[iii] which he thought would ultimately result in the dehumanization of society. He sought to establish the everyday experienced human world as our scientific foundation; the aim being to bring forth the full richness of our lived world.

Husserl defined the science of phenomenology as the study of the essence of conscious[iv] experience. His aim was the description and structural analysis of consciousness as it is given (i.e. how it appears) in experience: 'to the things themselves' (*zu den Sachen selbst*). Husserl was trying to dissect the dualism of *subject* (researcher/philosopher) and *object* (the 'thing' being studied) by looking at how things show themselves to us.[v] He was also trying to encourage us to leave aside our previous knowledge and investments in order to see phenomena as experienced: in his words: 'We should separate the purely descriptive examination of the knowledge-experience, disembarrassed of all theoretical psychological interests' (Husserl, 1970, p. 262).

Through phenomenological reflection, Husserl explains, we grasp that consciousness is **intentional** in the sense of always being directed towards something: consciousness is consciousness *of* something.[vi] The phenomenologist needs to study both acts of consciousness or the manner of being aware (**noesis**) and the objects of consciousness/awareness (**noema**) just as we experience them. (Of course Husserl was speaking as a philosopher and he was referring to philosophers' reflections on their own experiencing. Applied to research, the focus shifts slightly: researchers study participants' experiences of phenomenon. The 'subject' here is the researcher and the 'object' is the participants and their experiencing of the phenomenon.)

To engage this study of consciousness, Husserl asks phenomenologists to bring a special attitude to bear involving **reduction**(s). In this reductive attitude, phenomenologists rigorously '**bracket**' past/theoretical knowledge *and* abstain from positing the existence of the natural world around us. (Phenomenologists even bracket the idea that there exists a world independent of our experience. This means that phenomenologists can study things to do with memory, dreams and imagination just as well as studying perception of the 'real' world.) Phenomenologists are then asked to dwell repeatedly with and immerse themselves in the immanent experience of appearances (i.e. what is given) in order to discover emergent patterns of inter-related essences revealed in actual experience. (In research terms 'bracketing' helps the researcher remain constantly vigilant to the ways in which their personal intellectual baggage might distort the description of the phenomenon and it offers a way of systematically and rigorously identifying essences. The more the researcher can dwell iteratively in the data holding tight to the reduction, the more rigorous and trustworthy the resulting description will be.)

In Husserl's later works he highlighted the idea of the *Lebenswelt* (lifeworld) which manifests as a meaningful structural whole that is both shared and experienced by individuals from their own unique perspective. This lifeworld consists of certain invariant structures: we are all **body-subjects** – i.e. we all have sense of embodiment and sense of self; the life world entails various forms of **sociality** in that we relate to others in the world, we use language and we are joined by our cultural and ethnic history; and the life-world involves a sense of **spatiality** (we are inserted into the world that surrounds us) and **temporality** (we live in an unfolding present with a determining past and yet-to-be determined future). (See *Chapter 8* which expands on these ideas applied to research.)

If Husserl's ideas sounds too dry and the jargon threatens to derail your attention, it is worth remembering that Husserl's intention is to bring out the *full richness of our subjectivity as ways of discovering the world*. So a thing we love, becomes 'lovable'; a thing we dread is 'dreadful'. The goal is not to achieve some kind of objective account of the thing but how our lived experience of it appears to us, what it means. Sartre (1939/1970) makes this point when he acknowledges Husserl's revolutionary brilliance:

> Husserl has restored to things their horror and charm. He has restored to us the world of artists and prophets: frightening, hostile, dangerous, with its havens of mercy and love. He has cleared the way for a new treatise on passions which would be inspired by this simple truth . . . if we love a woman, it is because she is lovable. (Sartre, 1939/1970, p. 5)

The 'reduction' as a special shift in attitude

Husserl's notion of reduction(s) (in shorthand called '**bracketing**'), so critical to his methodology, is the one idea supporters and critics of phenomenological research today seem to grab hold of and either use enthusiastically or reject emphatically. Yet, all too often, the process is misunderstood and its application mangled out of recognition. Too often bracketing is simplistically used and the full import of the reductive *process* is missed. Because it is such an important and contested component of phenomenological practice, it is important to dwell further on what it means.

As phenomenologists, Husserl argues, we must work to free ourselves from prejudices and previous understandings and secure a level of detachment from our own history. This involves continuous struggle in which we strive in our description/analysis to honour what is given to us when encountering the phenomenon – encountering 'the things themselves' in their appearing. (This is similar to what we do in therapy when we try to see the world from our service users' point of view and temporarily set aside any preoccupations or inner turmoil we may feel.)

The term '**reduction**' was first articulated by Husserl as a radical, self-meditative process where the philosopher puts aside the *natural world* and world of *interpretation* in order to see the phenomenon in its essence. The process, he explains, involves a personal transformation and 'reorientation of the natural mundane attitude' (Husserl, 1936/1970, p. 258) where objectivity is constituted out of subjectivity. (In psychotherapy, we also do this, when we aim to loyally honour our clients' subjectivity, rather than trying to be 'objective'.) Thus, bracketing has been wrongly and simplistically interpreted as being objective, putting aside one's subjectivity. Instead, bracketing involves putting aside previous understandings in brackets to put them temporarily out of action, thereby reducing the field which commands one's special focus of attention. (Husserl was originally a mathematician so he uses bracketing in this mathematical way.) Prior assumptions about the nature of the phenomenon being studied are set aside leading to a gradual penetration of an essential residue which is purified of preconceptions.

> We can do nothing but reflect, engross ourselves in the still not unfolded sense of our task, and thus secure, with the utmost care, freedom from prejudice, keeping our undertaking free of alien interferences . . . and this . . . must supply us with our method. (Husserl, 1936/1970, p. 134)

For Husserl, the reduction delivers the philosopher to the 'groping entrance into this unknown realm of subjective phenomena' (1936/1970, p. 161). A number steps or procedures are involved including:

1) the epoché of the natural sciences;
2) the epoché of the natural attitude;
3) the transcendental reduction; and
4) eidetic reduction.[vii]

The first **epoché of the natural sciences** (Husserl, 1936/1970) brackets scientific theory and knowledge, and reduces the field of investigation to the lifeworld from the standpoint of the *natural attitude*. This means a return to phenomena as they are lived and experienced instead of beginning with scientific preconceptions. This step is more difficult than it sounds as we take so much scientific understanding for granted (such as that our mind and body are separate, that depression is a 'real' phenomenon, or that therapy is a good thing!)

> *All sciences which relate to this natural world*, . . . fill me with wondering admiration, though I am far from any thought of objecting to them in the least degree, *I disconnect them* all, *I make absolutely no use of their standards, I do not appropriate a single one of the propositions that enter into their systems.* [italics in the original] (Husserl, 1913/1962, p. 111)

The **second epoché of the natural attitude** brackets the reality of the natural, taken-for-granted lifeworld – i.e. bracketing ontological presuppositions that things really exist.[viii] (In research terms, if a participant says they see a ghost then judgemental questions about whether or not that ghost is 'real' are set aside.) The task, as Husserl points out, is to go beyond the natural attitude paradoxically in order to discover it (Husserl, 1936/1970). This epoché leads first to the *psychological phenomenological reduction* (the process we specifically engage when doing research using descriptive phenomenological methodology). This process, according to Husserl, involves more than simply critically purifying oneself of bias and prejudices, instead it involves entering a new *way of being*. 'The gaze made free by the epoché must likewise be . . . an experiencing gaze' (1936/1970, p. 153). 'We begin our considerations as human beings who are living naturally, objectivating, judging, feeling, willing, "*in the natural attitude*"' (1913/1983, p. 51).

Here Husserl wants to examine the phenomenon as a '*presence*' without attributing existence to it. Specifically, the focus is on subjective meanings, i.e. the meaningful ways the lifeworld presents itself and the subjective processes that constitute these presentations (e.g. through perceptions, emotions, beliefs).

In the third **transcendental reduction**, Husserl proposes an even more radical epoché which involves standing aside from one's subjective experience and ego, in order to be able to focus on transcendental consciousness. Here he seems to claim that the consciousness that constitutes the world can somehow be separated from the world. (It is worth stressing that this transcendental realm applies to philosophy and is less directly relevant to us as researchers. Giorgi (2009) and others recommend that meanings emerge from applying the phenomenological *psychological reduction* rather than the transcendental reduction – see *Chapter 6*. Unfortunately, misinformed critics are rather too quick to latch on to these particular ideas about transcendence to legitimate a wholesale rejection of Husserl's phenomenological project as being 'unrealistic'.)

Finally, in the **eidectic reduction**, also called **intuition of essences**, the invariant characteristics and meanings of the phenomenon are described. Here, the philosopher or researcher attempts to intuit consistent or fundamental meanings – the essence of what appears in our consciousness – without which a phenomenon could not present itself as it is. (We might say, for instance, that the experience of depression invariably involves a sense of bleak despair, dark thoughts, meaninglessness and hopelessness while sleeplessness is common but not invariable so would probably not be seen as part of the essence of depression.)

Husserl formalized a procedure to give rigour to the search for such essences called **free imaginative variation**. This procedure involves freely changing aspects of the phenomenon in order to distinguish essential features from particular, accidental or incidental ones. (So we might ask, 'If hopelessness was turned into a hopeful optimism, would depression still be depression?' If the answer is yes then 'hopelessness' would not be an essential structure or essence of depression.)

Through these reductive processes, Husserl showed us how to fundamentally alter our way of seeing akin to entering a new 'realm'. Turning the tables on the traditional scientific understanding of reduction as a narrowing or abstracting process, Husserl saw the reduction as a movement towards perceiving and reflecting in more complex, layered, expansive and all-encompassing ways. He continually emphasized the *radicality* of the reduction, which he saw as potentially transformative:

> Perhaps it will even become manifest that the total phenomenological attitude and the epoché belonging to it are destined . . . to effect . . . a complete personal transformation, comparable in the beginning to a religious conversion. (Husserl, 1936/1970, p. 137)

In summary, the phenomenological attitude involves the 'scientist' (philosopher or researcher) in *questioning* the natural attitude instead of taking it for granted. At the same time, Husserl recognizes how the lifeworld – including our involvement with others and the way we stand in a horizon of human civilization – constitutes us. It was precisely this lifeworld and historical horizon that became the focus of the work by Husserl's most infamous student – Heidegger.

Heidegger: Exploring the Nature of 'Being'

Martin Heidegger (1889–1976), another German philosopher, remains a controversial figure. He has been widely revered as perhaps the greatest twentieth century philosopher while widely reviled for being a Nazi.[ix]

He had started out as Husserl's student and assistant but soon steered the phenomenological project away from the study of consciousness, towards the deceptively simple question of what is meant by the verb 'to be'. Forging into hermeneutic, existential territory his central concern was how to approach – phenomenologically – the ontological question of human existence – *Being*.[x]

Below, I sketch a range of Heidegger's ideas as they have been so foundational to the existential movement and have particular relevance to psychotherapy. The ideas remain extraordinary today in that they demand we take a radical new look at being and the world. Heidegger created a whole new language of concepts, coining new words (or new meanings for old words) in order to look at ourselves with fresh eyes. The fact that these words have been translated into English doubles the interpretive challenge![xi]

Summary of key ideas

Dasein In his early, most influential work *Being and Time* (1927/1962), Heidegger described the human being as *Dasein* (literally 'there-being') or '**being-in-the-world**'. Instead of seeing ourselves in terms of being self-contained individual subjects, Heidegger pointed to our mode of Being: *Dasein* is existence itself. Specifically he emphasized human beings' immersion in, and openness to, the surrounding world. 'Self and world belong together in the single entity *Dasein*. Self and world are not two beings, like subject and object' (p. 297). In a more complicated move, he talks of human being's existence as *Ek-sistence* being a 'clearing' or 'opening up of being' – the opening (openness) in which beings can come to presence. Using a metaphor related to his home in the Black Forest, it is as if humans are a 'clearing in the forest' where things can be seen which cannot normally be seen in the shadow of trees.

For Heidegger, Being is fundamentally interlinked with **Time**. Time is an ever-present horizon for us. There is no fixed existence, said Heidegger, we are always 'becoming' – we live in our anticipations. For example, if we are engaged in a task in the present, we are also being pulled ahead envisaging that task completed. In our existence we are constantly projecting ourselves into the future, yet at the same time the 'who' we are becoming emerges from our past.

'**Thrownness**'   *Dasein* is 'thrown' into the (pre-existing) world of objects, projects, relationships, language, culture and history – a 'situatedness' which limits our freedom and our understandings. As we immerse ourselves in this world we become absorbed by familiar, ordinary, banal daily activities which mostly we just engage pre-reflectively, without thinking. Who we are is revealed through our way of being with worldly things and through our doing. Objects are ready-to-hand, to be used or produced in everyday experiential ways: one knows a hammer through hammering.

Part of the world we are thrown into is a world of other people – *Dasein* is inherently and inescapably social. The world of *Dasein* is a 'with world' (***Mitsein*** or Being-with). Even when we are physically alone or we ignore others, we remain in-relation through our everyday engagement in our common world. (As Heidegger pointed out, my glove is also the glove I bought from the clerk at the shop and fashion dictates its wearing.) In sharing our world with others we understand others and our Self: the 'I' is a derivation of Being-with and is formed on the basis of a mutual recognition (and thus empathy) in the intersubjective world. In sharing the world with others, just as my own existence is an issue for me, we also develop a care or concern (what he called ***Sorge***) for others' welfare.

'***Das Man***', **authenticity and existentialism**   Recognizing how it is impossible to exist without depending on others and without conforming to shared communal norms, Heidegger suggested our being-with-one-another dissolves us into a being *of* others where we risk becoming a 'they-self'. Here one exists as *das Man* (the 'they'). I dress myself conforming to prevailing fashions. If I rebel and adopt a counter-culture fashion I am still basing my appearance on 'they' as a negative guideline and/or embracing a new counter-culture 'they'. Using this term 'they', Heidegger described a certain 'everydayness' of how bland, petty conformity, averageness and anonymity comes to dominate our perceptions and actions as we unthinkingly – *inauthentically* – follow the herd. *Das Man* is anonymous, alienated from its authentic self – its selfhood – as it thinks and acts just like everyone else.

As we confront life's meaninglessness and the abyss of nothingness which awaits us when we die, we experience *Angst:* feel unsettled, alienated, homeless (**unheimlich** – literally not-at-home[xii]). We can flee from this radical insecurity and deny our existential anxiety by 'falling' into the attractions of a mindless, anaesthetizing 'they'. But Heidegger calls us to own up – authentically – to our self and situation; it is precisely this *being-towards-death*, he said, which gives life its intensity, urgency, meaning and potential for authenticity. I can be free to become myself once I face death and the pettiness of my life. 'The sense of void imminent makes my life pulsate for me with anxiety that is, more palpably, more keenly, more ardently...' (Lingis, 1989, p. 113). (Put in psychotherapeutic terms, van Deurzen-Smith (1997, p. 43) argues that we should 'welcome anxiety as an indicator of our willingness to be braced by the truth of the finality of our destiny'. Therapy is about 'facing up bravely to the wounds of living'.)

According to Heidegger, as we face up to the human condition and to our past, present and future choices, we are torn between authentic and inauthentic modes of living and feel a type of 'guilt'. Our conscience calls us to own up to our guilt and make our actions our own. Polt explains:

> Heidegger claims that we need a special moment of insight, the call of conscience, to alert us to these aspects of our existence, because everyday existence is absorbed in the present and avoids owning up to guilt. In the call of conscience, then, Dasein as care is silently calling Dasein as the fallen theyself, alerting inauthentic Dasein to the indebtedness and responsibility that are part of care itself. (Polt, 1999, p. 89)

Late Heidegger In *The Question Concerning Technology* and other later writings, Heidegger points out how, in our fast-moving modern world, we are absorbed by technology and come to understand things in the world as economic-physical resources to be exploited. He warns against submitting to the **totalizing** spirit of the technological age where everything is presumed to be improved by the application of science (a theme that Husserl had explored many years earlier). As we become objects to be used and manipulated, he says, we cease to be human; we become a 'One' rather than an 'I'. The greatest danger is that the 'technological revolution in the atomic age could so captivate, bewitch, dazzle and beguile man that calculative thinking may someday come to be accepted and practiced *as the only* way of thinking' (Heidegger, 1966, cited in Dreyfus, 1993, p. 305). Again, he calls us to claim more authentic ways of being.

The later Heidegger comes to view philosophy as being closer to poetry than to science. Both philosophy and poetry are sensitive to the richness of meanings and these can be brought to life within and through language (particularly Greek and German, according to Heidegger!). Artworks (in the broadest sense), claimed Heidegger, have the power to touch us and transport us out of the realm of the taken-for-granted. Art *unconceals* (reveals). Through art we can really notice the Being of beings. Through the 'saying' power of poetry Heidegger draws our attention to language as a 'house of being'.[xiii]

In his later works, Heidegger focused on the constitutive power of language. In *Being and Time* he focused on language as 'existential discourse', i.e. part of *Dasein*'s existential understanding/interpretation of the world. In his later work the emphasis shifted in a more radical direction to emphasize 'hearing' and 'listening-in' to language (as part of a bodying forth) which offers an unfolding openness and mystery of Being. Language and Being are entwined. 'To speak means to say, which means to show and to let [something] be seen. It means to communicate and, correspondingly, to listen, to submit oneself to a claim, addressed to oneself, and to comply and respond to it' (Heidegger, 1987/2001, p. 215).

The hermeneutic (interpretive) turn[xiv]

For Heidegger, language and understanding are inseparable – it is only through language (and thus interpretation) that our Being-in-the-world becomes manifest and can be understood. Heidegger described his approach to the study of human existence as 'hermeneutical' meaning that interpretive steps are taken between implicit pre-understandings and evolving current understandings; between the interpreter and that which is interpreted; between understanding the whole and its parts.

Existential, hermeneutic philosophers from Heidegger onwards have problematized Husserl's ideas of the reduction and bracketing by highlighting our embeddedness in the world. Understanding, they say, *depends on* us recognizing our pre-understandings and historicity. Our 'horizons of experience' (e.g. temporal horizons of our past experiences and future anticipations) are implicated and penetrate any perception of the world we may have. We experience a thing 'as' something – it has already been interpreted. Thus, to understand anything means to have first interpreted it. We cannot stand neutral, as though outside our current understandings.

In Heideggerian terms, interpretation is an inevitable, basic structure of our being-in-the-world: 'Whenever something is interpreted as something, the interpretation will be founded essentially upon fore-having, fore-sight, and fore-conception. An interpretation is never a presuppositionless apprehending of something presented to us . . . .' (1927/1962, pp. 191–192). However, Heidegger goes on to insist that we take control of our fore-conceptions and not allow them 'to be presented to us by fancies and popular conceptions, but rather to make the scientific theme secure by working out these fore-structures in terms of the things themselves' (p. 195). The point here is that understanding comes from prioritizing the thing to be interpreted rather than holding on to preconceptions. It is here that Heidegger offers a nod to Husserl's bracketing. See for example, how he explains the way to begin thinking about time:

> We would do well to disregard entirely and immediately what we believe we already know about time. We must also disregard the manner and the way in which we are accustomed to treat the theme of "time", for example, the distinctions between subjective and objective time, between cosmic and personal time, between measured and lived time, and between quantitative and qualitative time. (Heidegger, 1987/2001, pp. 38–39)

Beyond approaching something to be understood, carefully and systematically, Heidegger explains that a **hermeneutic 'circle'** is involved when working out fore-structures *in terms of the things themselves*. It starts by having a fore-understanding (which is a rough and ready approximation) and moves on to being open to discover something. Initial understandings are then challenged and this involves meeting a 'resistance' when interrogating experience. Through this there comes an interpretative revision of the fore-understanding. The hermeneutic circle thus moves between question and answer; between implicit **pre-understandings**[xv] and explicit understandings; between the reciprocal relationship between the interpreted and interpreter; between understanding parts and the whole. Understanding deepens by going round the circle again and again.

Through his extraordinary dense, poetic, enigmatic writings, Heidegger challenges us to go beyond our current understandings and probe the mysterious relationship between Being and language. He pushes us to a vision of Being as 'openness' concerned about itself and involved in an intimate participation with the world. By way of summary of his many different ideas, I offer a passage from Todres (2007) which suggests the style and spirit of Heidegger:

> For Heidegger, there is a mysterious relation between language and Being, in which the 'unsaid' lives always exceedingly as that which the said is about. Speech in a broad sense is pregnant with this excess . . . Being-in-the-world not only disappears into the 'unsaid' of world-happening, intimate with

excess, it also appears again in a historical gathering of what this means for living forward with others in situations . . . The enacting self as the shape of understanding is first 'wet through' by the insight of intimate participation and this can come to language in tentative ways. (Todres, 2007, p. 19)

It was Heidegger's life work to explicate the nature of Being and existence. Other philosophers, including Merleau-Ponty and Sartre expanded on these existential themes.

Merleau-Ponty: Exploring Perception and Body-World Constitution

The French existentialist philosopher Maurice Merleau-Ponty (1908–1961) was influenced by both Husserl and Heidegger. He was also a contemporary of both Sartre[xvi] and de Beauvoir (see below) as well as being strongly influenced by Karl Marx – throughout his life he was a committed radical, speaking out for political freedom.[xvii]

At the core of Merleau-Ponty's dialectical philosophy is a sustained argument for the foundational role that perception has in engaging with and understanding the world. The world, however, is something we live and engage in a bodily way. Consciousness, says Merleau-Ponty, is practical, perceptual and embodied; it is an act of the whole body engaged in – grounded in – the world which both constitutes us and is constituted by us.

Humans can never grasp the world in its totality, he says, expressing his more relativist leanings. We can only understand it as its being revealed according to the mode in which we inhabit it.

Perception is perspectival, open, and indeterminate: as we move, fresh perspectives open up and objects disclose themselves in new ways. We are an opening to the world, but each object, too, is in its own way both an opening and a way of hiding. (Packer, 2011, p. 187)

Summary of key ideas

In *Phenomenology of Perception*, Merleau-Ponty argues that philosophy and psychology have misunderstood perception as being created by our senses and as being a simple dissociated result of the impact of external stimuli. Drawing on Gestalt psychology[xviii] he insists on a holistic dynamic intermingling of sensory possibilities which describes the manner in which objects appear to us pre-reflectively in a worldly context – as we bodily live it in our everyday activities. Things in the world are known because the experience is connected to and simultaneously evoked in the lived body. So, for instance, I perceive a pen as graspable, to write with; a piano as something to play. I might *see* colours when I hear music; I might see a red carpet as a specific, soft, textured, woolly, cosy, red carpet; or I discover things as being 'tall' or 'short' on the basis of my bodily orientation to it. If my mobility is impaired, I face a world of 'restrictive potentialities'[xix] as things feel 'too low' or 'too far' and so on. In short, perception is more than the sum of the data transmitted to us by our senses.

'The body is the vehicle of being in the world', says Merleau-Ponty (1945/1962, p. 82). It is the 'horizon latent in all our experience . . . and anterior to every determining thought' (1945/1962, p. 92). Thus, Merleau-Ponty argues that the body not only connects us to the world, but also offers us the way to be in that world and to understand it.

Phenomenological theorizing of the body reveals a fundamental onto-logical (i.e. to do with being) distinction between the 'subjective body' as lived and experienced pre-reflectively, and the 'objective body' as observed and scientifically investigated.[xx] Merleau-Ponty (1945/1962) highlights this fundamental ambiguity of our body: while the lived body is that which is most intimately mine/me, it is also an object for myself and others; it is experienced from the inside and out.

The **subjective body** is the body-as-it-is-lived. It represents my particular view of the world as well as my *Being-in-the-world*. I do not simply possess a body, *I AM* my body (Merleau-Ponty, 1945/1962). My particular bodily style or bearing identifies my body as mine and it is this lived body that engages the world. I find myself in the world of my projects, daily activities and relationships and these are encountered as a context for the body's possible action. So food is to be eaten, a dog is to be walked, words are to be spoken, a lover is to be touched, a doorknob is to be turned. As we engage in our daily activities, we tend not to be conscious of our bodies and we take them for granted. This is our **habitual body**, the body that is 'passed-by-in-silence' (Sartre, 1943/1969).

Abram (1996) elaborates on our embodied consciousness when he in-sists that the experiencing body is not an enclosed object but an open, incomplete, participatory, sensuous dimension of *Being*. The body merges fluidly with the world. 'Considered phenomenologically – . . . as we actually experience and *live* it – the body is a creative, shape-shifting entity' (Abram, 1996, p. 47).

The **objective body**, in contrast, is the body that is known by the Other. We can observe and objectify another's body. We can peer at, leer at, admire, criticize, probe, investigate and dissect another's body. In so doing, we become aware of it as a contained, material, biological thing. We can also do this to our own bodies. This occurs most commonly in illness when we can no longer take our bodies for granted, when our bodies do not do what we expect them to do. Then we might focus on specific parts of our body: an aching stomach, a scar or a broken leg. As Toombs, a phenomenological philosopher who has multiple sclerosis herself, explains:

> Illness engenders a shift of attention. The disruption of lived body causes the patient explicitly to attend to his or her body *as* body . . . The body is thus transformed from lived body to object-body. (1993, pp. 70–71)

Beyond simply being a body subject or body object, however, phenomenologists stress the way our bodies are intertwined with the world, 'thrown into spaces and times that animate us as moving, sensing, emoting flesh of the world' (Smith, 2006, p. 1).

The intertwining of body-world: a radical ontology

In his last (incomplete, poetic and tantalizingly mysterious) work *The Visible and the Invisible*, Merleau-Ponty (1964/1968) offers a radicalized phenomenology of embodiment. Here he moves from an understanding of 'embodied consciousness' to 'intercorporeal being', suggesting that a kind of bodily experience and reflexivity eliminates the ontological dualism of body subject and body object. He pursues the twin metaphors of '**chiasm**' (crossing point such as between body-world, subject-object) and '**flesh**' (an ontological concept naming the elemental impermeability of our bodily inherence in the field of Being as a whole): we are the world that thinks itself – or 'that the world is at the heart of our flesh . . . once a body-world relationship is recognized, there is a ramification of my body and a ramification of the world and a correspondence between its inside and my outside and my inside and its outside' (1964/1968, p. 136).

Flesh is the fabric or 'element' of being (similar to fire, earth, water, air) in which both my body and things are given. 'The flesh we are speaking of is not matter', says Merleau-Ponty. 'It is the coiling over of the visible upon the seeing body, of the tangible upon the touching body' (1964/1968, p. 146). He uses a phrase flesh-of-the-world, replacing Heidegger's Being-in-the-world, to bring philosophy down to earth and capture our embodied way of being. The world and body are within one another and intertwined/ criss-crossed.

> Flesh of the world' speaks to an embodied connection to the spaces we inhabit deeply, primally, elementally. Flesh suggests water and its circulations, air and its respirations, earth and its conformations, fire and its inspirations . . . Movement arises not specifically in the body, but in the nexus and intertwining of bodily engagement with the world. There is a primacy to movement that registers in the living body in its carnal ties to the elements of the world's flesh. (Smith, 2006, p. 1)

With his use of such obscure words, Merleau-Ponty (1964/1968) seeks to expunge dualisms (such as subject/object; natural/mental; interior/exterior). Flesh describes both the body and the substance of the world. If humans are seen as inherent in the world then they cannot be reduced to categories apart from the world. So we are both subject *and* object, existence *and* essence. In pursuit of an ontological rehabilitation of the body, he argues for the notion of a reversible interpenetrating relationship – a 'double belongingness' – between the body as *sensible* and as *sentient*, seeing/perceiving and thinking.

He famously draws the analogy of touching hands – in which hands both simultaneously touch and are touched. The being who touches is necessarily touched by the being of that which is touched. Similarly, the seer and the seen reciprocate. When we are seen by the other we emigrate into that vision, we are seduced, captivated, alienated. The being of the seer is inevitably reflected back by the being of that which is seen.

The same intertwining applies between the 'visible' and 'invisible' (i.e. the seen and the thought) where the invisible is both *of* and *in* the visible while the visible and invisible are also mutually (reciprocally) transformative.

> Where are we to put the limit between the body and the world since the world is flesh? . . . The world seen is not "in" my body, and my body is not "in" the visible world . . . A participation in and kinship with the visible . . . There is a reciprocal insertion and intertwining of one in the other. (Merleau-Ponty, 1964/1968, p. 138)

Concepts like 'chiasm' and 'flesh' are challenging to say the least. If you are just starting out on your phenomenological journey perhaps it is sufficient to recognize that body and world are interconnected. Similarly, recognize how distinctions between inside-outside, subject-object, my body-being and your body-being, touching and being touched, sense and being sensed, perception and thought, and so on, are fundamentally and mutually entwined.

Other Significant Philosophers

Buber

Psychotherapists of existential, gestalt and relational persuasions might well be familiar with the work of Martin Buber (1878–1965) – a Austrian-born Jewish theologian,[xxi] educator[xxii] and existential phenomenological philosopher.

In his best-known work, a short philosophical essay *Ich und Du* (1923/2004), Buber writes of the more spiritual dimensions of human relationships as linked to the relationship between God and man [sic].

He talks romantically of the potential of the *I-Thou* **relationship** where each person is accepting of and open to the other; recognizing the I-ness of me and the you-ness of you. 'I become through my relation to the *Thou*; as I become *I*, I say *Thou*' (Buber, 1937/1958, p. 11). The *I-Thou* relationship is one of mutual regard; it is free from judgement, narcissism, demand, possessiveness, objectification, greed or anticipation. Persons respond creatively in the moment to the other, eschewing instrumental and habitual ways of interacting (as found in the *I-It* **relationship**).

The *I-Thou* relationship is mutually revealing because recognizing the value of the other's personhood helps one's own authenticity and personhood come into renewed being. In the authentic open relationship of *I-Thou*, each person gives of themselves without attempting to perform or control the impression being created. The direct experience of such 'presence' of ourselves with another, is both comforting (in showing us we are not alone) and threatening (because we are challenged to be *more*). There is poignancy in the connection with another, for instance, as we gaze into the eyes of a loved one.

Treating others as 'Thous' rather than 'Its', says Buber, allows us a way to overcome our moral dilemmas. The holocaust, for instance, according to Buber, is a particularly powerful and terrifying example of the ethical consequences of seeing others as 'Its' (Martin, 2009).

For Buber, our communication is not just conversation, it is a reciprocal exchange which opens up awareness; it is where we can grow through each other – ultimately having a conversation with God. Buber talks specifically of the value of dialogue in a relationship as a mysterious experience occurring **between** one person and another (Hycner, 1991).

> Where the dialogue is fulfilled in its being, between partners who have turned to one another in truth . . . The world arises in a substantial way between men [sic] who have been seized in their depths and opened out by the dynamic of an elemental togetherness. The interhuman opens out what otherwise remains unopened. (Buber, 1965, p. 86)

The meaning of Buber's notion of **interhuman** is to be 'found neither in one of the two partners nor in both together, but only in their dialogue itself, in this "between" which they live together' (1965, p. 75).

'All real living is meeting' (Buber, 1937/1958, p. 11).

Gadamer

Hans-Georg Gadamer (1900–2002) was a German hermeneutic-phenomenological philosopher best known for his magnum opus, *Truth and Method* (*Wahrheit und Methode*) (1960/1996). His central thesis focused on the conditions, challenges and 'art' of human understanding (*Verstehen*).

Following his inspirational mentor Heidegger,[xxiii] Gadamer focuses on the nature of the **hermeneutic** process. Stressing an active and historical/ cultural situatedness of all understanding, he uses the concept of '**horizon**' to describe one's location in history which both offers the possibilities of understanding and its limits. But, in order to learn something new or see the 'otherness' of something, we need to have an 'open mind'; to raise our gaze beyond our normal horizons and allow a dialogue between past and present, a 'fusion of horizons':

> The horizon is the range of vision that includes everything that can be seen from a particular vantage point . . . We speak of narrowness of horizon, of the possible expansion of horizon, of the opening up new horizons and so forth. (Gadamer, 1960/1996, p. 302)

His key message is that historical texts such as the Bible (or works of art/literature) can only be studied from the vantage point of today because it is impossible to understand entirely what the original authors intended. Meanings, says Gadamer, can only be understood from the vantage point of the interpreter – meanings will vary between different people of different interests, in their different situations. Our vantage point, replete with our own historical-cultural understandings and '**prejudices**', are both our openness and closedness to the world. The 'tyranny of hidden prejudices . . . makes us deaf to what speaks to us' (p. 270).

For Gadamer (1960/1996) the philosopher strives to strike a balance between: (i) keeping a scientific openness and attempting to escape from personal prejudices, and (ii) being aware of one's worldliness and embeddedness. If possible, he says, 'distinguish the true prejudices, by which we *understand*, from the *false* ones, by which we *misunderstand*' (1960/1996, pp. 298–299); the challenge is to separate out productive prejudices as we are unconsciously influenced:

> A person who believes he [sic] is free of prejudices, relying on the objectivity of his procedures and denying that he is himself conditioned by historical circumstances, experiences the power of the prejudices that unconsciously dominate him. (1960/1996, p. 360)

Challenging the value of 'method' – particularly scientific method – Gadamer asserts the only way to (partially) understand meanings is through language,[xxiv] namely conversation/**dialogue** to 'question and provoke' our pre-understandings. After asking the questions we should wait for the answer and keep open:[xxv]

> To reach an understanding in a dialogue is not merely a matter of putting oneself forward and successfully asserting one's own point of view, but being transformed into a communion in which we do not remain what we were. (pp. 378–379)

Gadamer's own words offer a good summary:

> The important thing is to be aware of one's own bias, so that the text can present itself in all its otherness and thus assert its own truth against one's own fore-meanings. (Gadamer, 1960/1996, pp. 268–269)

Sartre

Like Merleau-Ponty, Jean-Paul Sartre (1905–1980) was a French existential philosopher and Marxist (although more politically active and passionately vocal). He was also a literary critic and prolific writer of numerous plays, novels and short stories. Sartre was also known for his long-standing relationship with Simone de Beauvoir.

In his key existential work *Being and Nothingness* (1943/1969), Sartre uses phenomenological description to clarify the fundamental features of lived experience. He labels the objects, concepts and experiences perceived and conceived by consciousness as 'beings in themselves' (*être-en-soi*). He explains that humans are conscious of the subjective meanings these objects hold for us. Yet the self/consciousness – 'being for itself' (*être-pour-soi*) – has no 'essence' or essential characteristics. It is both no-thing-ness ('nothingness') and the foundation for human freedom (freedom to make choices, to construct meanings). 'Man [sic] is condemned to be free'.

For Sartre, the existential anxiety of consciousness in the face of its nothingness is allayed by what he calls '**bad faith**'. Bad faith is our refusal to take responsibility for our choices, instead we accept the social attributions of others by conforming to (self-)given roles. A waiter who so identifies with the role that he cannot imagine himself as anything else, has made himself into an object and has stopped making choices. He is in bad faith.

Sartre famously describes his 'Look' whereby he imagines that – moved by jealousy, curiosity, or vice – he spies on someone by looking through a keyhole:

> I am alone and . . . But all of a sudden I hear footsteps in the hall. Someone is looking at me! What does this mean? . . . I now exist as myself for my unreflective consciousness. It is this interruption of the self which has been most often described: I see myself because somebody sees me . . . Shame reveals to me that I *am* this being . . . (Sartre, 1943/1969, pp. 259–262)

In his *shame*, he is discovered, judged and objectified – he becomes an object to the other and sees himself thus. Yet it is through this relationship with others that reflective consciousness arises. Others are imperialists, says Sartre, more so the more intimate we get. No wonder Sartre so famously declared: 'Hell is other people'!

Levinas

Emmanuel Levinas (1906–1995) was a French existential-hermeneutic phenomenological philosopher and Talmudic commentator.[xxvi] Following Husserl,[xxvii] Heidegger and Buber, his particular contribution was to offer an interpretive description of the precognitive face-to-face intersubjective encounter.[xxviii]

In his first magnum opus, *Totality and Infinity* (1961/1969), Levinas develops his unique philosophy of ethics which is both shocking and radical in its message. His basic thesis is that human existence involves a Self-Other **relationship** at its heart. Levinas seeks to go beyond the traditional Heideggerian ontology (which he sees as ethically neutral)[xxix] and to engage an analysis of the 'face-to-face' relation with the **Other**. Thus, he prioritizes the Other and puts concern for the Other at the centre of his ethics.[xxx]

Diverging from Buber, Levinas explains that the relationship of Self-Other is not mutual – there is 'asymmetry'. The other is an elusive stranger, an absolute and infinite Other who never be fully possessed or understood. I might appreciate the Other's viewpoint and understand a little of how they see me but I cannot step out of myself to experience the Other as if I were them. The Other continually exceeds our image of them and any partial labels we might ascribe to them. The Other's 'alterity' (difference) is always much larger than we can ever know. Levinas calls this the '**infinity** of the face of the Other' (Kunz, 1998).

Levinas argues that humans uncritically absorb **totalizing** narratives from society in a complacent, self-absorbed, inauthentic, idolatrous slumber. It is the Other who wakes us up, challenging, disrupting and decentring us; reminding us of our responsibility and calling us to our Goodness. The Other is present in the *here* and this singular here-ness catches me off-guard. The **Face** (the concrete presence of the Other) says, 'I am Other' and commands not be reduced to and annihilated by simple categories and labels. Awareness of the Face causes devastating, traumatizing *violence* to the ego. In awe and awakened, I am called to Being:

> Encountering the Other brings about a violent awakening to the self. Exposure to the Other creates a denucleation and dethroning of the self's sovereignty and dismembers its sense of security and comfort. (Goodman & Becker, 2009)

Yet, in this recognition of the otherness of the Other, lies the beginning of peace and love, reminding us we have responsibility for life: 'Thou Shalt not Kill'. Power over the Other through an objectifying, diminishing gaze must not, asserts Levinas, be the defining feature the relationship (as it was with the perpetrators of the holocaust). Such totalizing is not just ethically irresponsible; it weakens me, sabotaging me into isolation (Kunz, in press).

Levinas charges us with the ethical responsibility to be open to the otherness of the Other despite the disruption it might cause to our complacent pre-conceptions. Thus, for Levinas, the 'interhuman' calls us into our alterity and, ultimately, transcendence (Kunz, 1998).

Levinas elaborates these themes in a later major work *Otherwise Than Being or Beyond Essence* (1974/1981) – a volume that pushes intelligibility to the limit in its sophisticated but obtruse metaphorical description of the enigma of being human.[xxxi] Here is a taste:

> The psyche is the form of a peculiar dephasing, a loosening up or unclamping of identity: the same prevented from coinciding with itself, at odds, torn up from its rest, between sleep and insomnia, panting, shivering. It is not an abdication of the self, not alienated and slave to the other, but an abnegation of oneself fully responsible for the other . . . In the form of responsibility, the *psyche in the soul is the other in me*, a malady of identity, both accused and self, the same (self) for the other, the same (self) by the other (pp. 68–69, cited in Kunz, in press).

De Beauvoir

Existential phenomenological philosopher, prolific author and Marxist-feminist social theorist, Simone de Beauvoir (1908–1986) modestly identified herself as the 'midwife of Sartre's existential ethics'.[xxxii] Yet her most famous work *The Second Sex* spearheaded the feminist movement with its critique of patriarchy and women's oppression as '**Other**'. The new, richly nuanced 2010 translation of this book shows de Beauvoir at her best and attests to her growing contemporary influence.

In an earlier book, *Pour Une Morale de L'ambiguïté* (*The Ethics of Ambiguity*, 1947), de Beauvoir lays out her existentialism[xxxiii] as the philosophy of her time – in her view, the only one to take the question of evil seriously. Exploring the human condition, she says we exist without guarantees but we have the 'truth' of our freedom which entails a responsibility to contest the terrors of a world ruled by the tyranny of power (which she experienced first-hand with the Nazi regime).

In *The Second Sex* (1949/1984, 2010) de Beauvoir reprises her earlier arguments with more concrete examples. She argues against the either/or frame of the woman question where women and men are seen as either equal or different. Instead she wants to argue for women's equality (asserting the immorality of using sexual difference to exploit women), while insisting on the reality of the sexual difference. As a **feminist phenomenologist** she seeks to describe the ways in which women experience their bodies. She examines the meanings of the lived female body while bracketing how these meanings affect women's place in the world. Taken-for-granted assumptions such as how women are the 'weaker' sex are bracketed and challenged, for instance, by her asking: What criteria of strength are used? Muscle power? Average body size? Why is longevity not considered a sign of strength?

Like Sartre, de Beauvoir believes that **existence *preceeds* essence**: 'one is not born a woman'; she is made into one. Over history, she argues, women have been considered abnormal, deviant, outsiders and less than the ideal of men. This attitude limits women's success; the assumption must be set aside and new choices made:

> Woman may fail to lay claim to the status of subject because she lacks definite resources, because she feels the necessary bond that ties her to man regardless of reciprocity, and because she is often very well pleased with her role as the Other. (2010, pp. xxiv–xxv)

Women need to move beyond the 'immanence' to which they were previously resigned, she says, and reach a 'transcendent' position in which they take responsibility for themselves and the world, choosing their own freedom.

Beauvoir died aged 78 of pneumonia. She is buried next to Sartre at Montparnasse in Paris.

Ricoeur

Paul Ricoeur (1913–2005) was a French philosopher who combined phenomenological description and hermeneutic interpretation following the tradition of Heidegger and Gadamer. A prolific writer himself, he touched on diverse subjects across the social sciences, writing on the nature of being, discourse and metaphor. Most significantly perhaps he articulated a comprehensive vision of the relation of time, history and narrative.

Throughout his texts he endeavours to make sense of the question 'Who am I?' He seeks to provide an account of the tensions and ambiguities that underpin our human-ness. However, as a hermeneutic philosopher Ricoeur insists that whatever is understandable arises in and through language – self-understanding is mediated by signs/symbols/texts – and therefore has to call for interpretation. The human embodied being both pre-exists language and is understood interpretively through language.

In his *Interpretation Theory: Discourse and the Surplus of Meaning* (1976) he develops the concept of '**hermeneutic arch**' where he considers the way interpretation begins with the pre-reflective experience but how, in order to reach an understanding of our being, we need to utilize interpretation. Unlike other hermeneutic phenomenologists, however, Ricoeur remains content to import different theories/sciences to explain experience as part of the hermeneutic task, for instance, he draws on both psychoanalytic ideas and narrative theory. Here he moves beyond a traditional phenomenological **hermeneutics of empathy**/meaning-recollection (bringing out the meaning of an experience) towards embracing a **hermeneutics of suspicion** (where meaning is hidden/latent and has to be extracted).

In his later works, *Time and Narrative* (1984, 1985, 1988) and *Oneself as Another* (1992), Ricoeur develops his ideas on metaphor and narrative positing that we construct stories to make sense of our lived experience – the plots of the narratives we tell give us our 'directedness', explaining our lives. He argues that any philosophy for understanding human existence must embed the analysis in a narrative of past–present–future, i.e. a temporal framework.[xxxiv] Further, '**narrative selves** will be multiple and contingent, historically and culturally specific' (Langdridge, 2007, p. 52).

For Ricoeur, the meaning of all texts (and that includes research interview transcripts) is relative. Texts need to be 'conceived in a dynamic way as the direction of thought opened up by the text' (1971/1979, p. 92) disclosing *possible* ways of looking at things. Texts can only be interpreted; they do not offer a window onto the speaker/author's subjectivity, they just offer a new way of seeing (Packer, 2011):[xxxv]

> When a text unfolds a new way of seeing a critique of how things are becomes possible, along with a critique of the illusions of the interpreter. (Ricoeur, 1973/1990)

With this message Ricoeur takes a step away from phenomenology – planting his feet firmly in hermeneutic territory as he moves towards a more discursive, post-modern, post-structuralist landscape.[xxxvi]

Gendlin

Another existential phenomenologist who can be located in the post-modern movement is Eugene T. Gendlin (1926–), an American[xxxvii] psychotherapist and philosopher following in the tradition of Husserl, Heidegger and Merleau-Ponty. Gendlin's contribution is to articulate the tension between the lived body and language – a debate perhaps better placed *beyond* in the 'post-postmodern context': 'Let us enter and speak from the realm that opens where all distinctions break down' (Gendlin, 1997, p. 269) towards more 'intricate understandings' that go beyond the lines drawn by both modernism and post-modernism, embracing both and neither.[xxxviii]

Humanistically orientated therapists may well be familiar with some of the work of Gendlin, particularly his collaboration with Carl Rogers on client-centred therapy and bringing to the fore the practice of *Focusing* (Gendlin, 1996).[xxxix] (Focusing involves paying attention to intuitive 'gut' feelings. Through a series of steps, the Focuser can find exactly the right words/images for capturing this bodily 'felt sense' perhaps having an 'Ahah!' moment where new ideas, solutions or actions suddenly become clear.)

Following Heidegger and others, Gendlin agrees that humans first act and interact pre-reflectively and then they interpret. The body lives and 'knows' the situation directly, he says. Yet, there is also an intimate relationship with language. Language is embodied and the body can be language. Our bodies open us up to the '*more*', while we can also speak from this '*more*'. There is a 'responsive order' in which body makes authentic sense of language and links language to an embodied world of meanings.

> Sometimes, the bodily depth of what one has lived through is 'more than words can say.' Yet such experience 'looks for' words. Sometimes, the language of what things mean changes bodily experience, and the words disappear. (Todres, 1999, p. 288)

Expanding on these ideas in *Experiencing and the Creation of Meaning* (1997), Gendlin formulates seven 'modes' in which felt meanings (bodily intuitions) and symbolizations (language, images) interact.[xl] The following is a simplified summary of his discussion:

Felt experiencing: involves paying silent attention to a vague, pre-verbal 'felt-sense' that there is something.

Recognition: when we recognize and know what some word/symbol means at an embodied unconscious level.

Explication: where we begin to put the felt sense into some words.

Metaphor: involves achieving new meanings by drawing on old experiences and new language. For instance, saying 'my head is pounding like a drum' creates a new felt meaning for the listener.

Comprehension: where understanding is further languaged and developed through illustrations; it is shown when we cry out 'Yes, that's it exactly!'

Relevance: where the accumulation of meanings through experience is put into context with other meanings and experience.

Circumlocution: operates as previous meanings are challenged and further meanings created, for instance, in dialogue.

There is always a '*more*' lying beyond the language we use to represent experience.

Reflections

I am conscious of the fact that any attempt to discuss phenomenological philosophy is a precarious act. Have I sufficiently 're-presented' the philosopher's ideas? To what extent may I have (mis-)appropriated, (mis-)interpreted and re-constituted ideas away from what was initially meant? I have tried to remain faithful to the spirit of what I have understood though I will admit my interpretations cannot help but be involved.

I am reminded of Merleau-Ponty's words which he spoke in his essay *A philosopher and his shadow* where, with touching respect, he dialogued with Husserl's ideas:

> I borrow myself from others; I create others from my own thoughts . . . There must be a middle ground on which the philosopher we are speaking about and the philosopher who is speaking are present together, although it is not possible even in principle to decide at any given moment just what belongs to each. (Merleau-Ponty, 1964/1968, p. 159)

Reading this chapter will have confirmed for you how the language used and ideas within phenomenological philosophy are cast in a broad and frequently opaque net. Some ideas are so obscure and radical that we simply cannot really grasp them unless we bracket out our everyday and scientific understandings. (Ironically, one needs to be a phenomenologist in the first place to understand them!) However, it is not always such hard work. In my own struggle to grasp these ideas, I have taken Heidegger's lead and approached phenomenological philosophy as a form of poetry-to-dwellwith. As I dwell with the words of these great thinkers, my soul can be stirred by the language and profound depth, passion, pain and wonder of what is being revealed.

The best way for us as practitioners to understand these dense, baffling philosophical ideas is to start applying them. But herein lies the difficulty. These philosophers were offering a philosophy, *not method*. It has been left up to successive generations of scholars and researchers to work out what the ideas meant and how to apply them. No wonder the world of phenomenology remains one of uncertainty, controversy and competing diverse interests (Finlay, 2009a).

I love all this philosophy, so I find it unsatisfactory when novice researchers lay claim to the ideas of great philosophers when they have only ever used secondary sources. Often philosopher's original words and ideas may be presented so simplistically that their meaning is lost; the philosopher's intentions warped.

Most novice researchers will not need to read the original tomes of course – indeed, I might even advise them to avoid the originals in the first instance! My challenge is to researchers who *say* they are doing Husserlian and/or Heideggerian phenomenology without ever having touched their writings. Why not, instead, come clean and say for instance, that 'I am following Giorgi's method based on Husserlian ideas' or that 'I am drawing on some existential-hermeneutic ideas' or that 'I am following xxxx who has applied Merleau-Ponty's ideas'? I also challenge researchers who lay claim to a mix of philosophies without recognizing contradictory positions in their approach and focus (Giorgi, 2008a). Philosophies cannot simply be lumped together!

The following chapter, and also those in Part II, shows the different ways that philosophy has been specifically applied in practice. The key lesson is to recognize the need to be anchored philosophically. Having glimpsed of the worlds the philosophers have opened up, are you pulled to go exploring in any particular direction?

Notes

i Further information about the work of these and other phenomenological philosophers can be found online. Two websites I particularly recommend are: http://www .phenomenologyonline.com/websites/websites.html#Philosophers – *the Phenomenology Online* website developed by Max van Manen; and http://www.phenomenologycenter .org/ – the website for the *Centre for Advanced Research in Phenomenology* (Lester Embree is the current President of the Board of Directors). I also recommend Orange (2010).

ii Husserl (1859–1938) was born in into a Jewish family in Moravia, then a part of the Austrian Empire.

iii **Positivism** is a philosophical perspective (paradigm) that celebrates the methods of natural science: objective observation, testing, and measurement of cause and effect. Positivists hold that concepts that cannot be proved empirically (through observation) are not worthy of scientific study. They tend to adopt a 'realist' view of the world as a permanent and stable reality. This view contrasts with the paradigm of **interpretivism** which holds that objective understanding is impossible as it depends on your perspective, i.e. knowledge is 'relative'.

iv Husserl's notion of essences has been misunderstood as being reductionist, essentialist, realist whereas his view of the essence of phenomenon is what appears in being lived through. His intention was to 'bring back all the living relations of experience' (Merleau-Ponty, 1962, p. xv).

v In making this move Husserl was avoiding both the 'realist' position which posits that all objects exist solely in themselves and the 'idealist' position which reduces objects to just being in our minds. However, some critics point to Husserl's proclaimed position as a 'transcendental idealist' revealing a tendency to go towards that pole even if he claimed he was going beyond idealism.

vi Intentionality can be directed to real/palpable objects (subject to time) and to ir-real/impalpable ones (that are atemporal) such as 'justice' or 'prejudice'.

vii The different stages and grades of the reduction are not always so clearly delineated. While in *Crisis* he mentions eight different reductions and in *Ideas I* he speaks of phenomenological reductions in plural, in *Cartesian Meditations* he runs transcendental-phenomenological reduction together (Moran, 2000).

viii This is not an attitude of scepticism. As Husserl (1913/1983, p. 61) says, 'I am *not negating* this "world" as if I were a sophist; I am *not doubting its factual being* as though I were a skeptic; rather I am exercising the "phenomenological epoché which also *completely shuts me off from any judgment about spatio-temporal factual being*".'

ix He also betrayed his mentor Husserl by breaking off contact with him when Husserl (a Jew) was excluded from his university by the Nazi Party. Heidegger's position remains controversial today as he consistently refused to repudiate the Nazi regime and his own suspect actions. Was his problematic relationship to Nazism and Nationalist Socialism a mistake or part of his philosophy? It is hard to judge. As you grapple with his work/writings, you will need to work out your own (authentic) position and the extent you are prepared to engage his philosophy.

x There is much debate in the phenomenological field as to the extent Heidegger diverged from Husserl's ideas. Often, the philosophies of these two giants in the field are set up as polar opposites with Heidegger being seen as offering a severe *critique* of Husserl. While he makes some implicit criticisms and challenges, I would say Heidegger is respectful and simply goes beyond Husserl's ideas into different territory. It should be remembered that Heidegger dedicated *Being and Time* to Husserl 'in friendship and admiration'.

xi To help you get to grips with the ideas you might first turn to various video recordings about Heidegger, e.g. you might check out: http://www.youtube.com/watch?v=tRm6dElRZqQ. Also, I can recommend reading *Zollikon Seminars: Protocols-Conversations-Letters*. This book provides a record of the profound exchange of ideas between Heidegger and psychiatrist Medard Boss (through conversations and excerpts from hundreds of letters that Heidegger wrote between 1947 and 1971). Reading the material from the seminars you get a flavour of Heidegger the teacher; from the personal letters to Boss, you get a sense of Heidegger the person.

xii In a number of papers, Svenaeus (2001b) applies these concepts of 'being-at-home' and 'not-being-at-home' to health and illness. In health, he says, we feel at home and take our bodies for granted. In illness we experience our bodies as uncanny, we feel 'not-at-home'. But there is also a paradox here as the homelikeness of health can constitute an inauthentic mode of living and comes at a cost while illness can help us actively grasp possibilities for living. This is why many people who have experienced life-threatening or chronic health conditions talk about positive transformative benefits.

xiii Heidegger critiqued the traditional view of language as being representative of inner thoughts/ideas or as being an expression of the world. Both these views mistake language as being rooted in the human subject.

xiv The field of hermeneutics can be seen as separate from, but overlapping, phenomenology. Traditional hermeneutics refers to the study of the interpretation of written texts such as the Bible. Modern hermeneutics encompasses everything in the interpretative process. Basically, the question asked is: 'Can a text be understood in terms of the author's original meanings or does it depend on the socio-historical positioning of the reader?'

xv Husserl, Heidegger, Gadamer and Merleau-Ponty all tended to use a different lexicon to describe the concept of presuppositions or previous assumptions. Husserl's use of 'apperceptions' or 'appresentations' is comparable to the 'pre-understandings' of which Heidegger, Gadamer and Merleau-Ponty speak (Dahlberg *et al.*, 2008). Heidegger also favours other terms such as 'fore-having' and 'fore-conception'. Gadamer uses the concept of 'prejudices' while Merleau-Ponty prefers the concept of 'implicit understanding'.

xvi Much has been written about the long-standing relationship between Merleau-Ponty and Sartre (see for instance, Stewart's 1998 edited volume about their 'debate'). Their lives intersected through the French existential movement and when they came together both as Marxist comrades and as co-editors of the *Les Temps Modernes* – a philosophical, socialist journal which came out of the Resistance movement. Their much-vaunted political break (heralded by Sartre's passionate polemic supporting the Soviet Union while Merleau-Ponty turned away with a more measured 'intellectual' approach) eventually led to a brief *rapprochement* (when Sartre officially broke with the Communist Party after the invasion of Hungary in 1956) before Merleau-Ponty's death in 1961. In their various writings divergences remain including Merleau-Ponty's critique of Sartre's isolated accounts of the self and radical claims for freedom.

xvii In his translator's Preface, McCleary (in Merleau-Ponty, 1960/1964) summarizes Merleau-Ponty's 'Husserlian-Marxian' view as one where Merleau-Ponty insists that: 'the only acceptable humanism today is the one which works concretely for man's effective and universal recognition by his fellow man. In order to do so, it must . . . constitute a common bond between all men . . . [and] create political structures which can hold power in check without emasculating it' (1964/1968, p. xxx).

xviii Gestalt focuses on the whole as being greater than the sum of parts. While Merleau-Ponty was critical of gestalt psychology, he supported their central tenet that perception always involves a continually shifting attention to figure and ground where particular parts of the field become more prominent at any one time. If I am with an anxious client, for instance, I might be attending to their words and bodily expression and then suddenly my awareness shifts as my own embodied sensation of my stomach clenching in tension becomes figural.

xix One of Merleau-Ponty's useful methods is to examine breakdowns in bodily being which bring to light routines/understandings which are taken for granted. For example, he discusses the case of Schneider, a war veteran, whose brain had been damaged by shrapnel damaging his perceptual and motor function.

xx Sartre draws our attention to a third ontological dimension of the body: **bodily self-consciousness**. At the level of the lived body, I do not have awareness of my body as a separate thing – I am my body. At a reflective level the body becomes an object for me as a subject. 'I exist for myself as a body known by the Other', he explains (1943/1969, p. 351). Here, the body comes into awareness and being when the person becomes aware of the regard of another (see the discussion on Sartre's 'Look').

xxi Buber supported the potential of Zionism for social and spiritual enrichment. In 1930 Buber became an honorary professor at the University of Frankfurt am Main but resigned in protest when Hitler came to power in 1933. When the German government forbade Jews to attend public education, Buber founded the Central Office for Jewish Adult Education and a few years later left Germany to settle in Jerusalem.

xxii As an educator, Buber believed that students grow through the direct encounter with the person of the educator who in turn, enters the phenomenological world of the student to experience and feel it. In this way we are challenged to grow through our relationships.

xxiii Unlike Heidegger, Gadamer was not a Nazi, preferring a more apolitical, low key approach where he seemed to compromise with the ruling regime.

xxiv Gadamer agrees with Heidegger that language accomplishes understanding. Words are 'worlded' while dialogue involves a transformative communion. Gadamer, and other hermeneuticists, recognize the complex, dialogical nature of human science research where researchers are active agents, actively making sense while being changed in the process as history and context come into play.

^{xxv} In a long-running debate, the critical theorist Jürgen Habermas challenges Gadamer's approach that we should become aware of preconceptions and that understanding-interpretation contributes to passing on our tradition. Instead, Habermas calls us to use interpretations to question preconceptions and to critically challenge ideology and dogmatic tradition.

^{xxvi} Levinas was originally born in Lithuania but became naturalized French in 1930. For further biographical information see: http://www.levinas.sdsu.edu/.

^{xxvii} Levinas brought phenomenology to France through translating Husserl's *Cartesian Meditations* and other works.

^{xxviii} I am grateful to George Kunz who recommended a number of papers to me which apply Levinasian philosophy to Psychotherapy: see the Seattle University web-site (http://www.seattleu.edu/artsci/map/Inner.aspx?id=7268&terms=levinas); also Orange (2010).

^{xxix} Levinas located 'evil' in the self or being, challenging Heidegger's more neutral ontology. His focus on evil and on the violence of our interpersonal relations takes on an added dimension when we understand that Levinas was an interpreter in the French army during the Second World War being fluent in both German and Russian. Later he became a prisoner of war, forced into labour but protected from the annihilation of Jews. However, most of his relatives were killed.

^{xxx} For Levinas, ethics has a special meaning. It 'involves the effort to constrain one's freedom and spontaneity in order to be open to the other person, or more precisely to allow oneself to be constrained by the other' (Moran, 2000, p. 321).

^{xxxi} Partly in response to criticisms by Jacques Derrida, his aim was to avoid his previous ontological language. The Other, for example, is now expressed as 'Otherwise than being' – beyond being.

^{xxxii} Contemporary commenters are now recognizing that rather than echoing Sartre's work, de Beauvoir significantly influenced his work. Until his death they always read, debated and critiqued each other's work before it was published.

^{xxxiii} This book is an elegant and accessible entry into French existentialism and Sartre's own *Being and Nothingness*. The book starts by recognizing the meaning-disclosing, meaning-making and meaning-desiring activities of consciousness as both insistent and ambiguous. First, consciousness is free to disclose/discover the meaning of being; then consciousness exists as the freedom to bring meaning to the world, to be the author of one's own meaning. De Beauvoir identifies each of these *intentionalities* of freedom with a mood, namely either joy or hope and domination where this latter intentionality becomes the ground of projects related to liberation or exploitation, respectively.

^{xxxiv} He distinguishes cosmological time (natural, infinite time), phenomenological time (lived finite time) and straddling between the infinite and finite, humans have created historical time (archives and stories told over generations).

^{xxxv} Packer (2011) notes that recorded/transcribed interviews that leave out critical non-verbal/situational information can actually have greater relevance and power. For Ricoeur, the goal is not a reconstruction of the speaker's subjectivity or what x means to them so much as to learn about their project and new modes of being. 'It is a process of interpretation that begins with the *tacit* understanding a researcher has reading the text ... Through attention to the elements of narrative ... this tacit understanding can be articulated ... and communicated. The effect on the researcher, the meaning *for them*, is explicated, along with *how* that effect came about' (Packer, 2011, p. 119). In other words, the researcher is presenting their own reading of the text rather than making claims about the participant's experience.

xxxvi Unlike other post-structuralists such as Foucault and Derrida who deny subjectivity and focus on discourse, Ricoeur insists on retaining 'subjectivity' which he anchors in the body and material world with narrative as a way of giving meaning to a potentially fragmented life.

xxxvii Gendlin was born in Vienna, Austria, in 1926. His Jewish family fled the Nazi invasion and immigrated to the United States when he was 13 years old. In the 1950s, he went to the University of Chicago and studied under Carl Rogers. He later became a professor of psychology and philosophy at that same university.

xxxviii The position *beyond post-modernism* challenges the extreme relativism, arbitrariness, particularism and cynicism which post-modernism potentially represents. A similar concept of 'postphenomenology' is offered by Ihde (1993): 'Postphenomenology is precisely the style of phenomenology which explicitly and dare I say "consciously" takes multidimensionality, multistability, and the multiple "voices" of things into account – to that degree it bears a family resemblance to the postmodern' (Ihde, 2003, p. 26).

xxxix There are many brilliant resources on the Internet detailing the Gendlin's biography, theories and the practice of Focusing. For your first stop I recommend: http://www.focusing.org/gendlin/. The full archive of Gendlin's online work can be downloaded from the Seattle University site: http://www.seattleu.edu/artsci/map/News_Article.aspx?id=19192. Then, check out Gendlin's live lectures on *Focusing* on youtube: e.g. http://www.youtube.com/watch?v=zmL4zjVi8Dk&feature=related; also see Krycka's introduction on: http://www.seattleu.edu/artsci/psychology/default.aspx?id=3492.

xl Applying Gendlin's ideas to research, we first see how the participant makes an effort to describe their experience. He or she tries out some words relying on a felt sense to tell him/her when the expression feels 'right'. The researcher focuses on being present, facilitating and being open to the inter-embodied experience where the researcher's own felt sense is activated in response to the participant's. Understanding is deepened through discussion. Then when it comes to analysis, the researcher again tries to be present to the '*more*' through words.

Chapter 5

The 'Phenomenological Attitude'

Our . . . journey requires us to be touched and shaken by what we find on the way and to not be afraid to discover our own limitations . . . , uncertainties and doubts. It is only with such an attitude of openness and wonder that we can encounter the impenetrable everyday mysteries [of our world]. (van Deurzen-Smith, 1997, p. 5)

Most phenomenologists would probably agree that the 'phenomenological attitude' is one of the more, if not the most, significant dimensions of phenomenological research. Following Husserl's ideas of the **reduction**[i] (also known as epoché), the attitude involves the researcher adopting a particular open, non-judgemental approach; one filled with wonder and curiosity about the world while simultaneously holding at bay prior assumptions and knowledge. Past understandings about the phenomenon need to be **bracketed** so that critical attention can be given to the present experience (Giorgi, 2009). The aim is to reach beyond the natural attitude of taken-for-granted meanings and understanding.

The phenomenological attitude evolved initially as a philosophical method and this means that researchers are continually challenged about how to apply it in practice. Debates and uncertainty abound regarding the extent to which 'bracketing' can and should be applied. Novice researchers often find this confusing, with good reason. A particular mistake is to see the phenomenological attitude as something to be engaged in, once and for all, at the beginning of research, perhaps thinking it an attempt to

Phenomenology for Therapists: Researching the Lived World, First Edition. Linda Finlay.
© 2011 Linda Finlay. Published 2011 by John Wiley & Sons, Ltd.

be rigorous, objective and to eliminate biases.[ii] The reduction is, in fact, anything but an exercise of objective detachment. Instead, researchers need to be fully and continuously engaged in the process of managing the intrusion of pre-understandings. Bracketing is a process whereby the researcher refrains from positing altogether and takes an open approach to the data.

The phenomenological attitude can be seen as a kind of dance between the reduction and **reflexivity**:

> Reductions can be intertwined with reflexivity and . . . in this process, something of a dance occurs – a tango in which the researcher twists and glides through a series of improvised steps. In a context of tension and contradictory motions, the researcher slides between striving for reductive focus and reflexive self-awareness; between bracketing pre-understandings and exploiting them as a source of insight. (Finlay, 2008, p. 1)

In this chapter I elaborate some of the 'steps' of this 'dance'. First, I describe the process of engaging '**scientific phenomenological reduction**' – the approach favoured particularly by descriptive phenomenologists.[iii] Phenomenologists less interested in a 'scientific' stance prefer to embody broader humanistic values of **empathic openness**. This way of engaging the phenomenological attitude is discussed next. The final section explores how phenomenologists might apply **reflexivity** as part of the reductive-reflexive dance and a case study example is offered.[iv]

Scientific Phenomenological Reduction

For Husserl, the reduction(s) (including epoché/bracketing) places the philosopher at the 'groping entrance into this unknown realm of subjective phenomena' (1936/1970, p. 161). It is a radical self-meditative process where the philosopher 'brackets' the natural world and any interpretations, in order to see the phenomenon as it is given, i.e. in its essence.

> [Phenomenological reflection] must suspend the faith in the world only so as to *see it* . . . It must question the world, it must enter into the forest of references that our interrogation arouses in it, it must make it say, finally, what in its silence *it means to say*. (Merleau-Ponty, 1964/1968, pp. 38–39)

However, there are important differences between a *philosopher's* reflections and the phenomenological *researcher's* approach to participants and a reflective analysis of descriptions of lived experience. For one thing, as researchers, we are not concerned with pure reflection; for another, we usually deal with other people's accounts. Pragmatic, instrumental compromise is needed and that means we must modify philosophers' ideas when applying them to empirical and psychological research (Giorgi, 1997, 2009; Giorgi & Giorgi, 2003).

A modified form of the reduction is called for – one that emphasizes an open, reflective stance without treading into Husserl's transcendental realm (which involves transcending the perspective of human consciousness and standing above one's subjectivity, i.e. viewing the world as a pure essential consciousness). Giorgi calls this the **scientific phenomenological reduction**[v] (see *Chapter 6*). In this reduction, researchers aim to be fully present to their participants and to what is being described. In order to be present, past knowledge and existential claims about what is being experienced need to be held in abeyance. What is bracketed then is previous knowledge (specifically theoretical or scientific understandings) of the phenomenon and the assumption that it 'really' exists.

Consider research on experiencing a ghostly visitation, for example: when my participant describes seeing a 'ghost', it is this *experiential given* which needs to be explored. I need to set aside any ontological claims regarding the reality and nature of ghosts. I bracket any spiritual beliefs I may hold along with any possible scientific explanations. I simply (well, not so simply!) try to focus on my participant's experience.

The phenomenological research project thus aims to focus on the psychological reality of the lived experience (its 'givenness') rather than the 'reality' (material or otherwise) itself.

In order to receive these intuitions about meanings of lived experience, researchers need to place themselves in the present moment and within the (scientific phenomenological) reduction. Researchers can be aware of theories/past experiences but these are probably best regarded as 'temptations' to be temporarily suspended in order to explore what meanings are emerging in the present (Giorgi, 2009). This is not an obliteration of the past, insists Giorgi, it is a heightening of the present. Past and present are held in tension in order to discern their respective contributions. As Giorgi advises (2009, p. 92), 'the demand is to remain open to the recalcitrant data and all of its contrary implications'.

Wertz (2005) similarly emphasizes a slowing down:

> The researcher strives to leave his or her own world behind and... empathically joins with participants ('coperforms' participant's involvements) in their lived situation(s) . . . This attitude involves an extreme form of care that savors the situations described in a slow, meditative way and attends to, even magnifies, all the details. This attitude is free of value judgments from an external frame of reference and instead focuses on the meaning of the situation purely as it is given in the participant's experience (2005, p. 172).

While most phenomenologists go along with the need to bracket truth claims and not let one's own prejudices get in the way, loud debates centre on what it is exactly that needs to be bracketed. Ashworth (1996), for instance, identifies three particular areas of presuppositions that should be set aside in order to get closer to the lifeworld:

1) scientific theories, knowledge and explanations (e.g. from natural science, psychology and sociology);
2) truth or falsity claims being made by participants;
3) personal views and experiences of the researcher.

Helpfully he then recognizes clear limitations to what can be bracketed:

> Certain assumptions are made which are certainly not at any stage bracketed. These include the belief that the research participant is a competent human being whose life-world is open to empathic understanding since it shares at least certain baseline meanings with our own life-world as investigators. (Ashworth, 1996, pp. 21–22)

Here, Ashworth calls attention to the prior understandings that underlie our communications with others. He shows us how researchers do not necessarily bracket assumptions about the shared intersubjective world and the existence of a social reciprocity of perspective. When researchers introduce their topic of research to participants as being about a certain lived experience, there is a shared focus and probably shared cultural meanings, and these are not set aside. (A practical illustration of this from my own experience is how I explicitly use my therapist skills of listening and reflecting back to facilitate a participant's description and I assume what they tell me reflects something of their experience. Further, my use of empathy with participants is based on an assumption that empathetic understanding is possible. These, and many other, unbracketed presuppositions lurk, mostly unnoticed.)

While accepting limits to bracketing, Colaizzi (1973) and others contest the idea that the personal views/experience of the researcher should be set aside. Self-reflection constitutes an important part of the reflection, they say.[vi] Hermeneutic researchers argue even more vociferously that researchers are implicated in what they study and cannot be 'set aside'. Similarly, researchers using their own first person experience use only self-reflection so there is no question of setting researcher subjectivity aside. The conundrum then, is how and when to include self-reflection and personal experience. Different researchers negotiate this process differently as demonstrated by the various approaches described in Part II.

Critics of phenomenology, and researchers resistant to the use of the reduction, often latch on to Merleau-Ponty's famous statement: 'The most important lesson which the reduction teaches us is the impossibility of a complete reduction' (1945/1962, p. xiv). But Merleau-Ponty is simply echoing Husserl's view and highlighting the radical challenge of the reduction given the way we are always in the world and how reflections are 'carried out in the temporal flux on to which we are trying to seize' (p. xiv). Research (any kind) is always partial and we are simply being invited to recognize that reflections (or research findings) are inevitably partial, imperfect, emergent and tentative. More meanings always hover at or just beyond the horizon. We can acknowledge the incomplete nature of the process and still strive to engage phenomenological reflections *from within the reduction*, appreciating its potentially transformative nature.

Openness, Empathy and Other Humanistic Values

Many phenomenologists – particularly those with hermeneutic sensibilities – prefer to move beyond the idea of bracketing per se and discuss the phenomenological attitude more broadly as 'openness'. Here the researcher is open to be surprised – even awed – by the research; prepared for preconceptions to be shredded; open to the possibility of a shift in understanding.

Explicitly **humanistic** principles and values are brought into play such as acceptance, empathy, holism, creativity, spontaneous self-expression and transcendence. Arguing against the experimental psychology tradition and in favour of a humanistic human science, Wertz draws on Husserl's call for a radicalization of the scientific spirit:

> We need a psychology of affirmation, not control; a psychology of witness and recognition, not test and measurement; a psychology of deep commemoration, not superficial prediction. Human presence, not a proliferation of instrumentation. Privacy, not intrusion. A psychology of embrace, not engulfment . . . This means human science. (Wertz, 1986/2000, p. 165)

Phenomenological researchers believe that what participants say about their own experience is their 'truth' and that is the starting point of any explorations. We accept (i.e. do not morally judge) our participants and assume that what is given in research is their reality – at least as they understand or wish to present it. Part of this acceptance is also acceptance of their socio-cultural background, 'taking seriously our respect of difference and diversity' (Finlay & Evans, 2009, p. 37).

> As soon as we begin to move and gesture in response to the presence of the human Other, we are held by our culture in the corresponding beholdenness of our bodies. In every human voice, there are echoes of the mother's tongue,

echoes of significant teachers, respected elders, close friends; and there are accents, too, which bind the voice to the history of a region, a culture, and generations of ancestors. (Levin, 1985, p. 174)

As phenomenological researchers, we pay close attention to our participants through 'curiosity, empathy and compassion'. We attempt to 'feel into' the Other, aiming to get a sense of what their lived experience is like. At the same time, differences between researcher and researched are 'preserved so there is sufficient distance to challenge and be critically analytical where appropriate' (Finlay & Evans, 2009, p. 38). The differences between researcher and researched mean that we can never fully know our participants. More than this, we have an ethical responsibility to respect and be open to the *otherness* of the Other. While we might try to acknowledge our potentially powerful, oppressive position as researchers, at the same time, we need simultaneously to hold ourselves to being humble and modest in our claims.

Dahlberg *et al.* (2008) explicitly discuss the idea of **openness** in their version of Reflective Lifeworld Research. They recommend researchers adopt an 'open discovering way of being' and develop a 'capacity to be surprised and sensitive to the unpredicted and unexpected' (2008, p. 98). One implication of this stance is that researchers are advised not to fix beforehand the methods they are going to use to study the phenomenon. In their version of openness, researchers dance between 'vulnerable engagement' and 'disinterested attentiveness':

Openness is the mark of a true willingness to listen, see, and understand. It involves respect, and certain humility toward the phenomenon, as well as sensitivity and flexibility. To be open means to conduct one's research on behalf of the phenomenon. (2008, p. 98)

Similarly, Churchill *et al.* (1998) propose an intuitive '**empathic dwelling**' towards 'feeling into' another's experience. Engaged as a first stage of their phenomenological method, this empathic dwelling is enacted alongside the epoché. Here, the researcher tries to stay with the participants' descriptions becoming ever more open to what is being communicated. In empathy, they say, '*I participate in the other's positioning himself or herself from a unique perspective within a situation*... While maintaining one's own position as researcher, one gradually allows oneself to feel one's way into the other's experience' (1998, p. 66).

Other hermeneutic researchers maintain an open stance and limit bracketing perhaps to shuffling half-steps. In their application of interpretative phenomenological analysis (IPA) for instance, Smith *et al.* (2009) emphasize the importance of engaging with the participant *more than* engaging with bracketing – although they acknowledge that attention to the former inevitably enables the latter.[vii] The role of bracketing is seen primarily as a way of acknowledging evolving preconceptions, hunches and theoretical predilections while engaging the hermeneutic circle where fore-structures are continually modified. However, an open attentive approach is still called for: 'Whatever my previous concerns or positions, I have moved from a point where I am the focus, to one where the participant is the focus . . . This requires an intense attentiveness to, and engagement with, the participant as he/she speaks' (Smith, 2007, p. 6).

In summary, phenomenological researchers engage bracketing to different degrees while holding on to a stance of non-judgemental acceptance, wondering openness and respectful empathic dwelling.

Reflexivity[viii]

In my own work, I too try to be empathically open and I strive to embrace holistic values of humanistic theory. But I also argue the need for researchers to have a critical (and embodied) self-awareness of their own (inter-)subjectivity, processes, assumptions and interests.

As researchers, we need to examine how our attitudes/values/behaviour impact on the research process and findings; how our subjectivity both opens up and closes down evolving understandings. It is not enough that we identify previous understandings and somehow bracket them. The process is much more difficult, continuous, iterative, layered and **paradoxical** (Finlay, 2008). We need – I believe – to *reflect reflexively* on meanings arising in our research and upon our role as (embodied) researchers in constituting those meanings. At the same time, we also need to guard against becoming too self-absorbed and caught up in self-indulgent introspection such that the focus of the research shifts away from the phenomenon on to the researcher. Equally we want to avoid situations where hyper-reflexivity results in objectifying ourselves and others.

In addition to bracketing and being empathically open, I suggest researchers engage in a dialectical process of **hermeneutic reflexivity**: a process of 'continually reflecting upon our interpretations of both our experience and the phenomenon being studied so as to move beyond the partiality of our previous understandings and our investment in particular research outcomes' (Finlay, 2003b, p. 108). This process involves more than introspective 'self-reflection' to acknowledge one's initial positioning and expectations at the beginning of research. Instead, it is used throughout research to critically evaluate research process and outcomes. Reflexive awareness of understandings, along with bodily/emotional intersubjective intuitions, can also shed light on a participant's experience (see, for instance, Finlay, in press) where I discuss the use of reflexivity in qualitative research interviews[ix]).

It is only recently that the term reflexivity has become particularly associated with the phenomenological method[x] although it has been a defining feature of qualitative research methodology in general for at least a couple of decades (Banister *et al.*, 1994; Finlay, 2002a, 2002b). Qualitative researchers appreciate that the researcher actively constructs the collection, selection and interpretation of data and that any results are *co-constituted* – a joint product of the participants, research and the social context.

While this particular understanding of the term reflexivity has not been traditionally drawn upon in phenomenology, the concept has long been central to the phenomenological project. Sartre (1943/1969), for example, distinguishes between: *unreflective consciousness* where the self is taken up with experiencing, forgetful of one's own agency; *reflexive consciousness* where the self and experience become the object of reflection; and *self-reflective consciousness* where the self becomes, reflexively, the aim of reflection.[xi]

Merleau-Ponty (1945/1962, 1964/1968) runs with these ideas when he talks of 'radical reflection' arguing that self-understanding consists – paradoxically – in recovering our unreflective experience. Reflexivity is a partial attempt to overcome subject–object dualism and to focus on intentional conscious lived experience in a self-aware way.

In his later work around the intertwining, Merleau-Ponty radicalizes these ideas, seeming to suggest that to understand something means to have related it to ourselves in such a way that we might discover there an answer to our question. 'The seer is caught up in what he sees, it is still himself he sees: there is a fundamental narcissism of all vision' (1964/1968, p. 139). Later he reminds us to ground reflection in the body by referring to a quasi-reflective redoubling: 'Reflexivity must be understood by the body, by the relation to self of the body, of speech . . . This flesh of my body is shared by the world, the world *reflects* it, encroaches upon it and it encroaches upon the world . . . ' (p. 246, 248).[xii]

It is easy to get lost in these seductively mysterious ideas so it is worth exploring what they might mean in practice. In Example 5.1, I discuss the way I applied the phenomenological attitude in practice during my research with Kenny on his lived experience of mental health problems. (His fuller story is given in *Chapter 12*.)

**Example 5.1   A case study applying the
'phenomenological attitude'**

At a key point in our interview, I noticed both Kenny and I were holding ourselves, arms tightly folded across our bodies, rocking. It seemed at the time, that in striving to **empathize bodily**, I might have been mirroring his experience (what Husserl calls imaginal self-transposition). I reflected on this powerful moment both during the interview (sharing my observations with Kenny) and after during the analysis phase. I nudged myself to be open and **bracket** my habitual interpretations of what this might mean. I tried to empathetically **dwell with** the meanings for Kenny. The posture seemed less 'defensive' and more a means to 'hold himself together', to stop himself 'falling apart'. Later in my analysis I tried to engage Husserl's **eidetic reduction** using the procedure of free imaginative variation. I asked myself questions and imaginatively varied possible meanings to distinguish incidental meanings from those particular to Kenny's lifeworld:

> 'Was my sense that he was trying to hold himself together revealed in other gestures or words? Are there instances where his holding gesture is a self-protective or self-nurturing one? As my analysis progressed it seemed that part of the structure of Kenny's experience was that he sought to isolate himself in his anxiety for fear of hurting others as well as keeping himself safe. So I asked: Did he only "lose it" when he was with other people?; Would he still "lose it" if others intruded into his bedroom?; and so forth. Reflecting through imaginative variation allowed me to see the pressures Kenny faced were primarily to do with the presence of other people. His bedroom was a sanctuary only because he could be alone there.' (Reproduced from Finlay, L. (2008). A dance between the reduction and reflexivity: Explicating the 'phenomenological psychological attitude', *Journal of Phenomenological Psychology*, 39, 1–32 (p. 27), with the kind permission of Brill Publishers.)

This brief example shows how a researcher might engage the **reductive-reflexive dance**, stepping away from initial assumptions and understandings, then moving in to reflexively interrogate them. Pre-understandings are challenged with each new thought and insight. 'The researcher makes interpretative revisions and the ground is re-covered. And the "dance" steps begin once more . . . ' (Finlay, 2008, p. 17).

Reflections

'No work can be consider[ed] phenomenological if some sense of the reduction is not articulated and utilized', declares Giorgi (1997, p. 240). I agree.

While I accept some hermeneutic practitioners do not engage Husserl's reductions to the letter, I believe all phenomenologists would agree about the need to return to phenomena as they are lived/experienced and about the need to be open to the phenomenon as given. All would agree that a continuous iterative disciplined struggle is involved if we are to become aware of, and then manage, evolving understandings.

So the question at stake is *how to apply* the phenomenological attitude in research practice. How do we engage a broader view, allowing us to freshly experience the phenomenon being studied? In this chapter I have suggested that it can involve a rigorous application of the 'scientific phenomenological reduction' *and/or* a looser empathically open, perhaps reflexive, engagement with the phenomenon. Precisely how it is engaged clearly depends on the researcher's aims, style and the methodology adopted (see the chapters in Part II).

My personal approach of choice is usually to embrace a fluid, dynamically paradoxical, dance between the reduction and reflexivity: between bracketing lingering pre-understandings and exploiting them as a source of insight; between being empathically, and naively open and self-critically aware; between detaching from lived experience and being involved with it; between going with the rhythmic flow of the dance while technically following set steps. Drawing on my therapy practice, my approach is also *relational* and involves an attempt to be empathically present with my participants while also engaging in reflexive embodied empathy (Finlay, 2005).

Whenever I have discovered something interesting, puzzling or surprising in research it has come about precisely because I have engaged this phenomenological attitude and was open to the possibility of seeing something new. For me, this is the excitement of phenomenology:

> The reward comes with extraordinary, though fleeting, moments of disclosure where the phenomenon reveals something new about itself and understanding acquires greater depth . . . For an instant or two, the researcher shares the rapture of the dancer: the sinuous embrace of something elemental, unexpected and almost beyond the possibility of being put into words. (Finlay, 2008, p. 29)

Notes

[i] Across his different writings Husserl variously posits numerous reductions including the *epoché of the natural sciences, epoché of the natural attitude, transcendental reduction* and *eidetic reduction.* He also pulled them together in writing about '*the* phenomenological reduction' (1913/1983, p. 66) – see *Chapter 4.* These early formulations have subsequently been elaborated in existential-hermeneutic directions (recognizing the philosopher's historical/cultural embeddedness) and further modified in various ways to be applied in

empirical psychological research. (See Finlay, 2008 for a more in-depth account of this history.)

ii The mistake here is to embrace this positivist approach which holds fast to the very scientific assumptions and attitudes that need to be bracketed! Inquiry is a 'continuous beginning' says Merleau-Ponty (1960/1964, p. 161) explaining Husserl's reduction.

iii Van Manen in fact proposes a '**hermeneutic reduction**' version which mirrors the process:

> One needs to reflect on one's own pre-understandings, frameworks, and biases regarding the (psychological, political, and ideological) motivation and the nature of the question, in search for genuine openness in one's conversational relation with the phenomenon. In the reduction one needs to overcome one's subjective or private feelings, preferences, inclinations, or expectations that may seduce or tempt one to come to premature, wishful, or one-sided understandings of an experience and that would prevent one from coming to terms with a phenomenon as it is lived through. (van Manen, 2002)

iv In focusing on these different facets of the phenomenological attitude, I am trying to highlight the different ways it has been articulated and applied in research practice. These ideas are further elaborated in the approaches discussed in Part II of this book. However, I think it is important to avoid polarizing the phenomenological field into descriptive and hermeneutic and reflexive variants. In practice there is much overlap. For instance, Wertz – a committed descriptive phenomenologist – is equally wedded to the principles of being empathically open. And how else is a researcher going to know what to bracket unless he or she is reflexive? While I'm separating out these different facets, as you read, try to hold the 'whole'.

v Giorgi (2009) explains that Husserl talked about the modified, non-transcendental version of the reduction as 'psychological phenomenological reduction'. However, as this approach can be used in all the **human sciences** (i.e. carried out by health professionals, sociologists, etc.) – not just psychology – Giorgi prefers to use the term '*scientific phenomenological reduction*'.

vi Colaizzi (1973) advocates a process of 'individual psychological reflection' (IPR) as an important first step of the research process. Here, the researcher brings to awareness preconceptions/biases while attempting to formulate the research question. The process also helps to define the parameters and possibly significant dimensions of experience which might be explored during data collection and again when analysing findings. Wertz (2005), too, finds the idea of researcher self-reflection consistent with a Husserlian application of the epoché of the natural attitude:

> This second epoché and analyses that follow from it allow us to recollect our own experiences and to empathically enter and reflect on the lived world of other persons in order to apprehend the meanings of the world as they are given to the first-person point of view. The psychologist can investigate his or her own original sphere of experience and also has an intersubjective horizon of experience that allows access to the experiences of others. (Wertz, 2005, p. 168)

vii In the early years of IPA's development, proponents were relatively silent about the application of Husserlian reductive methods. However, more recent work (Smith *et al.*, 2009) acknowledges the philosophical basis of IPA more explicitly and identifies an explicit role for bracketing.

[viii] The terms *reflection* and *reflexivity* are often used interchangeably and this can create confusion. I prefer to distinguish the two. For me, reflection can be defined as 'thinking about' something in general whereas reflexivity involves a more immediate, critical *self*-awareness (see Finlay & Gough, 2003). Reflexivity in research can thus be seen as being critically self-aware of one's impact on the research rather than reflecting more generally on the research and evolving meanings.

[ix] More specifically, in Finlay (in press), I propose five 'lenses' through which researchers can reflexively evaluate interviews: **strategic reflexivity** which looks through a lens focused on methodological/epistemological aspects; **contextual-discursive reflexivity** to examine situational and socio-cultural elements; **embodied reflexivity** to explore the researcher's embodied felt sense and the gestural duet between interviewer and interviewer; **relational reflexivity** for examining the intersubjective, interpersonal realm; and, finally, **ethical reflexivity** which aims to monitor processual aspects and power dynamics, enabling possible ethical implications to be articulated.

[x] Self-reflection has, of course, been a defining feature of phenomenology since the beginning of this philosophical tradition. More recently, different researchers have built upon this tradition, approaching the topic of reflexivity in different ways and drawing on different concepts. **First-person autobiographical** accounts (see *Chapter 10*) are implicitly reflexive. Reflexivity can similarly be found in relationally orientated, second-person perspective accounts (see *Chapter 11*). These approaches offer a kind of reflexive-intersubjective perspective. Churchill (2010a), for instance, has pioneered the use of the second person perspective where he is open to experiencing meanings in the other's expression that are not his 'own' but are shared with the other in a kind of 'empathizing perception'. 'When I am a true witness of the other's experience, I am entering into the vibrant field of meaning in which meanings begin to 'resonate' in my experience.'

[xi] Sartre argues that when we retrieve our attention and refocus it on our self, the self effectively becomes an object which we can describe in terms of characteristics. However, he regards this as 'bad faith' as our characteristics can be actively changed.

[xii] Subsequently, Merleau-Ponty (1964/1968) calls for a much more critical embodied **hyper-reflection**. He highlights the fundamental ambiguous divergence within the body which maintains that any thorough all-encompassing self-perception is impossible (e.g. hands that touch and are touched cannot be perceived in the same moment). Our (self-)reflective perceptions are always limited and ultimately 'miscarry':

> If my left hand is touching my right hand, and if I wish to suddenly apprehend with my right hand the work of my left hand as it touches, this reflection of the body upon itself always miscarries at the last moment: the moment I feel my left hand with my right hand, I correspondingly cease touching my right hand with my left hand. (Merleau-Ponty, 1964/1968, p. 9)

Part II
Phenomenological Research Approaches

Introduction to Part II

In this section, I aim to reveal something of the rich range of phenomeno-logical approaches, arising from different philosophical traditions, available in research practice. There are many ways to 'do' phenomenology, and researchers have diverse choices before them.

While any attempt to map the different methodologies is challenging and unlikely to be free of controversy, a useful starting point is to divide phenomenological methodologies into two broad categories – **descriptive** and **hermeneutic**. These follow the broad philosophical traditions of Husserl and Heidegger, respectively.[i]

I start by laying out the distinctions between these two broad orientations. I then seek to move beyond this traditional division or categorization by identifying four additional ways of doing phenomenological research which do not easily fit into the descriptive-hermeneutic dichotomy: lifeworld approaches; interpretative phenomenological analysis (IPA); first person accounts; and reflexive, relational approaches. This represents very much my own attempt at classification, and some readers may take issue with it. However, I have selected the particular approaches I have seen most frequently used in research practice today, and this I believe makes them of special interest to prospective researchers. Each approach, I suggest, has become a 'tradition' in its own right with its own particular emphasis, strengths and limitations.

Phenomenology for Therapists: Researching the Lived World, First Edition. Linda Finlay.
© 2011 Linda Finlay. Published 2011 by John Wiley & Sons, Ltd.

Table Box II.1 Summary of the six approaches discussed in Part II.

Approach	General aim/focus	Philosophical foundations and research tradition	Specific methods/procedures involved
Descriptive, empirical	To describe (in a broadly normative and scientific sense) the essence or structure of experiences as given in consciousness: the descriptions are anchored rigorously to the data without bringing external theory to bear	This approach is based on Husserl's project to reveal the essence of phenomenon employing the epoché, intentional analysis and eidetic reduction. Giorgi and others of the 'Duquesne School' have developed the philosophy into a method for psychology and the human sciences more generally	At least three participants are interviewed or provide written protocols. The researcher *brackets* past knowledge/presuppositions; the description is broken into *meaning units*; then psychological meanings are systematically extracted and *imaginatively varied* to obtain a rigorous account of the general structure of the phenomenon
Hermeneutic, interpretive	To evoke lived experience using interpretations: Lived experience is thematicized through language and refracted through philosophical, theoretical, literary and/or reflexive lenses. Human scientific concerns blend with the stylistic, artful realms of the humanities	Following the lead of Heidegger and Gadamer and other hermeneuticists, (such as Ricoeur and Levinas), a tradition has grown. It been applied in various fields of human/social science, health, pedagogy and the arts by diverse writers including Jager, van Manen and Todres	No specific method is laid down except for applying the *hermeneutic circle*. Research findings are understood to be intertwined with the researcher's interpretations and the context. The end result is a kind of aesthetic phenomenology with a poetic, metaphorical sensibility

| Lifeworld | Both descriptive and/or hermeneutic designs may be used to explore how everyday experience shows itself in the *Lebenswelt* or lifeworld, i.e. as embodied and lived through time/space and in relationships with others | Husserl's concept of 'lifeworld' was developed by Heidegger (through his concept of *Dasein*/ being-in-the-world) and others including Sartre, Merleau-Ponty, Schutz and van den Berg. Dahlberg and Ashworth are two contemporary proponents of lifeworld-led research who have evolved particular versions | In Dahlberg's Reflective Lifeworld Research five or more participants are interviewed (although other methods may be used). Data analysis moves dynamically between the whole and parts, with the researcher being sensitive to both the generalities and particularities of the phenomenon. An open, slowed down, **bridled** attitude to both the phenomenon and process of understanding is maintained as the researcher **searches for the essence(s)** through active reflection. |

Table Box II.1 (*Continued*)

Approach	General aim/focus	Philosophical foundations and research tradition	Specific methods/procedures involved
Interpretative phenomenological analysis (IPA)	IPA is a structured version of hermeneutic phenomenology which focuses on the individual's sense-making, i.e. offering *idiographic* accounts of people's perceptions and how they make sense of their experiences	Philosophical ideas from both *phenomenology* (e.g. Husserl and Heidegger) and *hermeneutics* (e.g. Schleiermacher and Gadamer) are foregrounded. Smith and his colleagues initially evolved the approach in the field of psychology to bridge discursive and cognitive approaches	Perceptions/experiences of around three to six participants are explored using semi-structured interviews and other methods. While IPA analysis is iterative and inductive, a **systematic** approach is recommended focusing first on **individual meanings,** then looking for patterns across the participants. **Interpretive/literary revisions** then take the analysis to deeper levels
First-person	Researchers use their own personal experiences to examine and describe the quality/essences of phenomenon. The form used can either be descriptive or hermeneutic	First-person approaches follow the path of the original philosophers like Husserl who pioneered phenomenology as the reflective study of structures of consciousness as experienced from the first-person point of view. The approach has been applied in wide-ranging narrative accounts of experience, for instance, in relation to health (see the work of Toombs), feminism (e.g. the work of Young) and ecology (e.g. the work of Abrams)	Researchers may include concrete **narrative** descriptions of significant events perhaps interspersed with theoretical discussion and/or literary flourish. **Personal reflection** thus becomes a springboard for broader, deeper analyses or new insights

| Reflexive-relational | In reflexive-relational approaches, data is seen to emerge out of the researcher and co-researcher relationship and as being co-created (at least in part) in the embodied dialogical encounter. Researcher reflexivity and researcher-participant (inter-) subjectivity is celebrated | While these approaches may draw on any of the philosophers' work the dialogical and ethical spirit found in the work of Gadamer, Gendlin, Levinas and Buber is specifically prized. Psychologists who have applied these ideas in practice include Halling, Rowe and colleagues in their *dialogal* approach and Moustakas in his version of **heuristic** research | Diverse methodologies nest beneath this umbrella category. With *dialogal research, a group of* phenomenologists investigate a phenomenon sifting through different perspectives collaboratively through **dialogue** with others. With *heuristic research*, methods and processes aimed at **self-inquiry, reflexive dialogue** and **creative synthesis** are employed. With *reflexive-relational research*, researchers attend to the layered embodied intersubjective relationship between researcher and co-researcher |

It is worth remembering that the boundaries separating one approach from another are often blurred in practice (for example, IPA is a form of hermeneutic phenomenology). Also, different approaches are sometimes combined in practice, although this must be done selectively, judiciously and with due respect for logical consistency. (Lifeworld analysis can be both descriptive and interpretive, for instance.)

As you read the following chapters, try to be aware of areas of debate and contention: for instance, between researchers favouring scientific approaches and those favouring more poetic forms; between structured and more fluid, open procedures; between idiographic and normative concerns; between traditional and post-modern presentations (Finlay, 2009a). Table II.1 summarizes the key concepts and issues involved.

To enable comparisons to be made between the six approaches I have used the same structure in each chapter of Part II. I start by explaining the **methodology in general** (discussing aims, approach and methods/procedures). Then I use three **Example studies** to show how the approach can be applied in practice. I do not provide detailed guidelines on the mechanics of the analysis required by each approach: for this you will need to review the source material indicated in the references. Instead, I indicate the steps taken and the kind of findings that can result. Each chapter concludes with a **reflection section** where I offer my personal evaluation of the value, challenges and potential pitfalls of each approach.

Whatever your personal take on the different approaches, I encourage you to dwell with the quotes and examples offered in the chapters as they demonstrate phenomenology better than my words ever could. Let the examples touch you; then you will get closer to understanding the 'truth' of phenomenology.

Note

[i] Arguably, the theoretical differences between the two philosophical traditions have been overstated (Finlay, 2008). Heidegger was Husserl's student and he built upon Husserl's ideas, about the lifeworld for example, despite taking his descriptions in a hermeneutic/interpretive direction. As Merleau-Ponty pointed out, the whole of Heidegger's *Being and Time* 'springs from an indication given by Hussserl and amounts to no more than an explicit account of ... the "*Lebenswelt*" ... Husserl ... identified as the central theme of phenomenology' (1945/1962, vii).

Chapter 6

Descriptive Empirical Phenomenology

The inexhaustible diversity, depth, complexity, and fundamental mysteri-ousness of lived experience always exceeds our knowledge. (Wertz, in press)

While all phenomenology is descriptive in the sense that it seeks to de-scribe rather than explain, a number of scholars and researchers distin-guish between *descriptive* phenomenology and *interpretive* (or hermeneu-tic) phenomenology. In this chapter, I explore this distinction further by looking more closely at what is meant by the category 'descriptive em-pirical phenomenology'.[i] In general, researchers working within this tra-dition stay faithful to Husserl's original project, seeking to reveal the **essence** of a phenomenon (also called essential general meaning struc-tures). They stay close to what is given to them in all its richness and complexity, and restrict themselves to 'making assertions which are sup-ported by appropriate intuitive[ii] validations' (Mohanty, 1983, cited in Giorgi, 1986, p. 9).

Amedeo (Andy) Giorgi, an American psychologist and the main pro-ponent of a thorough, Husserlian method applied to research, states the project thus:

Phenomenological psychology refers to a human-scientific project whereby one does concrete analyses of the psychological meanings of specific experi-ences by using steps consistent with Husserl's philosophical phenomenolog-ical vision. (Giorgi, 1997, p. 254)[iii]

Phenomenology for Therapists: Researching the Lived World, First Edition. Linda Finlay.
© 2011 Linda Finlay. Published 2011 by John Wiley & Sons, Ltd.

In scholarly works dating back to the 1960s, Giorgi provides helpful guidelines on how to translate philosophy into scientific method – a *human* scientific one rather than a *natural* scientific one. A prolific writer himself, Giorgi has also provided the impetus for what has become known as the **Duquesne Tradition** which has spawned hundreds, if not thousands, of research studies throughout the world (see e.g. Colaizzi, 1973; Fischer, 1974; Giorgi, 1985; von Eckartsberg, 1971; Wertz, in press).[iv] In this method, Giorgi articulates a rigorous approach involving the collection of concrete examples of psychological subject matter, systematic observation and rigorous analytic reflection on their meanings.[v]

In this chapter, I offer a brief account of the descriptive phenomenological method (based on the work of Giorgi and others), followed by three examples of research ranging from large to small-scale studies.

Methodology

Aims

The descriptive phenomenological approach seeks to describe and clarify the nature of the phenomenon being studied in a broadly traditional, normative and scientific sense. It aims to **describe the structure of experiences** and the manner in which they are given in consciousness. It does *not* attempt to interpret meanings by bringing external theory to bear.

> A descriptive analysis . . . does not go beyond the given . . . The descriptive researcher obviously sees the same ambiguities that an interpretive analyst would see but is not motivated to clarify them by bringing in nongiven or speculative factors. An interpretive analysis, from a scientific perspective, usually strives for an interpretation that is theoretically elegant or . . . relatively complete. A descriptive result is more inchoate; it dares not go beyond what is present. Gaps in the results are filled by obtaining more data, not by theoretical speculation. (Giorgi, 2009, p. 127)

Giorgi's attempt to evolve a more rigorous, methodical approach to the study of phenomena has on occasion led to confusion. Some scholars have interpreted his work as an attempt to be objective and to minimize subjectivity. Giorgi himself (1994) has rejected such a characterization, observing that 'nothing can be accomplished without subjectivity, so its elimination is not the solution. Rather how the subject is present is what matters, and objectivity itself is an achievement of subjectivity' (p. 205).

In aiming to describe the essential structures of experience (essences), descriptive phenomenologists follow Husserl's ideas of the epoché, intentional analysis and eidetic reduction to bring the pre-reflective lived 'world' to light. This search for essences has been mistakenly understood in essentialist terms as if talking about objective reality whereas Husserl and his contemporary followers grant meanings are more slippery and inexhaustible.

Approach

The descriptive phenomenological approach is grounded in the philosophies of both Husserl and Merleau-Ponty and is applied to the empirical human scientific project. Giorgi argues that four core characteristics hold across all phenomenological variations, including his own: the research is rigorously **descriptive**, uses the phenomenological **reductions**, explores the **intentional** relationship between persons and situations, and discloses the **essences**, or structures, of meaning immanent in human experiences through the use of imaginative variation (Giorgi, 1989).

Wertz (in press) summarizes the process:

> The empirical researcher collects naïve description in ordinary language from participants who have lived through situations relevant to the topic under investigation. The researcher then reflects on the person's intentionality with respect to their situation, holistically explicating the organization of constituent processes and meanings, including the person's embodied selfhood, emotionality, agency, social relations, and temporality ... When conducted methodically, this approach is characterized by meticulous and thorough description that achieves fidelity to psychological life. (Wertz, in press)

While Giorgi supports the need to have a 'certain openness and flexibility' (2008b, p. 42) when it comes to applying his specific method, he insists that criteria associated with scientific **rigour** need to be completely respected. Meanings that emerge from research must do so from applying the phenomenological **psychological reduction** (rather than the transcendental reduction) must be seen to be based on data, and must be achieved through a systematic process of free imaginative variation which enables the researcher to grasp and verify the essential or invariant processes and meanings. Put another way, researchers using his method need to apply ideas from Husserlian philosophy *consistently* and *logically*.

Giorgi is clear that his particular method is neither exclusive nor exhaustive and that it should not be considered as paradigmatic (Giorgi, 1975). But he is critical of researchers who claim their work derives from Husserl while failing to read or understand Husserlian primary sources and of those who evoke Giorgi's own name and method falsely, thereby misrepresenting his work. Box 6.1 shows some of the ways in which novice researchers can stray from Giorgi's key principles (2008a, 2008b).

Example 6.1   Misunderstandings and problematic applications of Giorgi's method

1) Novice researchers sometimes misread Giorgi's phenomenology as aiming to describe **individuals' subjective experiences**. First, the descriptive phenomenological approach is concerned with more general phenomena (e.g. the experience of grieving or the experience of having therapy) rather than individuals' experience per se. Secondly, the method focuses not on 'subjective experience' but on situations as experienced by human subjects. The focus is on phenomena, not individual experience.

2) While some novice researchers tend to cite big **philosophical names** to shore up their academic arguments, Giorgi counsels against casting the net too widely, for example, arguing that confusion rather than harmonious integration is likely to result. Researchers are likely to be better off choosing one methodology rather than attempting to meld together ideas from, say, descriptive, hermeneutic and heuristic approaches (Giorgi, 2008a, 2008b).

3) The use of **bracketing**. Novice researchers can fall into the trap of simply listing assumptions and biases at the beginning of a research project as their way of 'doing bracketing'. Unfortunately, this approach does not come near what is required in the phenomenological attitude. The other point to remember is that the reduction has to take place throughout the research process, not just at the start.

4) The use of strategies to **verify findings**. Another tendency among novice researchers, especially those favouring 'realist' approaches[vi] is to offer their initial findings to participants or peers in order to *validate* them. While such collaborative strategies may be justified on ethical grounds, they are somewhat misguided if the researcher is following the descriptive phenomenological approach. Giorgi argues that participants describe their experiences from the perspective of the 'natural attitude' given they are unfamiliar with either phenomenology or the phenomenological attitude. As a result, participants will not be able to see the research in the same way the researcher does. He also makes the point that while participants are experts in what they have experienced, they are less clear and categorical about the *meanings* of their experience. After all, their view 'now' of an experience which took place 'then' could well have changed since they first described it.

Methods and procedures

Giorgi recommends recruiting at least *three* participants to give a sufficient and necessary number of variations in order to come up with a typical essence. He argues that the differences between them make it easier to distinguish the individual experience from the more general experience of the phenomenon. Idiographic analysis (i.e. researching a particular individual case) may form part of the process of analysis but the eventual aim is to **explicate** (i.e. describe, unpack) the phenomenon as a whole, regardless of the individuals concerned. In the process, idiographic details may be discarded, or typified and generalized.

Descriptive phenomenology tends to be conducted using **retrospective descriptions** of people's experience, most often obtained through in-depth interviews and/or written *protocols*.[vii] Other qualitative data collection methods, such as videotaping and 'talking aloud' while engaged in a task, can also be used. Whatever the data collection method used, the aim is to get as *thick* a description from participants as possible. For example, participants might be guided to provide a description that starts prior to the event or experience being described. Then the participant is asked to detail in a concrete way, their own thoughts, feelings and behaviours as well as describing the environment and others involved.

Interviews are usually audio-recorded and transcribed, and these transcripts – or written description protocols – are then subjected to detailed analysis involving the following steps:[viii]

1) The researcher assumes the attitude of the **phenomenological reduction** while being sensitive to the specific phenomenon being studied. Entering into this attitude means: (i) bracketing past knowledge of scientific research/theory about the phenomenon in order to encounter it freshly, and (ii) considering what is given without believing it to be necessarily 'real' (existential assent of the phenomenon is withheld).

2) The description (transcribed or written) is read – within the phenomenological attitude – to get a feel or **sense of it as a whole**.

3) The researcher rereads the description (still maintaining the phenomenological attitude), this time breaking it up into **meaning units** to make the data more manageable. This involves marking every point at which there is a transition in meaning. These meaning units can be phrases, sentences or whole passages. The point is to reflect intensely on short passages.

4) **Psychological meanings** contained in the participant's everyday expressions are reflected upon and extracted: in other words, implicit meanings are transformed into explicit ones. Giorgi (2009, p. 131) cautions that these meanings are 'not just lying there fully blown, ready to be picked out'. Instead, the psychological meanings have 'to be detected, drawn out, and elaborated'.

5) The researcher synthesizes the analysis and determines the structure of the experience as a whole considering all the participants' meanings. A rigorous application of free imaginative variation (Husserl's **eidetic**

variation) involves freely removing or changing aspects of the phenomenon in order to distinguish essential features from particular or
incidental ones (Wertz, 2010).

Giorgi cautions researchers not to adopt these steps mechanically when
he says:

> The researcher should feel a certain shift in perspective depending upon
> whether he [sic] is researching learning, anxiety, or guilt . . . Phenomenolog-
> ical analyses are fully embodied, experiential analyses. (2008b, p. 42)

These steps need to be approached slowly and systematically, allowing plenty
of time for the researcher to reflect. Wertz (2010; in press) tends to write
an extended reflection on *each* meaning unit before synthesizing these into
his 'Individual Psychological Structure'. Further reflection and analysis is
then needed to identify the 'General Structure'. Put in other words, Giorgi's
steps should perhaps be seen as a structure that enables researchers to *dwell*
longer with their data. The sequence of stages extends the process, allowing
researchers to resist the temptation to close off the phenomenon too soon.
As Fischer notes, 'Once immersed in data, some of the researcher's insights
may come while driving to work, awaking from a dream, or reading a novel'
(2006, p. xxiii).

When writing up and reporting the research, a brief general description
or condensed summary is usually offered to describe the phenomenon as
a whole (i.e. highlighting its essence or structure). Such a summary aims
to evoke the experience for readers, who may be able to identify with the
findings, and simultaneously challenge them to move beyond their own
'natural attitude'.

If researchers have dwelt with their data methodically and applied the
reduction and eidetic variation systematically, they can have a measure of
confidence that their findings will reveal the essential structure of the lived
experience being studied as the following examples show. However, the
essential structure identified is *never* the final word.

Example 6.1   The experience of being criminally victimized

Aims
In a fine-grained, in-depth analysis of the experience of being criminally
victimized, Fred Wertz (1983, 1985; Fischer & Wertz, 1979) provides
insights into the methodology of 'psychological reflection', in effect elab-
orating the steps Giorgi articulated. In a succession of papers, Wertz
records the minutiae of each stage of reflective analysis, rendering the
process of applying descriptive phenomenology more transparent.

The original research, conducted by Fischer, Wertz, and other colleagues with support from a National Endowment for the Humanities grant, involved some 100 interviews. Wertz used one case study, that of Marlene, to demonstrate his approach to analysis. He starts by exploring Marlene's experience of being the victim of attempted rape but ends by offering an analysis of the wider experience of being criminally victimized. In the process, he reveals the stages involved in moving from a psychological individual (i.e. idiographic) analysis of Marlene's experience to a broader psychological understanding of the phenomenon (in this case, being a victim of crime, whether burglary, assault, attempted rape or whatever).

Wertz's approach to reflection and analysis can be summarized in the following overlapping, iterative stages. It should be remembered that these are considerably more spontaneous than their linear presentation suggests.

Method
Psychological analysis of the individual– analysis of Marlene's experience:

1) Empathic immersion in the world of description
2) Slowing down and dwelling
3) Magnification and amplification of the situation
4) Suspension of belief and employment of intense interest
5) The turn from objects to their meanings through psychological reflection involving:
   * utilization of an 'existential baseline'
   * reflection on judgement
   * penetration of implicit horizons
   * making distinctions
   * seeing relations of constituents
   * thematization of recurrent meanings or motifs
   * interrogation of opacity
   * imaginative variation and seeing the essence of the case
   * languaging
   * verification, modification and reformulation
   * using existential-phenomenological concepts to guide reflection

Psychological analysis of the general (nomothetic) – analysis across all the accounts:

1) Seeing general insights in individual structures
2) Comparison of individual descriptions
3) Imaginative variation
4) Explicit formulation of generality

Findings

Space does not permit the depth and detail of Wertz's many pages of extraordinary reflection, analysis and emergent understandings to be demonstrated. Wertz (in press) himself admits he has a particularly meticulous, reflective style of dwelling in fascination of intricacy. Phenomenology for him is a labour of love:

> I experience research as a form of love in which I immerse myself in other people's lives, which I find surprising and astonishing when I think carefully about. I am sensitive to the dark side of human experience, and I am drawn to the precious value and dignity of actual human lives. (Wertz, 2010)

I would strongly recommend readers to return to Wertz's original analyses; however, a flavour of his style and work can be gained from the following extract:

> Victimization is . . . an empty possibility with which we are not concerned in normal, routine daily life prior to its emergence. Being victimized is the dawning of a new configuration of meaning . . . He is delivered to a strange, unfamiliar, shocking, hardly believable new realm outside the usual norms of lived experience . . . Victimization does not make sense . . . and is shot through with uncertainty . . . The structure of 'criminal' victimization has three constituents . . . : 1) the self's agency is lost and one stands helplessly vulnerable, isolated, and immobilized, 2) all helpful community has receded out of reach, and 3) a detrimental other has entered the subject's preferred situation in the mode of destruction . . . There is an upsurge of protest, rage, and perhaps a readiness for retaliation, counterviolation, or revenge . . . The person attempts to get back on top of the situation, negate victimization in its own turn, and re-establish the preferred order . . . The subject does not simply return to the pre-victimization order, but continues to live through victimization . . . Surpassing these meanings may take time . . . In this process the person takes responsibility for victimization. This process involves three interrelated aspects: active ['sense making'] efforts, the world's assertion of predictable safeness, and the other's active helpfulness. Through this process victimization appears . . . overcomable. (Wertz, 1985, pp. 195–204)

This seminal research has played its part in teaching many doctoral students how to do research (myself included!). It has also been used to inform both policy and the design of a model of therapy which aims to help victims of crime (see Fischer, 1984).[ix]

Example 6.2   Living through the experience of positive experiences of psychotherapy

Aims

This research by Amedeo Giorgi and Nico Gallegos (2005) forms part of a larger study (see Gallegos, 2005) about the experienced value of psychotherapy and symptom relief. This particular study focused on the accounts of just three of the nine participants within the larger study, examining how clients live through some positive experiences in psychotherapy.

Findings

Using the descriptive phenomenological method, the general structure (essence) of the experience of psychotherapy is identified as a whole, then its constituent parts are foregrounded. The authors stress the point that these constituents should, ideally, be viewed as a gestalt as they overlap in complex ways (e.g. to be able to speak without fear of being judged relates to the therapist being both trustful and non-judgemental). However, they can be understood to be constituents of the structure because if any *one* was taken away, the structure would collapse and the phenomenon would no longer be described.

General structure: A positive experience in psychotherapy for long-term clients is one in which the client feels that there is a reduction in the problem that motivated the therapy in the first place. This occurs through the quality of relationship with the therapist which is experienced as safe, caring, trusting, non-judgemental and:

> ... when the personhood of the therapist resonates well with that of the client such that an atmosphere is created in which the client feels free to express his or her authentic vulnerabilities ... and feels that these ... are being heard appropriately. (Giorgi & Gallegos, 2005, p. 204)

Constituents: These are identified in Table 6.1.

The findings reinforce the idea that it is the relationship with the therapist that is most significant – a finding consistent with the wider literature (Finlay & Evans, 2009). On the basis of their research, the authors argue against evaluating psychotherapy simply in terms of outcomes such as symptom relief and against defining progress in terms of therapy being terminated. Importantly, such a stance challenges most of the 'outcomes orientated research' to which quantitative researchers are so attached.

Table 6.1 Key constituents of the general structure and examples from Participant (P) descriptions.

	Clients		
Constituents	*P4*	*P5*	*P6*
1) Therapist (T) resonates with client	T is sensitive and had a helpful style	T was role model for P5	T was good match for P6
2) Therapist is trustful	P4 had trust in T who always did what she said	T had sharp boundaries and never violated them	P6 can only trust T
3) Therapist is safe	T extended P4's safety zone	After testing P5 saw it was safe to talk to T	P6 said T exuded safety
4) Therapist cares	T cared for P4 in a way that helped P4 care for herself	T really cared for P5	Ts have to be caring
5) Therapist is non-judgemental	P4 could say anything to T without being judged	T viewed P5's experience non-judgementally	T listens non-judgementally
6) Therapist meets idiographic needs	P4 needed T with no fee who could visit at home	P5 wanted T to talk non-ordinary about depth issues	P6 needed to be emotional in sessions

---

Example 6.3   Dissociative women's experiences of self-cutting

Faith Robinson (1998) studied 11 women's experiences of self-cutting. They had been diagnosed by their therapists as having multiple personality disorder (dissociative identity disorder) but who were considered to be currently stable and as having well-developed therapeutic support systems.

Aims/method
Given the sensitive nature of the topic, Robinson designed her methodology to ensure participants felt treated with the greatest respect and seriousness. She wanted each participant to have complete control over the type, amount and source of data provided while ensuring her researcher's role was as non-intrusive as possible.

The initial data collection process was highly structured in that the participants were handed written instructions to produce an initial written description. They were asked to recall an experience of self-cutting and to describe their feelings. Then Robinson engaged follow-up interviews which consisted of a structured 'walked-through' part and an unstructured 'dialogue' part. For the walk-through, the protocols were read aloud phrase by phrase and the participant was given the opportunity to clarify or enhance her description and this became the 'protocol' which was later analysed. During the dialogue phase, the participant's stories were brought to life. Although these were not directly analysed, they clarified the participants' intentions.

Analysis proceeded slowly towards distilling raw data down toward the essential constituents following Giorgi's (1985) practice of moving from individuals' meaning units to providing a general essential structure. However, Robinson also notes reflexively her own painful emotional response to participants' stories. She found it necessary to systematically distance herself after each step of the process to re-establish her emotional, mental and spiritual balance.

Findings

Consider the following summary of the general essential structure of the phenomenon of self-mutilation and how the cutter's experience is one of dissociation with 'alters' (alter-egos) emerging. In this excerpt I take the liberty of flagging up different lifeworld dimensions in brackets to provide a link to *Chapter 8* which explicitly focuses on the lifeworld as part of engaging descriptive phenomenology:

Cutters are wanting a release of tension, a relief from their enduring pain, and a quieting of the chaos and noise [**project**]. They reach a place where it feels as if they will explode [**spatiality**] . . . It feels as if physical pain could take away their emotional pain. Alters emerge who seem responsible for the cutting [**sense of self**]. The actual cutting takes on a compulsive, habit-like, automated process. The cutter may or may not have knowledge of plans to cut beforehand [**temporality**] . . . Cutters shift into an altered mental state. They find a pleasurable space where they are feeling in total control of their life [**spatiality**] . . . The sight and feel of flowing blood has much symbolism for cutters. It represents life, the possibility of death, relates of 'things trapped' in the body, and survival [**discourse**] . . . Visible scars become a sign to the outer world of their pain, fear, and needs [**embodiment**]. Cutters experience much fear and shame after cutting. Their good feelings and relief are always temporary. They feel sad knowing cutting brings their greatest comfort and meets their love and nurturing needs [**mood-as-atmosphere**]. (Robinson, 1998, pp. 218–219)

Reflections

Giorgi has bequeathed an extraordinarily rich legacy spanning several decades and an influence revealed by the ability of the Duquesne approach to tend 'the flame of phenomenology within the hostile environment of North American empiricist psychology' (McLeod, 2001, p. 40). While Giorgi may have hoped for even greater influence for his phenomenological project within the discipline of psychology (where he sought to dialogue with experimental colleagues), his method continues to help shape the practice of phenomenological research across the world, particularly in the nursing field and in broader health care.

While the descriptive-empirical phenomenological method advanced by Giorgi and others has had a major impact on phenomenological research, it has also drawn criticism. Some of this derives from the misrepresentation of his work or from the out-of-hand rejection of key ideas such as bracketing. Giorgi's critics also include those who disfavour his commitment to scientific rigour and who find some of his accounts overly preoccupied with systematic but seemingly mechanical or 'soul-less' constituent analysis. This, so the argument runs, can result in a slightly dry intellectualized approach and overly concerned with dialoguing with the natural science community.

That said, where the descriptive method is applied with care and imagination, as in the examples above, existential dimensions of lived experience emerge in all their power and glory. I agree with Todres (2007) when he supports Giorgi's methodology while advancing the idea that attention should be paid to textural aspects as well as structural; where heartful as well as academic languaging is attempted.[x] Wertz (in press) similarly argues for the value of being both poetic (in terms of using evocative language) and objectively systematic.

For me, the debate surrounding descriptive phenomenology relates less to the issue of scientific rigour than to the relevance of a scientific project in the current 'post-modern' context, where qualitative and broader phenomenologically inspired research is exerting ever-growing influence. Today, even the most inveterate quantitative researcher can sometimes be found acknowledging the relevance of people's embodied subjective experience. The debate with positivist experimental psychology which gave Giorgi's project impetus is less pressing – *perhaps*. In this post-modern context, experiential 'narratives of the self' have proliferated and in the past couple of decades there has been a surge of interest in post-structuralist, reflexive and feminist writings. The move is towards less authoritative, self-critical texts, ones that explicitly acknowledge their partisan, partial and socially contingent character. Most qualitative researchers now attempt to account for their own role in the (co-)creation of knowledge. In an effort to enhance the transparency and trustworthiness of their research, they try to make explicit the ways in which intersubjective elements impact on data collection and analysis. Parody, irony and scepticism are evident in hyper-reflexive, relativist discursive forms and these are seen to be the choice to represent a fragmented post-modern world.

How does Giorgi's project of a rigorous scientific phenomenology relate to this new landscape? Is it possible – or desirable – to discover the 'essences' of phenomena, or does the post-modern landscape, with its distrust of any universal discourse, require researchers to relinquish such claims? Does the current *Zeitgeist*, supportive of qualitative/subjective forms, demand a more relativist, hermeneutic and reflexive sensibility? Or does Husserl's philosophy, as Giorgi argues, leave enough room for the idea of fluid meanings and the fact that every analysis is limited, unable to grasp the totality of the original experience?

Giorgi himself seems entirely accepting of different phenomenological approaches. How can there not be many variations given the multiplicity of players: different researchers, different disciplines and different primary philosophers? The issue for Giorgi is the extent these different variations link appropriately to the philosophical theory (Giorgi, 2006). And here he leads the way.

In my view, the ability of the descriptive phenomenological approach to offer both a methodological touchstone and a trustworthy route into Husserlian philosophy ensures its continued relevance. Applied well, it results in powerful, rigorous and applicable findings, particularly well-suited to current demands for evidence-based practice.

For me, the best descriptive research is textured and nuanced while demonstrating systematically reflective and reflexive engagement (wherein researchers explicitly confront and explore the impact of their own subjectivity). When this phenomenological attitude is operationalized appropriately and transparently, the credibility and trustworthiness of the research is increased. Ultimately, all that matters is being faithful to the phenomenon and describing it well.

Notes

[i] Often this approach is simply called 'descriptive phenomenology'. I am including the word 'empirical' to highlight the scientific sensibility implicated, i.e. that it is based on observation/empirical data. Other commentators such as von Eckartsberg (1998) call this approach 'empirical existential-phenomenological' and contrast it with the 'hermeneutical-phenomenological' approach.

[ii] Husserl does not use this term 'intuition' to refer to something elusive and implicit. Instead, he uses it technically to refer to experience and how any object is given to consciousness.

iii Giorgi (2009, p. 68) admits that he is 'operating within a phenomenological theory of science that has not yet been systematically articulated' but that it is 'implicit in the writings of Husserl' amongst others. With his background in experimental psychology (i.e. trained in the natural science approach), Giorgi does not want to reject science. He just wants to modify it so that it investigates the human side of human beings. For a fuller explanation of the relationship between phenomenology, science and Husserl's writings, I recommend Giorgi's (2009) latest book, *The Descriptive Phenomenological Method in Psychology: A modified Husserlian approach.*

iv Since the 1970s, the phenomenological movement has been kept alive in psychology by Giorgi and other psychologists in the American Psychological Association Society for Theoretical and Philosophical Psychology plus the Division of Humanistic Psychology. Their project has been assisted by the highly respected *Journal of Phenomenological Psychology* (previously edited by Fred Wertz; now edited by Thomas Cloonan) and the annual International Human Science Research Conference (Giorgi, 2010). More recently, other online journals such as *Phenomenology & Practice*, the *Indo-Pacific Journal of Phenomenology* and *Environmental and Architectural Phenomenological Newsletter* have opened phenomenology to a wider community by offering an accessible forum for phenomenological debate.

v Some commentators call this approach '**empirical**' because it is based on this scientific approach. However, Giorgi – who was first an experimental psychologist – argues that his descriptive phenomenological method, unlike many other qualitative methods, is *not* 'empirical' (or at least it is only partly empirical), because it uses 'imaginative variation' which may not be based in actual scientific observations. While there may be an empirical starting point, the analyses themselves need to be seen as 'phenomenological' rather than empirical. Put in other terms, empirical science is based on investigating 'real' objects rather than 'experiential' ones (Giorgi, 2009). Giorgi thus distances himself from empirical philosophy and natural science, insisting instead on *human* science methodology.

vi **Realism** is a philosophical perspective that holds it is possible to acquire objective knowledge about the 'world out there' which is seen to be made up of structures and objects which have a cause–effect relationship with each other. Realists believe that it is possible to measure and study the world fairly accurately – it just depends on applying the scientific method well. Realist approaches can be contrasted with **relativist** ones which hold that there are multiple meanings/understandings of the world and that what is 'reality' can only be apprehended through personal perception and/or language use. Phenomenologists tend to place themselves somewhere on the continuum between realism and relativism, arguing that it is possible to capture some meanings about how the world is experienced but these are emergent, partial and tentative.

vii A written protocol (description) might be a page long or run to many pages. Sometimes researchers will combine methods and use, say, protocols alongside interviews. (See Wertz, in press for an extended worked example.)

viii In his latest work, Giorgi (2009, pp. 128–131) identifies three main concrete steps: 1) read for sense of the whole; 2) determination of meaning units; and 3) transformation of participant's natural attitude expressions into phenomenologically psychologically sensitive expressions. He stresses that the 'important criterion for the descriptive approach is that one neither adds to nor subtracts from the invariant intentional object arrived at, but describes it precisely as it presents itself' (2009, p. 137).

ix The interviews were conducted in collaboration with the Pittsburgh Police Department in the United States. Part of the grant was to conduct two public forums where the researchers shared the findings with groups of people including former victims, police personnel, judges, politicians, community organizers and concerned citizens. They were quite well attended and enthusiastically received. The victims felt their experience was understood and the community leaders and members took their experiences very seriously in the discussions of practices and policies (Wertz, personal communication).

[x] Todres (2007, p. 28) suggests the idea of 'essence' might usefully be reframed as *'authentic productive linguistic gathering'* to keep experiencing alive and to allow new nuances of meanings to continue to emerge. 'Ongoing experiencing would suggest that what is "most general" about experienced phenomena can never be the final thing said about that phenomena.'

Chapter 7

Hermeneutic Phenomenology

A poetics of research . . . deepens research and makes it richer by attending to the images in the ideas, the fantasies in the facts, the dreams in the reasons, the myths in the meanings, the archetypes in the arguments, and the complexes in the concepts. (Romanyshyn, 2007, p. 12)

As a human science, phenomenology aims to be systematic, methodical and normative (Giorgi, 1997, 2009). At the same time phenomenology also pursues the intertwining of science with art, the imparting of a poetic sensibility to the scientific enterprise. Science in this sense blends with the stylistic realms of the humanities. It is this artful rendering of science which hermeneutic phenomenologists are drawn towards.

The extent to which phenomenology should be an **artistic or literary project** rather than a more strictly scientific one constitutes one area of debate within the phenomenological field. Another concerns the issue of **interpretation.** In hermeneutic phenomenology there is a shift in commitment away from description and towards interpretation.[i] While structural and textual constituents are pursued in both descriptive and hermeneutic approaches, greater attention is paid to *contextual* meanings in hermeneutic variants (Churchill, 2007, 2010b). Here, the researcher's interpretations are understood to be inextricably intertwined with the research findings and context while researcher–participant (inter-)subjectivity is embraced:

> The researcher engages a solo waltz . . . moving in and out of (pre-reflective) experience and reflection as the researcher engages multiple meanings

Phenomenology for Therapists: Researching the Lived World, First Edition. Linda Finlay.
© 2011 Linda Finlay. Published 2011 by John Wiley & Sons, Ltd.

emerging from the data. Different interpretations are tried out like dance steps. Eventually the researcher settles on particular meanings revealing possibilities that may excite, inform or point the way to future research. (Finlay, 2006c)

In this chapter, I offer a flavour of hermeneutic or interpretive phenomenology.[ii] I choose the metaphor 'flavour' deliberately as the taste, sensation and texture of hermeneutic analysis are better experienced than talked about. More than any other chapter, this chapter allows hermeneutic phenomenologists to speak to you directly through quotations from their work. I invite you to dwell with their words.

Three examples of research are presented to show the creativity of the hermeneutic approach and the breadth of its sweep.[iii] Every researcher presented here fashions a dance between phenomenological reflection, interpretation and theorizing; each with a different dance style. The first two examples show how **scholarly contemplation** (one of theory/practice and the other of a fictional book) can result in new understandings. The final one is **empirically orientated,** involving 20 co-researchers. As you read the three examples, consider which – if any – you are particularly drawn towards.

Methodology

Aims

The aim of hermeneutic phenomenology is to evoke lived experience through the explicit involvement of interpretation. Lived experience is thematicized through language and understood by being refracted through a variety of lenses – philosophical, theoretical, literary and reflexive.[iv]

Such an approach potentially stands in contrast to the scientific descriptive phenomenology project described in the previous chapter, where the focus stays firmly on the research data and the epoché is rigorously applied. That said, some descriptive phenomenologists – notably Wertz – argue that the best descriptions attend carefully to language to ensure the power, resonance and poignancy of experience is expressed. Artistic flourish is not the sole realm of hermeneutic phenomenology. In practice, 'description' and 'interpretation' (found in Husserlian versus Heideggerian approaches, respectively) might be best seen as a *continuum* with different researchers valuing more highly one or other side of the spectrum.

Approach

The hermeneutic phenomenological approach is characterized, to a greater or lesser extent, by four tenets: commitment beyond science and towards the humanities; explicit use of interpretation; reflexive acknowledgement of the researcher's involvement; and placing emphasis on expressive presentation – usually writing using myth and metaphor.

Commitment beyond science towards the humanities   Hermeneutic phenomenologists recommend engaging modes beyond the scientific: for example, art, literary prose, dance, poetry.[v] Jager (2010), embracing the poetics of later Heidegger, argues that researchers interested in the human condition need to think in terms that apply to our lived human world:

> An education remains only partial and incomplete as long as it concentrates exclusively on science and technology and on the conquest of a natural universe and neglects the religious, literary, musical, thoughtful, and artful practices that build a liveable human world. Science and technology certainly lightens the burdens of our daily life, but we should remain mindful of the fact that we come face to face and heart to heart with our friends and neighbor or with a work of art only by entering into a covenant and obeying the grammar of an inhabited cosmos. (Jager, 2010, pp. 80–81)

Hermeneutic phenomenologists seek methods that allow the concrete, mooded, sensed, imaginative, aesthetic, embodied and relational nature of experience to be revealed.

> In living a human life we come with the seasons, with dryness and wetness, with the rhythms of darkness and light, of going away and coming back, of continuities and great discontinuities, with its Janus-face of both potential anguish and renewal. Framing and permeating all this is finitude; there, in the possibility of not being, and there, in the fragility of flowers, in the beauty of a sunset, and in the passing of a smile. (Todres, 2007, p. 116)

Drawing on such ideas, Willis (2002) advances '**expressive phenomenology**' as an approach which portrays research findings using poetic and/or aesthetic representational forms. Expressive phenomenology seeks to slow down both researchers and readers so they 'dwell' with the lived experience (the phenomenon).[vi]

Explicit use of interpretation   Hermeneutic phenomenologists argue that interpretation is necessary because phenomenology is concerned with meanings which are often implicit or hidden. The notion of interpretation is thus concerned with unveiling hidden meanings of lived experience (as opposed to being a process whereby external theories or frames of reference are brought in, such as when offering a psychoanalytic interpretation of dreams). The fact that we make a transition from experience to a second-hand account of that experience indicates some level of interpretation is involved.

> Phenomenology is seeking after meaning which is perhaps hidden by the entity's mode of appearing... The things themselves always present themselves in a manner which is at the same time self-concealing. (Moran, 2000, p. 229)

Interpretation is needed, hermeneutic phenomenologists say, in order to bring out the way that meanings occur in a **context** related to the participant, the researcher and the research as a whole. Importantly, interpretation of meaning is seen to arise through the data gathering and analysis process rather than being imported from outside sources and imposed arbitrarily. There are several layers to the argument here and it is worth going more slowly to separate the strands. First, hermeneutic phenomenologists argue that any description of lived experience by participants has to be seen in the context of that person's life situation and projects. A participant with chronic fatigue may say, for example, 'I'm frustrated by my lack of energy.' This statement takes on all the more colour and significance if we know the person is a professional athlete. When a participant expresses anger towards their psychotherapist, as another example, it helps to appreciate significant transferences may be involved. The contextual interpretation here is pursued to better understand lived experience.

Secondly, interpretation is further implicated as researchers empathize with, and make sense of data by drawing on their own understandings (which arise out of their life experience). Researchers can never be impartial, objective 'machines'. Instead, we bring to the task of interpreting lived experience our own history, beliefs, prejudices and predispositions. Researchers who have had chronic fatigue themselves may well appreciate its lived experience differently from someone who has had no contact with the condition. A therapist interviewing other therapists will probably pick up professional 'in-jokes' which an outsider would not.

Thirdly, interpretations are filtered through a spatial–temporal lens and arise out of particular cultural and historical fields. Researchers will inevitably bring to bear contemporary ideas. (For instance, a Western researcher studying anxiety in the past might have talked in terms of 'neurosis'. Now notions of anxiety in a *Diagnostic and Statistical Manual of Mental Disorders (DSM)* context would be placed within a larger spectrum of anxiety disorder, most probably seen in terms of psycho-social stresses and adjustment reactions. In Thailand, that same neurosis might be seen as 'wind illness').[vii]

Finally, interpretations (both participants' and researchers') arise out of the research context which involves a meeting of persons in a particular, situated, shared space. In the process of understanding another's world, we attune empathically to them and this attunement occurs in a shared, embodied, intersubjective space. If our subjectivity is a tool for perception, then it is our intersubjective sharings that allow the possibility of empathy. Put in Heideggerian terms:

> In Being-with-one-another understandingly we do not revert to our own inner world; we remain curious and attentive to the others' 'inner' world, which is now a 'shared world'. (Churchill, 2010b, p. 163)

Research findings are likely to have been co-created in dialogue where another researcher would impact differently on the participant and is likely to hear a different story. A researcher who has struggled with chronic fatigue is likely to empathize and have a different embodied conversation with participants about their experience of the condition compared to one who comes at the subject more naïvely. (We cannot assume that the story would be deeper or better, however, as other taken-for-granted aspects could well remain unaddressed.)

Reflexive acknowledgement of researcher's involvement   Hermeneutic phenomenologists argue that as researchers we cannot help but bring ourselves into the research. All our understandings are inevitably based upon our situatedness (our unique personal history and circumstances) and current understandings and these constitute both our 'closedness' and our 'openness' to the world: they are the basis of our experiencing. Since our perceptions and experience necessarily come into play when we seek to access the experience of others, our role as interpreters must be acknowledged when we formulate findings. While we should still attempt to disentangle our perceptions and understandings from the phenomenon being studied by adopting the phenomenological attitude, we have to recognize that interpretation cannot be exorcized from the ongoing revelation of the thing under scrutiny and should probably be acknowledged.

To help us remain aware of this interplay, hermeneutic phenomenologists may explicitly be reflexive (although this may not be the actual term they use). In this context reflexivity can be defined as:

> (the) process of continually reflecting upon our interpretations of both our experience and the phenomena being studied so as to move beyond the partiality of our previous understandings and our investment in particular research outcomes. (Finlay, 2003b, p. 108)

Reflexivity involves an active evaluation of the researcher's own experience in order to understand something of the *fusion of horizons* between subject and object, to use Gadamer's metaphor (Gadamer, 1975/1996). Our understanding of 'other-ness' arises through a process of making ourselves more transparent. If we do not examine ourselves, we run the risk of letting our predilections and prejudices dominate our research findings. New understandings emerge from a complex dialogue between knower and known, between the researcher's pre-understandings and the current research process.

In practice, researchers vary in how much they bring reflexivity to the fore. Some simply acknowledge their social position and where they are coming from (for instance, being a middle class, female therapist interviewing working class, male clients). Others may engage sustained reflexivity, for example, perhaps writing up their research some findings using a first person or reflexive voice.

Attention paid to expressive writing using myth and metaphor
Hermeneutic phenomenologists give great attention to the way they express findings so as to evoke lived experience. 'Phenomenology' says van Manen (1990, p. 13), is a 'poetizing project; it tries an incantative, evocative speaking, a primal telling, wherein we aim to involve the voice in an original singing of the world'.

In a more recent work, he suggests that:

> Not unlike the poet, the phenomenologist directs the gaze toward the regions where meaning originates, wells up, percolates through the porous membranes of past sedimentations – and then infuses us, permeates us, infects us, touches us. (van Manen, 2007, p. 12)

Following what is known as the Utrecht phenomenological tradition, van Manen (1990, 2007) advocates the inclusion of an artistic dimension in the writing up of phenomenological research so as to 'stir our pedagogical, psychological or professional sensibilities' (van Manen, 2007, p. 25).

Similarly, Todres and Galvin (2008) point to the growing trend of articulating an 'aesthetic phenomenology' (or expressive phenomenology) which draws on more poetic forms of writing. They encourage researchers to find words that carry textural dimensions of experience forward.

Hermeneutic phenomenologists often utilize **metaphor** in the service of such description. A net may be cast wide across space and time, the cosmos and history, drawing on **myths** and parables. A certain musicality is called for. Consider the way Blouin (2009), below, first draws a distinction between pornography and eroticism, then offers a parallel with the divergence between natural and human science. To explore the human condition, he says, we need to evoke the human world of erotic encounter: it is only with the poetic, musical touch of *Eros* that everyday experience is revealed:

> In pornography, the other is grasped. In eroticism, he [sic] is evoked. The pornographic hand is a working hand trying to master a material body. The erotic hand is an evoking hand trying to vibrate to the sound of an ever escaping poetic body, that is to say a body filled with multiple stories . . . Pornography is the end of talk. Eroticism is talk being born again . . .
> Illuminating the world is then more then just an exchange of information of unmusical words. The words must be made to vibrate to the touch of Eros so these words become musical and reveal our mundane experience. Here we are again in the world of evocation, not of grasping and bringing under control for the cause of the all in all. In an erotic encounter it is not just two bodies colliding but two resonating bodies evoking the surrounding world. (Blouin, 2009)

Methods and procedures

In terms of methods to be followed, hermeneutic phenomenology is sparing in the guidance it offers would-be researchers. In fact, *there is no actual method* of how to do hermeneutic phenomenology. 'Method' seems almost proscribed by this approach. As Gadamer (1975/1996) argued in his magnus opus *Truth and Method*, method – particularly scientific method – is seen as incapable of guaranteeing 'true' understanding.

This is both bad news and good news for budding researchers! There is no template to model upon, and virtually anything goes providing the research retains its phenomenological intent and sensibility.

Perhaps the one process that can be identified as method is what has come to be known as the **hermeneutic circle**.[viii] This is the process of coming to understand the being of something (be it a 'text' or the 'phenomenon' or 'participant' in the research context) through moving iteratively between the whole and parts and back again to the whole. In the first instance, an interpreter's previous understandings[ix] will initially colour what they access when addressing the thing itself. But this meeting between interpreter and what is being interpreted in fact involves an ongoing dialogue where previous assumptions – now found to be partial or wrong – are revealed and challenged as new understandings are nudged into being.

Applied to research, the researcher caught up in the hermeneutic circle, moves back and forth, dialoguing dynamically between parts and the whole and interpreting iteratively. The 'part' may be a single word or extract within the 'whole' of a sentence or an interview transcript; it may refer to one interview among several; it may allude to a single episode in the whole of a person's life (Smith, Flowers & Larkin, 2009).

Arguably the best (perhaps only) way to learn about the hermeneutic approach is to model on good examples, such as those that follow. Notice how they open up a space for interpretive, literary, artistic and/or reflexive flourish.

Example 7.1   'Soulful space': 'freedom for wound'

Les Todres (2007) contrasts 'narcissism', which he sees as a flight from vulnerability (*freedom from wound*), with 'soulful space', which he offers as an existential possibility where vulnerability is embraced, enabling us to connect empathically with others (*freedom for wound*).[x] Almaas' psychoanalytic-essentialist ideas and Gendlin's existentialist understandings are used as theoretical touchstones to explicate the contrasts.

Todres' 'method' is perhaps best viewed as scholarly existential contemplation, using the myth of Narcissus as counter-point. In the Greek legend, Narcissus becomes enamoured with the surface image of himself in a pool of water. Enthralled, he extends his hand only to find that the image eludes him. Todres points to the psychological metaphor of how we can 'become alienated from the nourishment of our lived experience [and relationships] by turning ourselves into an image or object' (2007, p. 152).

In narcissism, Todres explains, there is shame: a painful self-consciousness born of viewing oneself critically from the outside. Strategies of 'self-sufficiency', 'seeking others as mirrors of an ideal self' and 'merging with a great or special other' are engaged. Expending energy to project a strong front, we puff ourselves up with grandiosity and attempt to be special. We are needy of others' affirmations while being exceedingly sensitive to their potentially injurious views. We flee from ourselves, leaving our vulnerabilities and longings behind, by identifying with an idealized other who is seen as 'strong'. In short, we occupy a place of 'deficient emptiness' which no true nourishment of human connection, participation and relationship can reach.

With the creation of 'soulful space', Todres suggests, there is a human openness where we feel 'touched': what he calls a *freedom for wound*.

> This beautiful wound is the human realm. It is the realm that Narcissus would reject. . . . It is the mellower wound of longing that is worn gladly as we look deeply at one another and care for one another as fellow carriers. The wound sings the song of separation and longing, and the

body . . . remembers . . . a soulful space where we can deeply meet . . . The treasure of the wound of longing is the taste of the beauty and poignancy of human participation; the essence of relationship, the 'we-feeling' in mutual vulnerability. (Todres, 2007, pp. 162–163)

In his explication, Todres invites us to let go and open ourselves to pain. He beckons us into a soulful space that mixes vulnerability with freedom.

Example 7.2   Examining the cycle of developing relationships

David Seamon (1993a) offers a phenomenology of relationships based on his reading of a fictional literary text by Doris Lessing, *Diaries of Jane Somers*. The novel describes the growing friendship between Jane Somers, a stylish, middle-aged, middle-class fashion editor, and Maudie Fowler, a proud, indigent, 90-year-old woman who eventually dies from stomach cancer. Over the years, these two women from such radically different worlds take complementary positions, variously embracing active and passive modes in their relating. Maudie helps Somers become a better person while Somers helps restore a sense of self-worth in Maudie. Seamon uses Lessing's account of this poignant, developing friendship as his empirical base from which to explore the phenomenon of relationships:

In *Diaries* I had this deep feeling that there was something in it to be found phenomenologically. At first I thought it was Lessing's remarkable descriptions of an elderly person's lifeworld, but as I worked more, I sensed there was some larger structure 'to be had'. Eventually, the 'mother' phenomenon appeared as 'relationship', and I was much struck by the (at first) odd implication that there must be some sort of 'search' before the right 'relationship-ee' appears. (Seamon, personal communication)

Seamon suggests a model of 'relationship cycle' which unfolds in seven stages: dissatisfaction, asking, searching, trying to accept, accepting, understanding and caring. He summarizes the model thus:

In the beginning phase of the relationship (stages 1–3 . . .), the common thread is *search* – a sense that there is something more beyond who and what one is. In time, a situation in the world outside the person offers itself, which in Somers' case is the encounter with Maudie Fowler. The relationship then moves into a middle phase that might be called *trial* because it involves efforts of mutual acceptance (stages 4 and 5). The trial stage holds the greatest danger of failure because the two parties may not bond. If they do, a relationship results that is founded in the fact that two have become one. The third phase of the relationship (stages 6 and 7) might be called *fruition*. The relationship is now secure and as much an entity as the two participants, who feel mutual understanding and responsibility. (Seamon, 1993a, p. 239)

After explicating the touching nature of the 'encounter and symphysis' (growing together) between Somers and Fowler, he suggests that his model of a relationship cycle may have broader significance for social policy and environmental design which, he argues, may be failing through being founded in 'connection' rather than 'relationship'. For example, while Maudie would have undoubtedly benefited from better housing, a bigger pension and home help, her central need was to be part of a larger relational human whole:

> Relationship cannot readily happen because professional and client... policy maker and people planned for [it] – rarely do these people and groups have a real stake in each other... Somers' extraordinary contribution to Maudie's world is that she returns to it a *certain kind of nearness* – the friendship of a person who likes Maudie for just being who she is. Somers becomes *close* to Maudie, and Maudie is no longer an isolated individual... A key design concern becomes the thorough understanding of ways in which the built environment can contribute to a sense of nearness, place and human togetherness. (1993, pp. 237–238)

Example 7.3   Explicating the phenomenon of 'existential migration'

Greg Madison (2005, 2010) explores the phenomenon of 'existential migration'. He contrasts economic migration or forced migration/exile to 'existential migration' which he describes as a chosen attempt to leave one's homeland and become a foreigner thus expressing something fundamental about one's existence. Drawing on the theoretical work of Heidegger and Gendlin, Madison studied this phenomenon both *empirically* (by interviewing 20 voluntary migrants about their experience and analysing the results) and *conceptually* (by weaving into his thesis numerous literary references).

In his explication, Madison challenges conventional understandings and meanings: for example, the equating of 'home and belonging' with safeness and familiarity. 'Home' may not be a geographical place, he argues. The strangeness of being 'not-at-home' can simultaneously offer a 'home', while feeling 'at home' can, in some situations, be deeply unsettling. In his thesis he showed that on returning to their original homeland for visits, such as at Christmas, participants often felt 'not at home' and sought a return to their travels or adopted country.[xi]

In his description, Madison (2005) suggests a number of themes, including self-potential, escape, freedom, belongingness, homelessness, return, the spirit of leaving, home and origin. Below is an extract from the analysis concerning the nature of 'Return':

> I think about returning almost every day. Sometimes I am clear that I would never return, sometimes I fantasise about it, yet other times I feel a dull homesickness, a kind of pull back to the only place that could ever have been home but now isn't. I think this signifies a desire for a kind of spiritual and psychological reconnection, a healing of the self in some way, and reconciliation where there was originally rejection . . . Home has changed, though deeply familiar it is also different, and I return as a stranger in a strangely familiar land . . . How could I stay here now and not succumb to the suffocation that led me to leave in the first place? How can I protect my fluid self, elaborated by all my experiences in the world, and withstand the demand to cement into the conventional? How can I balance my desire for home with my need for self-direction? (2005, p. 161)

Later Madison elaborates by drawing on the Heideggerian concept of *Unheimlichkeit* (not-at-homeness):

> Experiencing the primordial unheimlichness of Dasein is presumably not only 'fascinating' but simultaneously disconcerting, so it is not surprising that we inevitably 'fall' back in to the mundane and anaesthetizing world. The fact that our co-researchers seem to continue to look for 'home' in some form indicates that they, at least at times, seek the tranquil-lized 'at-homeness' that they are nonetheless unconvinced by. (Madison, 2005, p. 210)

Madison's analysis is further enriched by numerous literary allusions, among them the epilogue of J.R.R. Tolkein's *Lord of the Rings*. As the main characters return to the Shire homelands, Frodo, in conversation with the wise wizard Gandalf, is complaining about his shoulder wound. When Gandalf comments that 'Alas! There are some wounds that cannot be wholly cured,' Frodo continues:

> *I fear it may be so with mine . . . There is no real going back. Though I may come to the Shire, it will not seem the same; for I shall not be the same. I am wounded with knife, sting, and tooth, and a long burden. Where shall I find rest?* Gandalf did not answer. (1967, p. 323)

> As they near the Shire, one of Frodo's companions remarks on their entry back into familiar lands and how their adventures and former comrades from other lands are already fading from memory as if it was all a dream, to which Frodo responds, '*Not to me*', said Frodo. '*To me [returning home] feels more like falling asleep again*' (p. 333) (Madison, 2010, p. 181)

Reflections

It is ironic that phenomenologists (who champion the non-dualist cause) are often pushed to line up behind either the 'descriptive' or 'hermeneutic' camps. In practice the space between description and interpretation is ambiguous. If the phenomenological researcher aims to go beyond surface expressions and explicit meanings to read between the lines so as to access implicit dimensions and intuitions, is interpretation necessarily involved? Much depends on how the term 'interpretation' is understood: if you subscribe to the Heideggerian view, there are no such things as un-interpreted phenomena.

Van Manen (1990) suggests that when description is mediated by expression, including non-verbal aspects, action, artwork or text, a stronger element of interpretation is involved. However, drawing on Gadamer's ideas, he helpfully distinguishes between interpretation as pointing *to* something (interpretation suited to phenomenological description) and interpretation as pointing *out* the meaning of something by imposing an external framework (such as when offering a psychoanalytic interpretation).[xii] Wertz (2005) picks up the former sense of interpretation when he argues that "'interpretation" may be used, and may be called for, in order to contextually grasp parts within larger wholes, as long as it remains descriptively grounded' (p. 175). Following these scholars, I see description and interpretation as a continuum where specific work may be more or less interpretive. Hard and fast boundaries between description and interpretation would be 'antithetical to the spirit of the phenomenological tradition that prizes individuality and creativity' (Langdridge, 2008, p. 1131).

Rather than fixating on description versus interpretation, my interest in hermeneutic phenomenology is its passion and soul. It seems to me that if we are not drawn into new discoveries and shaken by seeing the world in a different way, then phenomenology has not achieved anything like its potential.

Of course, not all hermeneutic phenomenology necessarily resonates at a heart-soul level. Sometimes hermeneutic pieces can be so densely packed with philosophical concepts that they come across as distant or smug; they lose their ability to summon the reader into the experience.

I value the communicative power of research that challenges, unsettles and reverberates, that strikes a chord with our everyday experience of life. I want to be touched by the captivating, allusive power of research which evokes lived experience. For me, phenomenology achieves this best when it can draw on the arts, and in particular when it turns to poetry and literary references. Such aesthetic phenomenological writing turns reading research into an experience in itself. I agree with Wilkinson when he says:

> It is indeed timely to turn to poetry now, to correct the one-sideness of medicine, to correct the one-sided ministrations of psychological science, but also because, thus, we can enjoy a psychotherapy [or research practice] which is a creative servant of life and laughter and love. (Wilkinson, 2009, p. 236)

Notes

[i] Sometimes this shift is expressed as representing a move from Husserlian (descriptive) to Heideggerian (interpretive) styles. Scholars explain the interpretive pole by drawing on Heidegger's hermeneutic-existential philosophy in different ways. For example, Churchill (2007) discusses how a moment of experience is understood to be situated within an over-arching existentially individuated '*care* structure' (which includes the '*projects*' that animate it and '*facticities*' that situate it). The researcher's mode of *attunement* to this care structure occurs through a Being-with intersubjective space and inevitably involves interpretation. Todres (2007) cues into the poetic language of later Heidegger which explores the play of presence and absence that is Being itself where unconcealment of the 'world' is grounded in concealment of 'earth'. Poetry is seen here by Heidegger as the pre-eminent way in which Beings are revealed in their being.

[ii] Note the difference between 'interpretive phenomenology' as a general approach and 'interpretative phenomenological analysis – IPA' which is a specific hermeneutic method (see *Chapter 9*).

[iii] A myriad of variations of **hermeneutic phenomenology** flourish. To name a few, consider: the existential, hermeneutic approaches of the Dallas School (Churchill, 2003; Garza, 2007); the open lifeworld approach of Dahlberg, Dahlberg and Nystrom (2008); the dialogal approach of Halling, Leifer and Rowe (2006); the literary, contemplative approach of Jager (2010); the person-place-architecture phenomenology of Seamon (2010a; Seamon & Mugerauer, 1985); the Interpretative Phenomenological Analysis in use by Smith and his colleagues (Smith, 2007); the embodied enquiry approach of Todres (2007); and the lived experience approach of van Manen (1990).

[iv] For further information about the hermeneutic approach (and its overlap with descriptive phenomenology) see Max van Manen's website *Phenomenology Online* at: http://www.phenomenologyonline.com/inquiry/1.html.

v See for instance, the 'Psychology and Literature' issue in the *Journal of Phenomenological Psychology*, Vol. 32(2). Guest editor: Bernd Jager.

vi Willis (2002, 2008) also applies this approach to vocational education where he advances what he calls an 'evocative pedagogy'. This, he explains, is a non-didactic approach to vocational education which seeks to engage learner's hearts and minds through 'showing' as opposed to 'telling'. Learners are invited to dialogue though drama/literature/poetry to evoke responses that 'capture the imagination' and 'move' others emotionally, 'touching their soul'.

vii Such evolving understandings are picked up using the methodology of **metabletics**. Created by the Dutch philosopher and psychiatrist van den Berg, metabletics been called 'historical phenomenology'. More than tracing ideas through history in the Foucauldian tradition, metabletics is an attempt to give a phenomenological account of how Western humanity has moved into its present existence. Metabletics investigates the nature of phenomena of human life as experienced (in contrast to the unchanging world of science where knowledge is largely 'fixed'). For instance, van den Berg was interested in the way there is not just one field of psychiatry but many, according to points in history and related to particular cultures/countries. For readers interested in this field, I recommend the work of Mook (1999, 2006, 2008) who has applied metabletic investigation to the changing nature of family, childhood and 'neurosis', respectively.

viii Originally, hermeneutics arose in the context of interpreting old *texts*, for instance, the Bible. The question was asked whether we could really understand what the original authors meant or whether we inevitably bring in and apply our own contemporary understandings. Given the fact that the author is not available to check the precise intended meanings of the text, in the hermeneutic process, the interpreter tries to 'hear' the being of the text (Seamon, personal communication).

ix Heidegger uses terms such as 'fore-having', 'foresight' and 'fore-conception'. Gadamer favours his version of the concept of 'prejudices' while Merleau-Ponty prefers to use the concept of 'implicit understanding'. For the purposes of this book, I am choosing to gloss over the subtle distinctions between the different concepts and refer more generally to 'previous understandings'.

x In subsequent papers Todres (in press) argues the potential gift of both encountering existential *vulnerability* and of encountering existential *freedom*. He notes this latter gift offers us the creative option of new possibilities and a non-repetitive future. But this freedom is threatening as it is in tension with our need for security and comfortable routines. Todres calls us to claim our existential freedom: the temporal freedom that allows us to see with fresh eyes, and the personal freedom to take responsibility for one's life as uniquely one's own.

xi Other phenomenologists, notably Seamon (2010a), Relph (1976) and Jacobson (2009), offer further insights into the nature of 'home' and 'place', acknowledging that many people may not be able to escape their geographical lifeworld. Seamon (2010b, p. 674) argues that:

> On the one hand, a sustaining home can be said to afford and reflect 'existential insideness' (Relph, 1976, p. 55) – i.e., the home and the world in which it finds itself is typically experienced without self-conscious awareness yet, in its lived nature, sustains a sense of individual and familial well-being and worth. On the other hand, the home that, for whatever reason, undermines a sense of individual and familial well-being and worth can be said to afford and reflect 'existential outsideness' (ibid., p. 51) – i.e., a

sense of separateness and alienation from the home or from the wider world in which that home finds itself.

[xii] Ricoeur similarly distinguishes between: (a) the '**hermeneutics of meaning-recollection**' which aims for greater understanding of the thing to be analysed in its own terms, where meanings are brought out; and (b) the '**hermeneutics of suspicion**' where deeper interpretations are needed to challenge surface accounts (Ricoeur, 1970).

Chapter 8

Lifeworld Approaches

Everything is finally outside, everything, even ourselves . . . It is not in some hiding-place that we will discover ourselves, it is on the road, in the town, in the midst of a crowd . . . a man among among men [sic]. (Sartre, 1939, cited in Moran & Moony, 2002, p. 384)

The lifeworld – *Lebenswelt* – is the **taken-for-granted** world as experienced; it is how our body and relationships are lived in time and space. The lifeworld is the meaningful subjectivity of the experienced world; the 'world that appears meaningfully to consciousness in its qualitative, flowing given-ness; not an objective world "out there", but a humanly relational world' (Todres, Galvin & Dahlberg, 2007, p. 55). The lifeworld points us to the *intentional* relationship between conscious, meaning-making human subjects and the external taken-for-granted, meaning-giving world.

A focus on the lifeworld involves a return to phenomena as they are lived pre-reflectively and prior to engaging scientific understandings. In the lifeworld we are immersed in our existence, engaged in our daily activities. As we act in the world – doing, being, experiencing – mostly we do not reflect on what our experience means as we are in the '**natural attitude**'. Lifeworld just happens, it unfolds.

Given this definition, it would seem then that all phenomenology is concerned with the lifeworld. (As Ashworth, 2006 acknowledges, Giorgi's descriptive approach and van Manen's hermeneutic one are both 'explications

Phenomenology for Therapists: Researching the Lived World, First Edition. Linda Finlay.
© 2011 Linda Finlay. Published 2011 by John Wiley & Sons, Ltd.

of the lifeworld'.) However, an *explicit* focus on lifeworld offers a valuable orientation.

In my view, lifeworld approaches overlap with, but are sufficiently distinct from, the phenomenologies described in *Chapters 6 and 7* as they have developed their own methodological style and focus. Because of this, I have chosen to give them a dedicated chapter.[i] Three of the main proponents of this approach are Karin Dahlberg in Sweden who, with her colleagues, developed the *Reflective Lifeworld Research* (RLR) approach; Peter Ashworth in the United Kingdom who has advanced using '*lifeworld fractions*' heuristically in his version of Sheffield Phenomenological Psychology; and David Seamon in the United States who over the last thirty years has advanced the cause of the '*geography of the lifeworld*'.[ii]

This chapter sketches some different ways of doing lifeworld-centred research. First, contrasts between the Dahlberg, Ashworth and Seamon approaches will be drawn out. Then, three examples are offered to show the methods involved and the potential richness, resonance and relevance of findings.

Methodology

All phenomenologists would probably agree that the lifeworld is universally present and an inevitable structure of being. Where different approaches to phenomenological research methodology vary is in the different views about how to access the lifeworld and what elements are prioritized.

Dahlberg's 'Reflective Lifeworld Research'

The overall aim of reflective lifeworld research is to describe and elucidate the lived world in a way that expands our understanding of human being and human experience. The focus is on the way that everyday taken-for-granted lifeworld meanings are implicit:

> Reflective lifeworld research in particular seeks to know <u>how</u> the implicit and tacit becomes explicit and can be heard, and <u>how</u> the assumed becomes problematized and reflected upon. (Dahlberg, Dahlberg & Nystrom, 2008, p. 37)

Reflective lifeworld research uses descriptive and hermeneutic design to explore how everyday experience shows itself as lived. The approach requires a phenomenological attitude of openness and willingness to see the phenomenon in new ways. Researcher's previous beliefs, knowledge, theories are '**bridled**' (the term preferred over bracketing), i.e. reined in from having an uncontrolled effect on evolving understandings. The stance adopted by the researcher is a kind of 'active passivity' where the phenomenon is allowed to show itself at its own pace, in its own way. More than a process of bracketing assumptions and previous understandings, bridling involves a whole process of understanding where the researcher embraces a restrained, systematic, open, scientific and careful way of examining the phenomenon. Put in other terms, bridling aims for a slowed down way of looking *forwards* towards understanding, rather than looking backwards at bracketing pre-understandings.

Typically, five or more participants are interviewed.[iii] Open questions are asked such as 'Could you tell me about your experience of x?' Through sensitive, flexible questioning, participants are encouraged to reflect in a focused but spontaneous way. Other data-gathering methods may also be used such as narratives, participant observations and the use of various creative forms as supportive data. More important than the method is the approach which favours detailed accounts of lived experience and works to avoid pre-conceived clichéd answers.

The process of analysing the data moves dynamically and iteratively between the whole – the parts – and the whole ('tripartite structure'), with the researcher being alert and sensitive to both the generalities and particularities of the phenomenon. An open, bridled attitude to both the phenomenon and process of understanding is maintained. The researcher **searches for the essence(s)** of the phenomenon through active reflection and questioning as suggested by Gadamer (1975/1996). For Dahlberg (2006) an 'essence' is a phenomenon's style, pattern or way of being. Expandable and openly infinite, essences can never be fully captured or explored. It is the *nuances* rather than any sense of fixed core that researchers aim to find.[iv]

The eventual description offered by the researcher aims to illuminate the most abstract, invariant meanings (i.e. the essence) along with constituents of the meaning. These essential meanings are said to characterize the phenomenon in general in that without them, a different phenomenon would be involved.

With its use of an open phenomenological attitude which restrains previous understandings, its systematic search for essences, and the firm anchoring in the philosophies of Husserl and Merleau-Ponty, reflective lifeworld research is twinned with the *descriptive phenomenological method*. Reflective lifeworld research is broader in its focus, however, as it attempts to theorize evolving understandings and the relationship between researcher and participant *hermeneutically*, engaging more interpretive possibilities. Further, the descriptive phenomenological method arose in response to the field of positivist empirical psychology, while reflective lifeworld research arises out of an explicit ethical, '**caring science**' approach.

In Europe over the last decade, there has been a discernible, topical and vibrant phenomenological trend to apply a lifeworld awareness to health care. Dahlberg, Todres and Galvin (2009; also, Todres, Galvin & Dahlberg, 2007), for instance, argue the value of revisiting a humanizing philosophy which they call '**lifeworld-led care**', as opposed to patient-led or person-centred, health care. They argue that consumerist orientations in patient-led care obscure attention being paid to persons' broader life including health and well-being needs.

Ashworth's descriptive approach to 'heuristic lifeworld dimensions'

Where Dahlberg's research approach emphasizes the search for nuanced essences, Ashworth favours idiographic sensibility.[v] For Ashworth, the lifeworld can be used to give a heuristic, practical, discovery-orientated structure to see the particulars of an individuals' experience, and that these can be described. He argues that empirical research can be strengthened and enriched by an explicit lifeworld analysis.

> Lifeworld has essential features and is a human universal, and it is through the evocation of this structure that a particular empirical lifeworld can be described. (Ashworth, 2006, p. 38)

Ashworth emphasizes the need, at least in initial stages, to stay with the **individual lifeworld**, taking an insider perspective. Here researchers focus on this particular person's experience of x (and this experience may be potentially different from another's experience of x). Later it may be possible to see generalities. For Ashworth, presupposing a researcher will find general themes is 'an avoidance of the epoché'(2006, p. 37). As part of applying the **epoché**, he says, we should be sceptical that general essences and psychological universals may be found at all.[vi]

The only universals we can assume at the start of research are that essential features of the lifeworld exist, encompassing: embodiment, selfhood, spatiality, temporality, sociality, mood-as-atmosphere, project, discourse, freedom and historicity.[vii] He calls these features '**fragments**' to emphasize their interlinking, interpenetrating meanings.

Ashworth identified these fragments through drawing on a wide range of phenomenological literature including the philosophical work of Husserl, Heidegger, Sartre, Merleau-Ponty, as well as that of Alfred Schutz (a sociological phenomenologist[viii]). Numerous authors have since attempted to point to some essential features of the lifeworld including van den Berg (1972), Valle, King and Halling (1989) and van Manen (1990). Ashworth's particular contribution is in insisting on the value of an idiographic description and the comprehensive detailing of the fuller range of specific 'fragments' identified across the literature.

Seamon's hermeneutic 'Geography of the Lifeworld'

We are bound by body to be in place. (Casey, 1993, p. 104)

Seamon is a phenomenological geographer who focuses on everyday taken-for-granted environmental experience, i.e. people's first-hand involvement with the geographical world. He uses a phenomenological-hermeneutic approach to explore environmental and architectural issues and how environmental design offers a vehicle for 'place-making'.[ix] He applies the concept of lifeworld to the field of geography, directing our attention to the **spatial dimension** and meaning of **place** (for instance, how we might feel safe or threatened, enclosed or exposed, included or excluded, free or trapped, at ease or stressed, and so on). Here, understandings of space are related to places we inhabit while meanings of place are derived from their spatial context. The central aim of his approach is to explore and interpret the mutual relationship between human beings and their **material/social world** through examining behaviour, experience and meaning in a descriptive, interpretive manner as they happen in their everydayness. (www.arch.ksu.edu/seamon/Seamon_reviewEAP.htm).

Lifeworld, for Seamon, focuses primarily on spatiality involving embodied–geographical–social intersections related to:

(a) a person or group's unique *personal situation* – for example, one's gender, sexuality, physical and intellectual endowments, degree of ableness, personal likes and dislikes; (b) a person or group's unique *social, cultural, and historical* situation – for example, the time and place in which one lives, economic and political circumstances, religious and societal background, technological infrastructure; (c) a person or group's situation as it involves their being typical human beings sustaining and sustained by a typical human world – for example, the lived fact that we are bodily beings who are always and already 'emplaced' physically in our world. (2009, p. 668)

In his seminal PhD work *A Geography of the Lifeworld* (Seamon, 1979), Seamon focused on 'everyday environmental experience' – people's first-hand involvements in their everyday places, spaces and environments. Groups of volunteer participants met weekly to examine and discuss their experience focusing on themes such as movement patterns, emotions of place, the meaning of home, and decisions about where to go and when. Synthesizing some 1500 personal observations, and taking a corroborative intersubjective approach to validation, Seamon produced three overarching, generalized themes: *movement, rest* and *encounter*.[x] Suggesting this structure offers an integrated way to envision human environmental experience and to attention to design and policy implications, his project is to explore whether (existentially speaking) we might evolve a better relationship with our lived geography.

As a hermeneutic phenomenologist, Seamon does not offer a specific method as such. Instead, across his numerous writings he picks up issues of interest and 'riffs off' the work of other writers, striving always to explicate that ambiguously layered, essential connection between person and place, spatiality and lifeworld.[xi] Drawing on a wide range of philosophical and theoretical sources[xii] including the work of Heidegger and Merleau-Ponty, he weaves a tapestry of the intertwining of person and environment (Seamon, 1993b).

The relevance for therapists of the work of geographical phenomenologists like Seamon is that it engages our appreciation of both existential concerns and issues around designing spaces for disabled individuals.[xiii]

Example 8.1   Experience of surviving out-of-hospital cardiac arrest

Anders Bremer, Karin Dahlberg and Lars Sandman (2009) employ reflective lifeworld research and interviews to describe nine patients' experiences of surviving out-of-hospital cardiac arrest (OHCA). Struck by the sudden threat to life itself, the survivors were thrown off the natural course of their lives. Out-of-hospital cardiac arrest is described as:

> A sudden and elusive threat, an awakening in perplexity, and the memory gap as a loss of coherence. Survival means a search for coherence with distressing and joyful understanding, as well as existential insecurity exposed by feelings of vulnerability. (Bremer, Dahlberg & Sandman, 2009, p. 323)

The essence, and some of the constituents of the phenomenon, are captured in the following passage:

> The awakening from unconsciousness . . . means loss of control, incoherence, and a sense of exposure . . . The growing understanding can be shocking, afflicting, and without comprehensive answers, demanding identity, coherence, and meaning to be re-created out of a re-evaluation of body subject, health, and previous life. The body, and thus life, appears vulnerable, insecure, and restricted. Existence is constituted by fear and insecurity that vary in time, space, and context, but also by surprise, gratitude, and joyfulness of continued life . . . Anxiety and insecurity appear at the thought of bodily deterioration, vulnerability, and the finiteness of

life. Anxiety and guilt arise, focusing on how death or bodily limitations will affect the lives of significant others...

By confronting threats against well-being and existence, confidence and joy of life are strengthened. Returning to everyday activities gives existence some stability, and clarity, and contributes to a sense of coherence. There is a turn toward a changed life with new characteristics, where well-being and meaning emerge through valuable human relationships. Wellbeing and suffering get new meanings and coherence, which can be found when everyday existence incorporates the life threat that, at least temporarily, has passed by. (Bremer *et al.*, 2009, p. 328)

The study shows survivors' emotional needs suggesting ways prehospital emergency professionals might provide support. Specifically, the authors suggest post-resuscitation care might focus on helping survivors to understand the connections they find important so that attention is given to well-being as well as illness.

Example 8.2   The lived experience of being a person with dementia

Peter Ashworth, in collaboration with Ann Ashworth (Ashworth, 2006; Ashworth & Ashworth, 2003), describes one woman's particular and unique lifeworldly experience of dementia. No claims are made to the typicality of her experience although Ashworth accepts there may well be commonalities with lifeworlds of other individuals with dementia.

The study is based on deep reflective observation rather than interview or other data gathering means. Findings are presented using the structured framework of the interlinked 'fractions of the lifeworld'. I paraphrase and summarize the findings below to show some of the potential breadth and depth of the fractions approach to analysis.

Self – The person with dementia is a 'Self' with a particular point of view but somewhat inclusive boundaries of ownership where the self is no longer associated with particular objects (e.g. my slippers). She exercises agency indirectly by requesting others to act and it can be frustrating when responses are not immediately forthcoming. If carers carry on with their own activities, she experiences a lack of 'presence' and has no 'voice'. While she presents herself as an invalid, on occasion applause and praise (when she proudly recites a well-remembered lengthy poem for instance) can invoke a positive self-view.

Sociality – Others may only have an active existence when present with her in the here and now – perhaps summoned into existence by her call. Mostly, others are an absorbing loci of activity or their presence provides an opportunity to perform a more lively (and preferred) self. Sometimes the others' behaviour is experienced as malicious or anxiety-provoking such as when a carer's expression of puzzlement is seen as 'scowling'.

Embodiment – Embodiment just 'is'; it is not overlaid with meanings. So bodily embellishment (e.g. tidied hair, clothing) is now missing from her lifeworld. Still, embodiment occupies considerable attention in the form of hypersensitivity, discomfort or irritation such as when feeling cold or when the shower spray elicits protests. While her body is typically made feeble by lack of direction, a purposive strength and vigour returns with the use of artefacts (such as a walking stick or when another person adopts an inviting ballroom dancing stance).

Temporality – The world, for this person with dementia, is entirely in the here and now with little talk of the future. The *nowness* of existence is shown in the way that discussion of future plans, such as when a carer is coming, is understood as just about to happen. However, moment to moment living can be erratic as shown when words elude or in the way that a movement started to answer a current need may have the moment stolen as the reason for the activity is forgotten. The past is spoken about as a tense in which current events must be spoken. The narrative structure of events and shared past experiences are not recalled. Certain markers of the temporal structure to the day are rigorously enacted with rituals (such as filling a kettle before getting into bed) although without regard to actual clock time.

Spatiality – She can no longer rely on space: a boundary or threshold such as a locked door can make itself felt treacherously and unaccountably. Space no longer radiates around her as known and familiar. Changes in space, such as the re-routing of a bus service, can shrink her world further.

Project – Projects become detached from contemporary life in that there is no longer concern to do, strive, possess, achieve. Past positive accomplishments no longer figure. Projects of dependency and disability now dominate:

> She refers frequently and with great rhetorical skill, to a disability sustained because of a childhood illness . . . apparently satisfied to assert her fundamental illness and dependency . . . Medical consultation are engaged eagerly . . . With studied dignity, she frequently asks to be taken to hospital. (Ashworth, 2006, p. 222)

Discourse – She adopts the style of dependent disabled person often performing a 'hurt child' by calling on the carer (sometimes called

'Mam') to look at her 'sore place'. With a flourish she declares she is 'eighty-two' and had 'infantile paralysis', thereby indicating she cannot be expected to take any initiative.

Mood-as-atmosphere[xiv] – Her lifeworld is 'mooded' and endowed with particular meanings: the frequently referred to but reference-less 'They' are oppressive; an unrecognized son-in-law is viewed with suspicion; unfamiliar unboundaried space offers a dizzying sense of fretful endlessness; a containing environment feels frustratingly restrictive, and so on.

In his discussion, Ashworth suggests carers may benefit by attending to the lifeworld of a person with Alzheimer's disease. The person with dementia acts in terms of a meaningful lifeworld and this world can be entered by carers in interaction. In attempting to grasp the lifeworld of the patient, carers may be enabled to see the personhood of the patient better which helps to make their own project of caring more bearable and satisfying. Care and respect is thus based on understanding rather than being based on the simple call to remember the person is an adult with rights.

Example 8.3   An existential analysis of lived space applied to domestic violence

The following analysis of *lived space* identifies how modes of place can be experienced as 'insideness' (where a person or people feels at home and at ease) or 'outsideness' (where they feel alienated and separate). This analysis – taken from the work of the phenomenological geographer Edward Relph (1976) and elaborated by David Seamon (2010a) – highlights how different individuals can experience the same physical space in different ways.

Relph's (1976) Modes of Insideness and Outsideness (cited in Seamon, 2010a)

Existential insideness – a deep unselfconscious immersion and identification with place; feeling 'at home' and having a sense of belonging, a deep identification with and attachment to a place.

Existential outsideness – a sense of being a stranger and outsider; experiencing oneself as 'out of place'; the place seems oppressive, unreal, alienating and/or not 'home'.

Objective outsideness – thinking about the place as an object as when studying a place or planning a development in the environment.

Incidental outsideness – experiencing a place as simply a background for activities such as when driving through a place.

Behavioral insideness – attending to the appearance of place such as when giving directions or familiarising oneself with a new town.

Empathetic insideness – encountering a place in a new way and being open to it in order to understand it more deeply.

Vicarious insideness – experiencing a place second-hand through accounts of others (e.g. through film or literature).

Seamon goes on to discuss and apply these ideas to the topic of **domestic violence**. He argues that domestic violence is a situation where a place that typically fosters a deep sense of existential insideness becomes one of existential outsideness. Strategies to help victims must therefore be centred on how to help them gain existential insideness. He challenges the view that post-modern society can ignore place in policy, design or in popular understanding, arguing that such a position is potentially devastating existentially.

I attended a conference session on negative and traumatic images of place . . . One example was how family violence regularly generated homes where people felt victimized and insecure. The postmodern conclusion was to call into question the entire concept of home and place and to suggest that they might be nostalgic notions that need vigorous existential and political modification – perhaps even substitution – in our postmodern society.

In fact, the problem here is not home and place but a conceptual conflation . . . The victim's experience should not be interpreted as a lack of at-homeness but, rather, as one mode of existential outsideness, which in regard to one's most intimate place – the home – is particularly undermining and painful . . . There are many domestic situations today that habor violence and abuse, but they should not be associated with 'home' nor should the experience of 'home' be blamed for the violation . . .

Domestic violence is a situation where a place that typically fosters the strongest kind of existential insideness has become, paradoxically, a place of overwhelming existential outsideness. The lived result must be profoundly distressing and distructive.

The short-term phenomenological question is how the victims of such experience can be helped to regain existential insideness. The longer-term question is what qualities and forces in our society lead to a situation where those responsible for the continuity of the home's existential insideness transform that place into an everyday hell. Something is deeply wrong, and one cause of the problem may be the very problem itself – the growing disruption of places and insideness at many different scales of experience, from home to neighborhood to city to nation. (downloaded from http://www.arch.ksu.edu/seamon/Relph.htm October 2010; Seamon & Sowers, 2008)

Reflections

If the field constituting lifeworld approaches is diffuse in the way it over-laps with other forms of phenomenology, the explicit focus on lifeworld dimensions offers phenomenology a clear, pragmatic framework that is well anchored in phenomenological philosophy (and so justified). The frame-work is one that guides methodology and upon which researchers can hang their understanding.

It is moot whether 'lifeworld approaches' can and should be regarded a specific methodological variant. All phenomenological analysis should be engaged in a project to grapple with existential domains of the lifeworld. Artificially separating out a specific approach to the lifeworld could be seen as '*methodolotry*', deifying method at the expense of content. In the end, I would say that what is important is to adopt an appropriate phenomeno-logical attitude and to do good phenomenological description, acquiring insights and knowledge that moves the field forward. The question at stake is the extent the approaches discussed here offer a helpful tool, focus or style towards broader/deeper reflection.

Leaving aside questions about whether lifeworld approaches can be dis-tinguished from descriptive or hermeneutic phenomenology in general, I find it useful when analysing data to think specifically in terms of lifeworld dimensions. Peter Ashworth supervised my PhD research and my introduc-tion to phenomenology was through his structured approach which, as a novice researcher, I found really helpful. I also appreciate the rigour with which Ashworth applies the epoché, modestly keeping to an idiographic account and holding back from making general claims in the first instance. With this professional socialization it is hard for me to be critical and step away from taking an idiographic approach and using lifeworld dimensions as a way to organize my thinking.[xv] I acknowledge, however, that some might criticize this strategy as being insufficiently ambitious in terms of establish-ing essentialist or general understandings which, they would say, is the point of phenomenology. Dahlberg's reflective lifeworld research (amongst other variants) perhaps answers this challenge, although some weaker studies in this field run the risk of uncritically embracing a *realist* approach and claiming too much certainty when offering general accounts of essential structures of experience.

In my view, explicit lifeworld analyses are valuable in emphasizing how body–others–world are interpenetrated, whatever the phenomenological approach. However, the phenomenological depth and richness obtained can be counter-balanced by the way the specific lifeworld headings (e.g. embodiment, identity, temporality, spatiality) may overly structure and constrain the analysis. Care needs to be taken by researchers to stay open to lifeworld experience *as a whole*. The fragments provide a framework – what Ashworth calls 'analytical moments of a larger whole' (2003, p. 151) and they should not be used mechanically. The work of Seamon provides a model: he takes spatiality as his starting point but wraps in other lifeworld dimensions as part of 'theoretical adventuring'.

The strength of a lifeworld perspective is the opportunity it opens up to highlight the ambiguity and ambivalence of different dimensions of peoples' lived experiences. As Dahlberg *et al.* (2008, p. 94) warn, however, researchers need to be 'careful not to make definite what is indefinite'. The best lifeworld research is characterized by its capacity to present the paradoxes and integrate polarities demonstrating holism (Dahlberg *et al.*, 2008).

Notes

[i] Others may prefer to see the field of what I am calling 'lifeworld approaches' as a *subset* of the descriptive phenomenology project given the common ground of anchoring methodology to Husserlian concepts. Husserl's original project was to examine philosophically the lifeworld as the tacit, reflective foundation of objective science. Husserl argued that the lifeworld could be engaged methodologically via the epoché of the natural sciences (Husserl, 1936/1970) where scientific theory/knowledge is bracketed, reducing the field of investigation to the lifeworld from the standpoint of the 'natural attitude'. Simply put, a focus on the lifeworld returns us to the natural attitude.

[ii] Like phenomenology in general, the respective lifeworld approaches of these scholars embrace a continuum of descriptive and hermeneutic approaches variously. Dahlberg *et al.* straddle both '**descriptive-hermeneutic**' interests; Ashworth is explicitly '**descriptive**', eschewing undue interpretive researcher attention; and Seamon is avowedly '**hermeneutic**'.

[iii] Dahlberg *et al.* recommend that informants of different ages, genders, cultures contribute, to ensure the data gathered is richly varied. Variation within the sample is more important than the question of number. Therefore a careful *snowball approach* to sampling is ideal.

[iv] The idea that 'essences' can be discerned in phenomena has been critiqued from a number of quarters. Mostly, critics reject the notion that social phenomena can be fixed somehow and constituent parts identified as if phenomenology had a realist agenda which claims it is possible to offer a definitive account. However, this view misunderstands the phenomenological project which aims to capture the *nuances* of experience. As Dahlberg (2006, p. 16) explains, 'Husserl discusses universal essences, but he also talks about open essences in relation to his understanding of the lifeworld as infinite . . . Essences leave open possibilities for further exploration.'

[v] In his early work, Ashworth was more essentialist and gave less weight to the specifics of individual accounts, e.g. Ashworth (1997).

[vi] **Idiography** is of great interest to us as psychologists, says Ashworth (personal communication), but it will be quickly passed over by philosophers. Ashworth forges a link between idiography and essence through the idea that individual accounts can be

considered instances of free imaginative variation (see *Chapter 6*). From there, he suggests the essence (i.e. that which can be intuited as the meaning of the set of possible instances) will emerge. His concern is to insist on not forgetting the actual lifeworld embedded-ness when pursuing essence.

vii Ashworth notes that Heidegger and Medard Boss (who translated Heidegger from philosophy to psychiatry) put forward a further existential of 'being-towards-death' (see, for instance, Lingis, 1989). Ashworth suggest that the notion of being-towards-death introduces a more speculative element. He rejects it as a universal 'fraction', preferring to avoid going down this more 'interpretive' route.

viii Alfred **Schutz** spearheaded the phenomenological sociology movement. His final publication (posthumously co-authored with Luckmann, 1973) *The Structures of the Life-World* represents a complex and comprehensive restatement of themes Schutz addressed throughout his life. After offering a more general account of the life-world and its relation to the sciences, Schutz acknowledges various stratifications, such as provinces of meaning, temporal and spatial zones of reach, and social structure. Perhaps his most enduring message is that everyday life is interpreted through a shared (socially derived) stock of knowledge (meanings, categories, constructs and '*typifications*').

ix See, for instance, his Environmental and Architectural Phenomenological Newsletter online at http://www.arch.ksu.edu/seamon/eap.html. See also a list a papers at http://ksu.academia.edu/DavidSeamon/Papers.

x For Seamon, '**movement**' relates to Merleau-Ponty's ideas about the role of the body and the habitual nature of everyday environmental behaviour. '**Rest**' acknowledges people's attachment to place. '**Encounter**' examines the many ways people make contact with their surroundings. Bringing these together Seamon suggests that:

- people become bodily and emotionally attached to their geographical world;
- this nexus of attachment is at-homeness;
- at-homeness sustains a taken-for-granted pattern of continuity, expectedness and order;
- as people move and rest in their geographical world they also encounter it;
- encounter varies in the degree to which people are part of or apart from their world.

xi To give an example, Seamon (2010b) uses the work of the American writer Louis Bromfield to shows how house and inhabitants can mutually reflect, sustain or unravel each other.

xii Seamon writes in the tradition of a group of scholars including Relph (1976), Norberg-Schulz (1985, 1996), Thiis-Evensen (1987), Casey (1993) and Mugerauer (1994). His philosophical orientation is towards the work of the German poet/writer/philosopher/scientist Goethe and the French phenomenological philosopher/historian Bachelard.

xiii See Seamon (2002b) for an analysis relevant to designing for the disabled. To give another example, Allen (2004) critiques early social geographies of disability that treat individuals with impairment as being 'disadvantaged'. Drawing on Merleau-Ponty, Allen argues the value of recognizing the habitual body in space. He shows how visually impaired children routinely exercise agency and navigate their spaces in various creative and positive ways.

xiv Ratcliffe (2008) talks about **existential feelings** as background orientations through which experience is structured and which are involve our bodily relationship with the world, e.g. 'feeling trapped in a situation'; 'feeling fulfilled'; 'feeling safe and secure'; 'feeling distant'; 'feeling of depersonalization'. They are more than affect/emotion in that they are not directed to something like feeling angry or in love. Instead they are woven into our perception, bodily being and experience of the world.

[xv] While these are my foundations, I have since elaborated the phenomenological attitude to encompass reflexive dimensions (Finlay, 2008) and I argue there is a need to attend to the relational dynamics of the data-gathering process (Finlay, 2009b). The lifeworld of researcher along with the researcher-researched context seem to me to offer the potential of additional understandings.

Chapter 9

Interpretative Phenomenological Analysis

> Without the phenomenology, there would be nothing to interpret; without the hermeneutics, the phenomenology would not be seen. (Smith *et al.*, 2009, p. 37)

Interpretative Phenomenological Analysis (IPA) is a specific hermeneutic version of phenomenology whose use has burgeoned rapidly over the last decade. Its starting point was a paper in which Jonathan Smith (1996) argued for an experiential approach that could enter into dialogue with mainstream psychology.

Currently, IPA is proving popular in the field of health psychology, particularly in the United Kingdom. With its many papers focusing on existential and illness experience IPA also comes highly recommended for many other fields, including counselling psychology, occupational therapy and physiotherapy (see Channine, 2009).[i] The structured approach and qualitative orientation offered by IPA seem to appeal to psychotherapy and health care researchers alike. Between 1996 and 2008, 293 papers presenting empirical IPA studies were published (see Smith's review in Smith, in press; see also http://www.psyc.bbk.ac.uk/ipa/references2.htm).

In this chapter, I offer a brief account of IPA methodology, together with three examples of IPA research in action.

Phenomenology for Therapists: Researching the Lived World, First Edition. Linda Finlay.

Methodology

Aims

Like other forms of phenomenology, IPA seeks to understand lived experience. In common with other **hermeneutic** approaches, IPA researchers utilize interpretation and accept the impossibility of gaining direct access to participants' experience. They recognize that any exploration must necessarily implicate the researcher's own views as well as interactions between researcher and participant.

What separates IPA from some other hermeneutic approaches is its focus on the **individual** and the way studies often prioritize explorations of participants' **sense-making.** IPA seeks *idiographic* accounts of people's views and perceptions: how participants themselves as individuals make sense of their experiences.[ii] The researcher then gathers these accounts to propose a general description of the phenomenon.

Typically, IPA research asks how individuals in *x* situation experience or understand process *y*. For example, a researcher might ask 'How do clients experience the ending of therapy?' or 'How do patients view their treatment protocols?' The questions are exploratory, open-ended and focused on meanings and processes rather than outcomes.

The three touchstones of IPA methodology are:

1) A reflective focus on subjective accounts of personal experience;
2) An idiographic sensibility;
3) The commitment to a hermeneutic approach.

Engaging in a reflective focus on **personal experience,**[iii] IPA assumes a model of a person as a sense-making creature. Many IPA projects tap into this by asking about individuals' views and engaging their reflections on life decisions and choices. However, it is not sufficient to operate at just a cognitive level focusing on people's attitudes. Instead, IPA seeks the *meanings* of experience which include embodied, cognitive-affective and existential domains.

The **idiographic** sensibility of IPA is revealed in researchers' commitment to understanding experiential phenomena from the perspective of particular individuals in particular contexts. It is also shown by the depth and detail of the micro-level analysis offered. Such micro-analysis may be viewed as an end in itself or it may form part of a sequence of similarly detailed analyses of other cases. Usually, IPA researchers start by analysing each case separately but this is followed by the search for patterns *across* cases. Ideally, convergences (shared themes) and divergences (particular ways themes are played out for individuals) are highlighted.

The **hermeneutic** commitment of IPA is captured in its use of the 'double hermeneutic' (Smith & Osborn, 2003, p. 51) – a term that seeks to describe the process whereby participants make sense of *x* while researchers make sense of participants' sense-making. IPA always involves researchers' own interpretations as they try to make sense of what is being said *while remaining grounded in the interview text*.

Importantly, the interpretations are understood to operate at different levels. At the first level, emergent themes are identified where the researcher aims to reconstruct the original experience descriptively in its own terms. Then the researcher might interject interpretive flourishes, perhaps by constructing a narrative or by bringing in metaphors (usually initiated by participants). The researcher might then introduce further layers of interpretation by drawing on theoretical ideas such as 'multiple selves' or perhaps by importing psychoanalytic or other theoretical perspectives as a way to understand the text. Care needs to be taken, however, when importing outside theories to do so *because the data invites it* rather than researchers playing with their pet theory. It is easy to get this wrong and make the energy base of the research theory and not the data (Smith, personal communication).

Through these different layers of interpretation, the IPA researcher aims to straddle both an 'insider' and 'outsider' approach to research through being both 'empathic and questioning' (Smith *et al.*, 2009, p. 36).

Methods and procedures

In practical terms, IPA is not a prescriptive approach. Smith *et al.* (2009) urge researchers to be creative and flexible rather than slavishly follow the 'method'. This flexibility within IPA methodology is shown in recommendations about sample size. Three to six participants is considered a reasonable size to provide sufficient comparisons without researchers getting overwhelmed with data. Smith *et al.* (2009) recommend three participants as the default size for undergraduate or Masters level as it takes time to do the required depth analysis. For doctoral studies the numbers may increase but it would not be impossible to use just one substantial case study supported by additional smaller studies with more participants.

Most IPA work is conducted using in-depth interviews, although other qualitative data collection methods can also be used. The interviews enable the participant to provide a full, rich account while allowing the researcher the flexibility to probe interesting areas that emerge. Interviews are always audio-recorded and transcribed verbatim, with any significant non-verbal behaviour such as laughter or pauses duly noted. The transcripts are then subjected to detailed qualitative analysis aimed at eliciting the key experiential themes in the participant's talk.

Many IPA researchers use semi-structured interview schedules. This has the advantage of allowing researchers to reflect carefully about what they are asking and how to phrase any particularly sensitive questions. However, interviews still need to be led by participants' concerns and so open questions are considered best. For example, the researcher might ask: 'Could you tell me about . . . ?' or 'What do you mean by . . . ?' or 'How does that make you feel?'

IPA analysis is iterative, inductive, fluid and emergent, although Smith *et al.* (2009; Smith & Eatough, 2007) offer a helpful step-by-step data analysis guide for novice researchers:

- *Step 1* Reading and re-reading – immersing oneself in the original data.
- *Step 2* Initial noting – free association and exploring semantic content (e.g. by writing notes in the margin).
- *Step 3* Developing emergent themes –focus on chunks of transcript and analysis of notes made into themes.
- *Step 4* Searching for connections across emergent themes – abstracting and integrating themes.
- *Step 5* Moving to the next case – trying to bracket previous themes and keep open-minded in order to do justice to the individuality of each new case.
- *Step 6* Looking for patterns across cases – findings patterns of shared higher order qualities across cases, noting idiosyncratic instances.
- *Step 7* Taking interpretations to deeper levels – deepening the analysis by utilizing metaphors and temporal referents, and by importing other theories as a lens through which to view the analysis.[iv]

The results of the analysis are presented as a full narrative or discursive account.[v] This may be organized into themes, with quotations from participants included to make the evidentiary base of the claims transparent. (An example of how this is achieved in practice is shown below.)

Smith (in press) offers advice about how to ensure a high quality study:

Interviewing is a critical part of the process and can require considerable time to develop expertise. Equally important to a high quality IPA analysis are rigour and systematicy as well as the quality of the interpretative work done. Thus the paper needs to be plausible and persuasive in terms of the evidence presented to support the claims made and the writing needs to be bold and confident in presenting the interpretation of that unfolding evidence trail.

**Example 9.1   Exploring meanings of HIV-positive,
gay men's relationships**

Paul Flowers carried out an extensive IPA study of gay men living in
Scotland who have been diagnosed with HIV. Unstructured interviews
with 16 HIV-positive gay men (a relatively large IPA study) began with
the question: 'What do relationships mean to you?' Analysis revealed a
number of themes around the management of risk and sexual decision-
making, particularly regarding unprotected anal intercourse.

One important finding was how unprotected anal sex tended to be
engaged in largely within the context of deeper relationships, as this
extended extract indicates:

> **Jack:** ... I wanted to please him, I wanted to, I suppose it was
> something that I could give him that ... I felt nobody else could, I
> suppose that was my way of trying to show him how much I care.
> **Interviewer:** So what ...
> **Jack:** I shouldn't have done but ...
> **Interviewer:** ... What were you giving him, to show him how much
> you cared?
> **Jack:** I was giving him myself, um I was giving him what he wanted,
> I didn't realize that at the time but um ... I was giving him my
> unprotected sex, which had never been an option in my mind
> before ...

The extract above illustrates the simultaneous engagement with HIV
risk reduction on the one hand and relational, romantic dynamics on the
other. Clearly for Jack the romantic dynamics shaped the sexual activity.
He describes his willingness to engage in unprotected anal intercourse
as making a 'gift' of himself ... At times it is almost as if actions are
speaking louder than words ... Jack who was infected by his long-term
partner, goes on to emphasize the difference between having sex and
'making love'. ...

> **Jack:** ... I had complete pleasure throughout my whole body, I was
> making love. I was in love with him, I felt that he was in love
> with me. (Reproduced from Smith, J.A., Flowers, P. and Larkin, M.
> (2009). *Interpretative Phenomenological Analysis: Theory, Method
> and Research*. Los Angeles, CA: Sage (pp. 138–139), with the kind
> permission of Sage Publication.)

Flowers notes that findings like these challenge traditional health psychology models which focus on health beliefs and rational approaches
to risk. Participants like Jack highlighted a range of powerful, complex and variable meanings clustered around 'giving of the self as a gift
to demonstrate commitment, love and intimacy' as well as 'using the

potential threat to the self to do likewise'. (Smith *et al.*, 2009, p. 142). This suggests that HIV risk behaviour is actively used to accomplish relational ends. Contrary to 'common sense' perception, individuals may be acting in a rational manner: being rational about their life choices rather than the health risks their behaviour may involve.

Example 9.2   One woman's account of personal meanings of dialysis treatment

Jonathan Smith examines *one* patient's experience of the psychological impact of haemodialysis treatment for kidney failure (Smith *et al.*, 2009). The extended case study of Carole draws on metaphors and dream interpretation to evoke how both the disease and the dialysis appear to undermine Carole's identity. Single case studies like this one make it possible to capture lived experience in detail. Smith *et al.* (2009) argue that such cases can then enter into dialogue with other findings and wider theoretical constructs in the literature.

Carole, aged 44 years, had been dialysing in hospital for 6 months before the start of this research. The semi-structured interview took place before one session. Carole was asked such questions as 'What do you do when you are dialysing?' and 'How does dialysis affect your everyday life?'

In the following extract, Smith *et al.* (2009) suggest a theme entitled, 'It's waiting to hurt me'.

> Carole appears to project her current trepidation about dialysis onto the machine itself:
>
>> **Interviewer:** How do you think of the machine?
>> **Carole:** I think I find it quite harsh [ ] It's stuck up there or down there I think it's sort of waiting for me (laughs) waiting to hurt maybe and keeping me prisoner to it.
>
> A presentation of the machine as malevolent seems to symbolize the entrapment Carole feels. Her sense of passivity and helplessness is turned, in the account, to her being a victim of the machine. Further, while recognizing the good the dialysis machine is doing her, Carole is acutely aware of its invasive nature:
>
>> It's sort of intrusive cos it's got these sharp needles of the thing that attaches you to it [ ] with the needling [ ] It can be quite painful and it's yeah that intrusion of metal into a very soft part of yourself. (Reproduced from Smith, J.A., Flowers, P. and Larkin, M. (2009). *Interpretative Phenomenological Analysis: Theory, Method and Research.* Los Angeles, CA: Sage (p. 126), with the kind permission of Sage Publication.)

Interestingly, during the interview Carole recounted a dream, or rather a nightmare, in which a devil spirit had rushed into and through her, causing great pain. The symbolic parallels with her dialysis are almost irresistible as the authors suggest below:

> **Carole:** ... When it rushed through it was alike a nervous um an electric shock. And it was very painful this sort of rushing through. And then it would call my name again sort of very quietly I thought I was safe and it would call – I knew it was going to happen again. (p. 128)

... Dialysis treatment has, for Carole, come to mean restriction, entrapment, a lack of control, passivity, invasion, and fear. These are not descriptions of the treatment itself, but rather of how Carole construes the meaning of the treatment for her at this stage in time. And it is these particular constructions that play into the undermining of her sense of identity that Carole experiences ...

The dream sequence is powerful in its own right but its meaning is strengthened when one recognizes it as contributing to the whole – the understanding of the personally debilitating impact of dialysis for Carole. And of course the horror of the dream becomes even more vivid when one realizes that much of what it seems to be about is the dialysis treatment. (Smith *et al.*, 2009, pp. 130–131)

Example 9.3   The contribution of visual art-making to the subjective well-being of women living with cancer

Frances Reynolds and Kee Hean Lim (2007) explored women's views about the contribution of art-making to their sense of well-being in the context of living with cancer. Participants were recruited through invitations placed in national UK art magazines. Twelve women participated in semi-structured interviews, each lasting between 1 and 2 hours, and their accounts were then analysed thematically.

Art-making was found to support subjective well-being in four main ways:

1) Creative activities helped the women to focus outwards on positive experiences rather than inwards on the destructive nature of cancer. As one participant said, 'While you're doing something, you're not dying. Literally.' (2007, p. 6).
2) Art-making enhanced a sense of self-worth by providing opportunities for achievement and challenge.
3) Art-making offered interest and helped the women to maintain a social identity beyond being a cancer sufferer.

4) For a minority, the use of art became a means of symbolizing the cancer experience and enabling the expression of fear, grief and hope.

This qualitative study suggested that art activities had strengthened the participants' sense of subjective well-being. The participants described gaining a 'sense of vitality' from their ongoing participation and their awareness of their own artistic development. Art-making offered the women an opportunity to focus positively on normal everyday identities and relationships rather than remain preoccupied with illness.

Discussing these findings, Reynolds and Lim (2007) argue that the study has important implications for art therapists and occupational therapists. In demonstrating the powerful positive effect of doing art for these women, such research adds to the growing pool of qualitative evidence supporting occupational therapy practice.

Reflections

The strength of IPA lies in its ability to identify meanings and develop understandings which emerge out of sustained interpretive engagement. For the most part, these understandings are rooted in the participant's 'sense-making' and lifeworld. At other times the interpretive (re)vision leads to more abstract sense-making which foregrounds the researcher's voice or wider theoretical or cultural issues (Eatough, 2009).

As the examples show, IPA studies have the potential to offer rich narratives or descriptions of embodiment, emotion, cognition, language and the culture or context. When the interpretive layers are done well, the imagery and insights offered are powerful. The systematic approach taken also increases the rigour and robustness of findings, allowing researchers to contribute with more confidence to the evidence base in both health care and psychological fields.

Novice researchers need to avoid the pitfall of treating IPA like straightforward, mechanical qualitative thematic analysis uncoupled from phenomenological theory. Such an approach can result in reductionist analysis of one aspect, thereby missing the opportunity to describe meanings and experience more holistically. Often, novice researchers focus overly on cognitions and sense-making at the expense, for example, of exploring embodied lived experience. Without a holistic focus on lived experience, the study is probably best considered phenomenologically inspired rather than phenomenology per se. Also researchers may fall into the trap of being over-reliant on simply re-presenting participants' words and perhaps accepting them as 'fact' or 'reality'. Instead, the researcher needs to 'work' the analysis and appreciate that findings are interpretations of a range of possible meanings as fitting the hermeneutic nature of the methodology.

Pitfalls aside, I often recommend IPA as a phenomenological method of choice for novice qualitative researchers who need structured support to engage their research. The clarity and accessibility of written accounts describing how to do IPA, combined with the sheer volume of practical empirical examples now available, makes IPA a safe and attractive route.

Of course, the field is still young. It was only in 2009 that the first textbook outlining this approach was published. Over time, a more sophisticated, theoretically informed, resonant body of research will surely evolve, ensuring IPA takes its rightful place alongside the best of what hermeneutic phenomenology can offer.

Notes

[i] Some recent PhD research studies using IPA relevant to therapists include: Avis (2010), Cronin-Davis (2010), McGreevy (2010) and Puig (2010). Three studies I particularly recommend which model how to do IPA are Eatough and Smith (2006a, 2006b) and Bramley and Eatough (2005).

[ii] From its inception IPA has focused on cognition and 'sense-making'. IPA originally arose in critique and dialogue with the social cognition experimental perspective dominant in mainstream psychology in the United Kingdom. Arguing against the view of cognition as separate thinking functions, IPA scholars see cognition as more intuitive, dynamic, emotional, embodied and multi-dimensional in its concern with people's engagement with the world. A cognitively oriented study focused solely on participants' thoughts and opinions is, arguably, insufficiently committed to the phenomenological – and therefore IPA – project.

[iii] Smith *et al.* (2009, p. 189) helpfully distinguish between types of **reflective activity** that both participant and researcher might engage in during their sense-making, moving beyond the pre-reflection and reflection distinction phenomenologists usually talk about. Smith *et al.* offer four types: 'pre-reflective reflexivity' (minimal level of awareness); 'reflective glancing at pre-reflective experience' (intuitive, undirected reflection on experiencing); 'attentive reflection on the pre-reflective' (fuller attention on the experience); and 'deliberate controlled reflection' (conscious phenomenological reflection).

[iv] The systematic, iterative process listed here has parallels with the analytic stages of descriptive phenomenology (see *Chapter 6*) except at this later, more interpretive stage. However, a significant difference between these two methods is that descriptive phenomenology directly follows a Husserlian approach to the reduction including explicit use of the epoché and imaginative variation (see *Chapter 4*).

[v] While IPA and discourse analysis are both linguistically based and concerned with close readings of transcripts/texts, their focus and rationale are quite different. Discursive approaches home in on the conversational features and linguistic resources participants are drawing upon to account for their experience (and therefore construct that experience). IPA, in contrast, analyses what participants say in order to learn how they are making sense of their experience and the connections with embodied emotional dimensions.

Chapter 10

First-Person Approaches

The reality of lived experience is there-for-me because I have a reflexive awareness of it, because I possess it immediately as belonging to me in some sense. (Dilthey, 1985, cited in van Manen, 1990, p. 35)

In a reflexive narrative, Kiser (2004) offers an autobiographical existential analysis of his experience of having a psychotic episode. He describes the episode as involving such internal devastation that it: 'leaves in its wake scars like canyons that can never be erased . . . When the wasteland of nothingness came to claim me yet again, I was utterly helpless and undone (Kiser, 2004, p. 433).

Work like this, where researchers use their own experiences to examine the quality and essences of phenomenon, exemplifies first-person approaches. Such approaches follow the path of the original philosophers like Husserl who pioneered phenomenology as the reflective study of structures of consciousness as experienced from the first-person point of view.[i]

In contemporary practice, there are many wonderful literary accounts of lived experience that draw on **personal reflection** rather than participants' descriptions. In health care research, for instance, this involves an individual's narrative of what it is like to live with a disability.[ii] Researchers also engage a first-person approach when they employ **reflexivity** within a broader study and critically focus on their personal experience of the phenomenon or research *process*. (This version of providing first-hand

Phenomenology for Therapists: Researching the Lived World, First Edition. Linda Finlay.
© 2011 Linda Finlay. Published 2011 by John Wiley & Sons, Ltd.

accounts is discussed more fully in *Chapter 11*.) Other types of first-person description can be found by turning to **literature**.

In this chapter, I offer a brief outline of what first-person, autobiographical approaches involve. Three examples are then offered. The first is a classic study: Toombs gives an account of her life with multiple sclerosis. In the second one, I offer an autobiographical account of living with pain. The third example moves away from ill-health/disability and examines the 'normal' experience of pregnancy. Space does not permit adequate exploration of the individuals' narratives and I would strongly recommend you seek out the original sources of all the autobiographical studies referenced to hear the fuller stories.

Methodology

Aim and approach

The aim of first-person approaches, as with any phenomenology, is to provide a rich, thought-provoking description of lived experience.

There is no set methodology laid down. Mostly, writers offer written autobiographical narratives which include concrete descriptions of events perhaps interspersed with theoretical discussion. Equally, it is possible to use other creative, self-expressive media such as reflexive writing, photography, poetry and painting. [Here phenomenologists can learn from the range offered in autoethnography.[iii] An accessible example is offered by Bains (2007), a practising psychotherapist, of her personal experience of racism on a webpage.]

Method

Van Manen (1990) gives advice on how to approach first-person accounts:

> I try to describe my experience as much as possible in experiential terms, focusing on a particular situation or event. (van Manen, 1990, p. 54)

These direct, concrete descriptions then become the 'data' with which to work further. They can become the basis of more generalized phenomenological analyses. Some researchers will even interrogate their personal diary account as if it was a 'transcript' from a participant.

Researchers often include concrete descriptions of significant events perhaps interspersed with theoretical discussion and/or literary flourish. Personal reflection thus becomes a springboard for broader, deeper analyses or new insights. To give an example, consider the way Broyard (1992, pp. 4–5) offers his experience of cancer using the surprising metaphor of intoxicating desire:[iv]

> When my friends heard I had cancer, they found me surprisingly cheerful and talked about my courage. But it has nothing to do with courage, at least not for me . . . I'm filled with desire – to live, to write, to do everything. Desire itself is a kind of immortality . . .
>
> The way my friends have rallied around me is wonderful. They remind me of a flock of birds rising from a body of water into the sunset. If that image seems a bit extravagant or tinged with satire, it's because there's something comical about my friends' behaviour – all those witty men suddenly saying pious, inspirational things.
>
> They are not intoxicated as I am by my illness, but sobered. They appear abashed or chagrined in their sobriety. Stripped of their playfulness these pals of mine seem plainer, homelier – even old. It's as if they had all gone bald overnight.
>
> Yet one of the effects of their fussing over me is that I feel vivid, multicoloured, sharply drawn. On the other hand – and this is ungrateful – I remain outside of their solicitude, their love and best wishes. I'm isolated from, them by the grandiose conviction that I am the healthy person and they are the sick ones. Like an existential hero, I have been cured by the truth while they still suffer the nausea of the uninitiated . . . I'm infatuated with my cancer. It stinks of revelation.

The challenge for researchers using first-hand experience is to engage personal reflection and revelation, not just as an end in itself but as a springboard for more general insight into the phenomenon of concern. Rather than showing 'straightforward, unreflected absorption in the objects of experience', says Toombs:

> the phenomenological approach involves reflection *upon* experience. The task is to elucidate and render explicit the taken-for-granted assumptions of everyday life and, particularly, to bring to the fore one's consciousness-of the world. (1993, p. xii)

In Example 10.1, for instance, Toombs writes of her experience of living with multiple sclerosis and describes her experience of navigating airports. This is the start of a broader discussion about her changing relations between self–body–world, her bodily intentionality, shame, and so on. In another of her works, *The Meaning of Illness*, she describes her bodily experience as part of a wider critique of the objectifying medical/professional gaze and the need for more healing relationships where she urges physicians towards better understandings of patients' lived experience (Toombs, 1993).

Example 10.1   Living with multiple sclerosis

S. Kay Toombs, academic and phenomenological philosopher, has written extensively about her lived experience of disability which she explores through her own experience as a person living with multiple sclerosis for over 30 years. In the following extract she describes the restricted interactions with the surrounding world forced upon her as a wheelchair user.

> On arriving at a small regional airport to begin a professional trip, I look for a parking space that is wide enough to lower the wheelchair lift so that I can get out of my handicapped equipped van. There is no handicapped parking . . . Once in the terminus I go to the airline check-in counter. In my battery operated wheelchair I am approximately three and a half feet tall and the counter is on a level with my head . . . I must crane my neck and shout in order to be heard. The small commuter plane arrives and there are steps leading into the cabin. Since I cannot walk, I must be carried on board . . . In the terminal building I am outside the security checkpoint. However, it is not possible to go through the security gate . . . I am taken to the side (once again in full view of everyone . . .) and my whole body from armpits to fingertips, from the top of my head to the base of my spine, from groin to ankle, from under my chin and over my breasts and abdomen, is . . . 'frisked' . . . by an airport employee. I leave and go to the restroom. Although the door is wide enough, the 'handicapped accessible' stall is too short to accommodate the length of my battery-operated wheelchair. I must, therefore sit in it with the door open. (2001, pp. 251–252)

Beyond the practical impediments, Toombs graphically draws our attention to the way **shame** is her constant companion as she navigates her way through the world.

> Feelings of shame inevitably accompany the changes in body that elicit negative responses from others. Every time I have had to adopt a new way of getting around the world, first a cane, then crutches, then walker, and finally a wheelchair, I have experienced feelings of shame. (2001, p. 257)

Toombs also intersperses more general discussion in her narrative, for instance, discussing how the loss of an upright posture links to philosophical notions of the transformation of the body and disrupted bodily intentionality and lived relations with others (Merleau-Ponty, 1945/1962).

> To live with multiple sclerosis is to experience a global sense of disorder – a disorder which incorporates a changed relation with one's body, a transformation in the surrounding world, a threat to the self, and a change in one's relation to others. (Toombs, 1995, p. 12)

Example 10.2 A personal account of pain experience

In 2004, I (Linda) fell down some steps and smashed my shoulder (a complex fracture of head of humerus). I had no inkling then that it would change my life, nor of the trauma that would be involved. Three major surgeries over 3 years were probably the least traumatic aspects of the process towards shoulder replacement and a new way of life. Each surgery was followed by a period of intensive rehabilitation involving ever more complex exercises and agonizing stretching which, at its heights, consumed 5 hours a day. I would scream with pain as my physiotherapist or husband forced my arm into impossible positions. Domestic and work responsibilities had to be curtailed while I hung by a thread to a modicum of activity and my life projects – hanging on to 'me'. Against the odds, I have regained almost full movement and strength in my arm. Most of the pain has receded. I still remember the months of my pain-world, however.

The following narrative of those early days has been constructed retrospectively from memory and from odd notes and writings I produced at the time. I share it now to give physical therapists, who work in taken for granted ways with patients in pain, a greater appreciation of what it is like from the 'inside'. I write, too, for the millions of patients in remedial clinics around the world who are casually instructed to do exercises without being given sufficient emotional support to face the trauma of the process . . .

I'm aware of layers of different types of pain. There is the more surface burning/pulling/stinging pain around my surgery wound. At a deeper level there are the throbbing pulsing waves coming from traumatic damage that cry from deep within. Then, there is the acute spasm fire-pain which violates me when I move. The tearing of fibres make me want to cry out, and sometimes I do. Always there is the continual, lingering dull ache of pain that resides away from my shoulder – my back in particular, aches constantly. Pain killers promise oblivion but never deliver.

Burning, throbbing, spasm . . . .. These words don't capture the experience, the layers, the colour, the flavour, the noise, the assault . . . Brown, black, red, grey . . . Molten lava with hard black crusty edges and endless grey ash beyond . . . A poisonous lemon fire-water with bitter aloes codeine-fuelled aftertaste . . . The high-pitched screech of an electric saw on metal, a pneumatic drill which will not be silenced.

Times of movement are the worst. Any dreaded movement is preceded by a sense of vertigo. An anxious anticipation of pain to come and the struggle within to resist. Forcing myself, I throw my body into movement. A faint threatens as I am overwhelmed with screeching, sheering pain. Can the body bear this level of agony? As movement ceases, the screeching turns to fire-y ache. Somehow I welcome its constancy with a glimmer of relief which knows the worst has passed (is past), for now.

The horizon of anxiety is a continual presence: fear shrouds the pain. A helpless anxiety gnaws. What does the pain mean? Should I stop exercising? Am I doing myself damage? What of the future? Can I endure this another minute, hour, day, week, another month, year, years? I scare myself. When I think about it, the pain gets louder, the red-blacks darken.

Time slows; there are only periods of more or less pain. With the distractions of the day some relief is to be had; at night a lonely black fear of endless waiting descends. Pain keeps me awake yet I'm bone weary from coping with the pain and too dopey to wake properly.

Being scared, or resisting the pain, only makes it worse. Somehow observing its forms – tolerating it and letting it be – brings its own curiosity. It's as if I'm in a prison with a potentially violent enemy or torturer. I resolve to know him. If we're locked here together for life I need us to build some kind of companionable relationship – one not based on fear. 'Come,' I say to the pain, 'Time to exercise'.

. . . I am diminished. Tears come to my eyes unbidden. A new shadow 'disabled shame-self' has replaced me: weak, vulnerable, handicapped, dependent, pathetic, needy . . . I become more reclusive and withdrawn . . . The spectre of uselessness and disintegration haunts me and I am tempted to give in, give up. But I don't. Instead I exercise harder . . . *Just exercise.*

I re-learn the meaning of pain. Once it meant, 'stop'. Pain meant something was wrong and the body was protecting itself, signalling for me to stop doing whatever it was that I was doing. Now, it just is: pain is the body and pain is the world . . . I learn a new way of moving in my world . . . I am alert to possible harm . . . and [self]protective, shielding my body from external threat . . . Yet I also I cause the pain in me. From somewhere I find the courage to invite pain in even *more* . . . *Just exercise Linda, just exercise . . .*

Example 10.3   Pregnancy as embodied subjectivity and alienation

Iris Marion Young (1984) takes an explicitly **feminist perspective**[v] – in the phenomenological tradition of Simone de Beauvoir – and explores the experience of pregnancy from the pregnant subject's viewpoint (her own and that of other women). She argues that discourses on pregnancy throughout Western culture tend to omit such subjectivity.

In the extract from her essay below, Young gives an account of what seems to be a reflection on her own lived experience of being pregnant. She explains how the experience reveals a body subjectivity that is herself but in a decentred mode of not being herself. Boundaries between self–other, body–world are both permeable and fluid:

As my pregnancy begins . . . I experience it as a change in my body . . . My nipples become reddened and tender, my belly wells into a pear. I feel this elastic around my waist, itching, this round, hard middle replacing the doughy belly with which I still identify. Then I feel a little tickle, a little gurgle in my belly, it is my feeling, my insides, and it feels somewhat like a gas bubble, but it is not, it is different, in another place, belonging to another, another that is nevertheless my body ... Pregnancy challenges the integration of my body experience by rendering fluid the boundary between what is within, myself, and what is outside, separate. I experience my insides as the space of another, yet my own body ... The boundaries of my body are themselves in flux. In pregnancy I literally do not have a firm sense of where my body ends and the world begins. My automatic body habits become dislodged, the continuity between my customary body and my body at this moment is broken ... I move as though I can squeeze around chairs and through crowds as I could have seven months before, only to find my way blocked by my own body sticking out in front of me, but yet not me ... As I lean over in my chair to tie my shoe, I am surprised by the graze of this hard belly on my thigh. I do not anticipate this touching of my body on itself, for my habits retain the old sense of my boundaries ... The belly is other, since I did not expect it there, but since I feel the touch upon it, it is me. (Young, 1984, pp. 48–50)

Young shows us how the dichotomy between self–other/self–world can dissolve and how this process can be positively experienced in pregnancy. However, she goes on to critique the way conceptualizations and practices of contemporary medicine can alienate the pregnant subject from her bodily experience. Medical definitions, Young argues, can reduce a pregnant woman to having a 'disorder' while objectifying medical relations and instrumentation in the medical setting alienate and reduce a woman's control over her body and experience.

Normal procedures of the American hospital birthing setting render the woman considerably more passive than she need to be. [Plus] the use of instruments provides means of objectifying the pregnancy and birth which alienate a woman because it negates or devalues her own experience. (Young, 1984, pp. 56–57)

Reflections

Personal accounts of the lived experience of health and well-being, illness, disability, pain, emotional trauma, and so forth, are often poignant and powerful. Such accounts offer us therapists, a way to get 'up close and personal' to specific experiences, to better understand and empathize with what our patients and clients may be going through. They challenge our blind-spots and taken-for-granted assumptions. Reminding us of our own fragile existence, they can resonate and touch us.

These accounts also have a value in that they offer an empowering 'voice', a way that individuals can express, work through and share their existential journeys with others. Often the journeys described focus on some transformational component and these can be inspiring to both self and other.

More than giving voice, however, first-person accounts invite others to 'witness' – and be enriched by – stories of the individual's struggle/achievement. Willis (2010) picks up this point when he invites readers to engage a 'listening reading' attitude which involves reading with a reflective, attentive, empathic silence allowing authors to speak to the imagination, heart and soul.

But personal accounts also run the risk of being self-absorbed and self-indulgent. They can be unduly preoccupied with clichéd banalities of everyday life. Researchers taking the first-person route need to keep the purpose of their study and the phenomenon in mind. As van Manen (1990, p. 54) puts it: 'the phenomenologist does not want to trouble the reader with purely private, autobiographical facticities of ones' life'.

Reflexive revelations in the research context probably have greatest value when one's own experiences shed light on others' experiences, i.e. when the account goes *beyond* the personal.

Notes

[i] The use of introspection and personal reflection, however, has a much longer history in philosophy and inquiry into the human condition. In the West, it can be traced back to the Greek Stoics in the third century BC who believed in non-dualism, formal logic, rationalism and naturalistic ethics. They developed personal examination, confession or self-disclosure as a tool for increasing self-knowledge. In the East, non-dualist philosophies, spirituality and reflective-meditative practices go back even further. The term 'phenomenology' began to be commonly used in philosophy after Hegel's seminal work *The Phenomenology of Spirit* (1807). Later in the nineteenth century, Brentano (Husserl's teacher) advanced the notions of phenomenological philosophy as an exact science and 'descriptive psychology'.

[ii] There is a tradition where authors offer deeply personal accounts of their illness experiences using autobiographical *narrative* research methodology (e.g. Robert F. Murphy's *The Body Silent* where he recounts his life as a quadriplegic). While not explicitly utilizing phenomenological methodology, they can be regarded as phenomenologically inspired as they offer a rich, descriptive accounts of lived experience.

[iii] *Autoethnography* is a version of autobiography which has developed from ethnography, anthropology, sociology and cultural studies. Combining the personal and cultural analysis, it aims via reflexive writings and other creative media to challenge traditional structural/historical power relations by describing cultural conflicts and the process of becoming Othered. See, for instance, Ellis (2008) and Chang (2008).

[iv] I am grateful to Peter Willis for drawing my attention to this wonderful work as well as introducing me to the practice of 'listening reading'.

^v In her book *On Female Body Experience: 'Throwing Like a Girl' and Other Essays*, Young offers a feminist account of a whole range of female bodily experience. Drawing on authors such as Simone de Beauvoir and Merleau-Ponty, she provides concrete analyses of a range of everyday experiences. Young's descriptions in essays like 'Throwing like a girl', 'Menstrual meditations' and 'Breasted experience', give expression to experiences that have been invisible and unspoken in the Western philosophical tradition and culture. She argues that women's experience is often stigmatized, devalued, relegated to the 'private sphere' of the Other (i.e. men). In bringing female experiences and modes of embodiment to light, she performs a critical function, pointing to the way female embodiment has been restricted and categorized through social norms.

Chapter 11

Reflexive-Relational Approaches

I have that quality of attention so that I may be with you, alongside you, empathizing with you: and yet not losing myself in confluence with you because the dialogue between us both bridges and preserves our differences. (Reason, 1988, p. 219)

Excerpt from a research interview:

Linda (researcher): I'm seeing your travelling when you were younger in a different light now. It sounds like you were really running away from home.
Pat (participant/co-researcher): Yeah.
Linda: But you've made something of yourself and you feel proud(?).
Pat: [nods] Now I'm putting them together.
Linda: So it is like two sides of you coming together: your childhood side and your adult side are now coming into one, instead of being split. [after a pause] I'm feeling very emotional like I'm about to start crying.
Pat: And I'm the same.
Linda: [after a pause] Feels profound. I think I'm beginning to understand something of your mixed feelings.
Pat: You definitely have! . . . When you were talking earlier I was puzzled and wondered *did I say it or did she*? . . .

In this brief dialogue, we can see that both Linda and Pat are mutually impacted and touched by the other. Together they unfold Pat's story. The co-creation is so subtle that Pat notes how hard it is to know where you end

Phenomenology for Therapists: Researching the Lived World, First Edition. Linda Finlay.
© 2011 Linda Finlay. Published 2011 by John Wiley & Sons, Ltd.

the Other begins. *Did I say it or did she?* 'To the extent that I understand, I no longer know who is speaking and who is listening' (Merleau-Ponty, 1960/1964, p. 97).

In reflexive-relational approaches to phenomenological research, data is seen as emerging out of the researcher and co-researcher[i] relationship and as being co-created (at least in part) in the embodied dialogical encounter. Reflexive-relational phenomenologists believe that when doing research much of what we can learn and know about another comes through dialogue and arises within the *intersubjective* spaces between researcher, co-researcher and the phenomenon being studied. This dialogue (verbal or non-verbal) forms the basis for reflection on both self and other. In this opening 'between' lurks ambiguity and unpredictability together with the possibility of true meeting; anything can – and does – appear. 'The joint phenomenological endeavour attunes, deepens and enriches' (Grant, 2005, p. 576).

Diverse methodologies nest beneath this umbrella category of 'reflexive-relational approaches'.[ii] Three of the most relevant for therapists (particularly psychotherapists) are explained here: **dialogal, heuristic** and **relational-centred**.[iii] While quite different in their respective style and emphasis, they remain linked in their commitment to the phenomenological project and they all grapple – explicitly or implicitly – with both reflexive (i.e. self-aware) and relational dimensions. All three approaches have been influenced by the work of phenomenological philosophers, most notably Buber, Levinas, Gendlin and Gadamer concerning self-other understanding, ethical relating and the healing power of dialogue (see *Chapter 3*).[iv] Buber (1937/1958) for instance, maintains that understandings of the Other – and thus ourselves – are to be found within the fullness of our open relationships when we engage in authentic, mutual, respectful dialogue.

In this chapter I sketch the differing methodologies of the three approaches and offer an example of each from research practice. As you read, notice how each values the *transformative* potential of the research process and how each foregrounds reflexivity and relational elements in varying ways.

Dialogal Research

The dialogal (sometimes called dialogical) approach was developed by Steen Halling, Jan Rowe and their colleagues in the United States (see, for instance, Halling, 2005,[v] 2008; Halling & Leifer, 1991; Halling, Leifer & Rowe, 2006). In this approach, a *group* of phenomenologists investigate a phenomenon through **dialogue** which takes place among researchers, between researchers and co-researchers/participants, and also between researchers and the phenomenon studied. Individual researchers share their experiences of the phenomenon, interview others and then negotiate layered meanings **collaboratively** in the group until finally some consensus is reached. Working with others, says Halling (2008), is potentially transformative, allowing each individual to reach a creativity and understanding that exceeds what the individuals are able to accomplish on their own.

These ideas arise out of the philosophical-theoretical tradition following the dialogal existentialist philosophy of Buber, the hermeneutic philosophy of Gadamer and the dialogal phenomenology of Stephan Strasser and Emmanuel Levinas.

Aims and approach

Apart from the fluid dialogically led approach, the method engaged follows many of the principles of 'descriptive phenomenology'. Researchers remain faithful to the phenomenon studied and the focus on **description** gives direction to the research. As with the descriptive phenomenological method, dialogal researchers make reflexive efforts to identify and **bracket** assumptions in order to focus more systematically on the phenomenon.[vi] (The bracketing process in the dialogal method involves researchers writing about their own experiences reflexively and then sharing these in the group). A further similarity is that both methods seek implicit meanings underlying the words/actions of participants.

While traditional descriptive approaches utilize the technique of 'free imaginative variation' varying the phenomenon *imaginatively* to arrive at what is essential to it (its essences), the dialogal method uses a kind of **'empirical variation'** where researchers sift through different perspectives in *dialogue with* others.

Halling (2008) argues for the value of dialogue for personal growth:

1) The multiplicity of perspectives allows for seeing the phenomenon in new ways.
2) It is easier for a supportive collaborative group to move beyond impasses where a lone individual may get stuck.
3) The group can be a resource where one word from one person can spark ideas in another with ideas cascading in an 'intermingling of receptivity and creativity, of discovering truth and creating truth' (Halling, 2008, p. 168).

In dialogue and being open to the other, presence, companionship, intimacy, truth and understanding can be found (Halling, 2005).

The spirit of this approach is captured by Gadamer's work on 'conversation' and how we can become 'carried away' in opening to the other, says Halling (2005): 'The more fundamental the conversation is, the less its conduct lies within the will of either partner . . . Conversation has a spirit of its own and . . . the language used in it bears its own truth within' (Gadamer, 1975/1996, p. 345).

Method

Although involving systematic steps, the dialogal method cannot be applied as a mechanical technique. Because it is based on dialogue, the reflexive, iterative, relational nature of the research process invariably takes it in unexpected directions. Primarily, the method relies on an attitude of openness and a preparedness to engage with others.

The basic method involves a small group of researchers working together, typically four to six people. At every stage the group negotiate how to proceed, for instance, when they make decisions about process, sort out the division of labour, review the literature and interpret the data. Researchers start by bringing the topic into focus by reflexively writing about their own experience of the phenomenon which they then share with the group. On the basis of this discussion, they formulate the interview question(s) and go out individually to interview participants (recording the interviews by audio- or videotape[vii]). Subsequent analysis of all this 'data' focuses both on the personal and outside description. Through the whole project, the process is guided by a continuing intense focus on the topic and the 'presence' of the phenomenon in the room, so to speak.

'Ongoing focus on the phenomenon', says Halling (2008, p. 166), 'allows it to take on a life and presence within the group rather being something abstract'. The topic can become palpably alive, creating its own challenges within the group. For example, Halling (2008) describes how in group study on the topic of 'despair', they found it hard to stay focused, paralleling the despair process. It was only after they reflexively supported each other that their trust and openness grew allowing the discussions to move forward and the dialogue deepen. A further challenge is the need for group members to respect and be open to others, accepting the diversity of views constructively by treating them as a basis for further exploration rather than taking any disagreements personally.

Heuristic Research

The word 'heuristic' comes originally from the Greek word *heruiskein* which means to discover or find. Heuristic research, as developed by Clark Moustakas (1990) in the United States, is a way of engaging in scientific search using methods and processes aimed at **discovery** through engaging **self-inquiry** and **dialogue** with others to find underlying meanings of human experience. It can be understood as a reflexive version of descriptive phenomenology that engages self and participants in dialogue about the experience being studied. Justifying this approach, Moustakas draws on the ideas of Carl Rogers: 'It is only by referring to the flow of my experiencing that I can sense the implicit meanings' (1969, p. 23).

Aims and approach

Moustakas considers heuristic methodology to be a systematic form of inquiring into human experience. In addition to drawing on Husserl's philosophy, Moustakas has been influenced by the research and theories of many writers including Buber's (1937/1958) exploration of dialogue; Maslow's (1956) research on self-actualization; Roger's (1969) work on human science; Polanyi's work on tacit dimensions; and Gendlin's (1962/1970) analysis of experiencing.

Where this approach diverges from other empirical, descriptive phenomenological approaches is in its implicit hermeneutic shift and focus on researcher self-search and personal transformation.[viii] Moustakas explains:

> Throughout an investigation, heuristic research involves self-search, self-dialogue, and self-discovery; the research question and the methodology flow out of inner awareness, meaning, and inspiration. When I consider an issue, problem or question, I enter into it fully... I search introspectively, meditatively, and reflectively into its nature and meaning... I may be entranced by visions, images, and dreams that connect me to my quest...
>
> If I am investigating the meaning of delight, then delight hovers nearby and follows me around... Delight becomes a lingering presence; for a while, there is only delight. It opens me to the world in a joyous way and takes me into a richness, playfulness and childlikeness that move freely and effortlessly. (1990, p. 11)

Method

With Moustakas's method, as with dialogal research, there is a fluid merging of introspection, data collection and analysis. The researcher travels on their experiential voyage (exploring participants' and their own inner experience) engaging in six interrelated phases:

- **Initial engagement** – the researcher immerses his/herself in a deep questioning about the topic/research in order to waken an intense interest and passion in the research subject.

- **Immersion** – the researcher begins to live, sleep, breath the research question to intimately appreciate its effects.
- **Incubation** – the researcher engages intuition awaiting tacit knowing to percolate to consciousness.
- **Illumination** – the researcher reviews all the data acquired from his/her experience and that of the co-researchers in order to identify implicit meanings.
- **Explication** – the researcher aims to familiarize him/herself more deeply with the layers of meaning and pull together key themes.
- **Creative synthesis** – now thoroughly familiar with the data, the researcher forms a creative synthesis which takes the form of a narrative depiction using verbatim examples or it may be expressed through other creative means such as a poem, story, drawing or painting.

Through these stages the researcher engages in reflexive dialogue. Moustakas makes this point when he explains the process of explication:

> The heuristic researcher utilizes focusing, indwelling, self-searching, and self-disclosure, and recognizes that meanings . . . depend upon internal frames of reference. The entire process of explication requires that researchers attend to their own awarenesses, feelings, thoughts, beliefs, and judgments as a prelude to the understanding that is derived from conversations and dialogues with others. (1990, p. 31)

For example, in his explication of loneliness, Moustakas describes how his interest in the topic began at a critical time in his life when deciding whether or not to agree to doctors' recommendations of major heart surgery for his daughter which could result in her death. 'The urgency of making a critical decision plunged me into the experience of feeling utterly alone' (1990, p. 91). From engaging an initial self-search he came to an intuitive grasping of the phenomenon of loneliness which he further clarified and refined by studying others' experiences and by searching the literature.

More recently, Sela-Smith (2002) has proposed an adaptation of Moustakas's method called **heuristic self-search inquiry**. She calls researchers to focus in more committed ways on *I-who-feels* and one's own subjective experience. In critique of Moustakas's approach she suggests his phenomenological shift, from the personal to researching others and the phenomenon more generally, can lead to some disconnections and insufficient exploration of the tacit dimension. She asks for the subjective elements not to be resisted or cast aside too soon in a rush to create general themes out of other people's stories. She argues the value of researchers surrendering to their experiential feelings and letting go into the unknown, what she calls the 'last frontier':

As we become conscious of the last frontier, the interiority of the self as experience by the self, we may learn how to consciously transform both the internal experience and the outside world. (2002, p. 86).

Relational-centred Research

The specific form of relational-centred approach I would like to put forward in this section has arisen out of collaboration in the United Kingdom between Ken Evans and myself (Finlay & Evans, 2009). Our approach – which is new and evolving – represents a *general orientation* for any qualitative exploration but it can also be applied specifically to the phenomenological project (see, for instance, Finlay, 2009b; Finlay & Molano-Fisher, 2008).

This approach argues that we need to attend to the embodied inter-subjective relationship between researcher and researched as this is our primary access to understanding an Other. Further, it is through the ***being-with*** another that both researchers and co-researchers have the potential for new learning and growth (Finlay, 2010a). (Dialogal and heuristic researchers would probably agree with this statement but would tweak it: dialogal researchers would emphasize phenomenological understanding arising through dialogue, while heuristic researchers would highlight the value of self-understanding.)

A range of theoretical concepts, straddling different traditions, underpin relational-centred research. At its core, existential phenomenological philosophy highlights consciousness as embodied intersubjective intentionality (e.g. Merleau-Ponty, 1945/1962). Ideas from the psychotherapy field are also embraced, including gestalt theory (e.g. Hycner & Jacobs, 1995), intersubjectivity theory (e.g. Stolorow & Atwood, 1992) and relational psychoanalysis (e.g. Mitchell & Aron, 1999).[ix] Collaborative, creative and action orientated feminist methodology, celebrating a focus on emotional dimensions and reflexivity as a source of insight, have additionally informed our emerging approach (e.g. Fonow & Cook, 1991; Stanley & Wise, 1983).

Aims and approach

Given their explicit use of reflexivity and focus on embodied relational dimensions, relational-centred phenomenologists may be best regarded as practicing a **hermeneutic** variant of phenomenology. They lean towards contingent, relativist understandings arguing that meanings arise in co-created contexts. (This contrasts with the epistemological positions of both dialogal and heuristic researchers which tend to be more critical realist, even essentialist, and less explicitly interpretive.)

This relational-centred approach was developed specifically for therapists although it can be applied more widely). Both Ken and I have a backgrounds in gestalt/phenomenological, existential and integrative psychotherapy practice and we wanted to bring to the fore a way of doing research that would suit therapists. We sought to parallel the process of relationally orientated counselling/psychotherapy, arguing that research data does not 'speak for itself' but is born within the *between* of the researcher–co-researcher encounter where they intermingle in 'pre-analytic participation' (Merleau-Ponty, 1964/1968, p. 203). Hycner (1991) explains this concept in reference to the therapy relationship (although we believe the principles apply equally to research):

> If we take seriously the concept of *between* there is a reality that is greater than the sum total of the experience of the therapist and client. *Together* they form a totality that provides a context for the individual experience of both. (Hycner, 1991, pp. 134–135)

Ken and I suggest that relational-centred researchers have a responsibility to build a bridge to the co-researcher, using their own special awareness, sensitivity, skills, experience and knowledge (Evans & Gilbert, 2005; Finlay & Evans, 2009). Central to our relational approach is the understanding that the research relationship involves an interactional encounter in which *both* parties are actively involved. As we see it, research does not involve a participant subject talking to a passive, distanced researcher who receives information. Instead, it emerges out of a constantly evolving, negotiated, dynamic, co-created relational process to which both researcher and participant co-researcher contribute (Evans & Gilbert, 2005). The process involves a way of being *with* rather than doing *to* where the relationship is 'continually established and re-established through ongoing mutual influence in which both [researcher and co-researcher] . . . systematically affect, and are affected by, each other' (Mitchell & Aron, 1999, p. 248).

'It takes courage to sit with uncertainty and not-knowing, and be open to what is emerging in the "now" of the embodied dialogical encounter' (Finlay & Evans, 2009, p. 39). The researcher's approach is one of **openness** where we pay close attention to the other with curiosity, empathy and compassion. When we intertwine with another in an encounter, we may well find ourselves surprised and touched by the connection we make and the transferences/counter-transferences we experience. Any 'here and now' moment contains something of the 'there and then' and meanings are layered (and not necessarily entirely in conscious awareness).

Method

There is no pre-set, structured method for relational-centred research except that researchers attend to having as open an **empathic presence** as possible and to be **reflexive** about what may be happening in the embodied **intersubjective** space between researcher and co-researcher.[x]

All the methods of data collection and analysis discussed in this book would lend themselves to this research approach providing a relational-centred dimension is added. Data could be gathered from a range of sources: interviews, focus groups, participant observation and other experiential-cum-therapeutic activities such as engaging in 'family sculpts' or 'two-chair work'. The data is then analysed thematically, narratively, reflexively or creatively with a phenomenological focus on exploring a person's embodied selfhood/self-identity and their lived relations with others. Taking a relational and development perspective, particular attention is paid to exploring the individual's existential needs and *being-in-the-world*, including their 'creative adjustments' (the defensive strategies they have developed in order to cope with past relational difficulties).

Analysis also focuses on the emergent dynamics of the research relationship where both researcher and co-researcher can be seen to be mutually impacted by the other. This impact might be conscious or unconscious – perhaps revealed in embodied emotional ways, dreams and images. An example of this might be when a researcher feels unaccountably irritated with a co-researcher and then realizes counter-transference may be in play and the irritation co-created.

With relational-centred research, relational dynamics between researcher and co-researchers are taken seriously and explored reflexively (Finlay & Gough, 2003). But this needs to be done without the researcher becoming excessively preoccupied with their *own* experience of the encounter (Finlay, 2002a, 2002b). Reflexivity in this approach is used to keep communication channels open towards acknowledging emotional and relational dynamics as well as possible political tensions arising from the different social positions of researcher and co-researcher (in terms of power, gender, class, race, age, ethnicity, culture and so forth) which may invest extra power/control in the researcher (Hertz, 1997). In the spirit of collaborative feminist methodology, reflexivity is used to disinvest the researcher's authority and to 'mute the distance and alienation' which comes from objectifying those being studied (Wasserfall, 1997, p. 152).[xi]

Example 11.1   Dialogal research – the experience of forgiveness

Steen Halling, Jan Rowe and their group (Halling, Leifer & Rowe, 2006) carried out a series of studies on forgiveness, first addressing forgiving another and then self-forgiveness.[xii] They wrote out accounts of their own experiences and then analysed these along with the stories of groups of graduate students and other participants (which had been audio-recorded and transcribed). The dialogic process was extended and intense, even including a day-long retreat.

They asked basic questions like: 'Can you tell us about the time during an important relationship when something happened such that forgiving the other became an issue for you?' On identifying themes in the individual stories, they compared narratives to look for common themes. Slowly, a tentative structure of 'forgiving another' evolved. The process was an iterative one returning regularly to the narratives, transcripts, literature and the co-researchers' own experience to flesh out the analysis.

The profoundly collaborative process was shown to be transformative for everyone involved. Interestingly, the research did not stop at a single study but grew organically. For instance, over the course of a decade, Halling asked students participating in seminars on the psychology of forgiveness at Seattle University to write their own descriptions, further deepening his understanding. As Halling emphasizes, 'forgiveness is an elusive and intricate phenomenon; there is always more to it than I or any other researcher can say about it' (2008, p. 84).

Findings

The process of forgiving another involves loosely delineated stages that engage existential life world themes such as embodied self-identity, temporality, spatiality and relations with others. First, forgiveness arises in a certain context. Over time there is a changing view of the other and a reclaiming of self. Finally, with a focus on the bigger picture, the world feels transformed and there is a movement towards transcendence.

> The process begins when one perceives oneself as harmed by another . . . It occurs within the context of a relationship involving another who has deeply affected one in a hurtful way . . .
>
> The need for forgiveness arises when someone has acted in such a way as to bring about a fundamental disruption to the wholeness and integrity of one's life. Initially . . . there is a tearing of the fabric of one's life, one's world. The injury . . . violates the person's sense of self . . . The future, as it was anticipated before the event, is irrevocably changed . . .
>
> One experiences the injury as a blow inflicted by the other . . . Oftentimes an acknowledgement of responsibility, an apology from the other person, is thought to be necessary for healing . . . The ongoing experience of hurt entails a preoccupation with the injury . . . Along with anger, there is frequently a desire for revenge or retribution . . . some sort of partial balancing of an injustice . . .
>
> . . . There is a sense of clinging to the hurt and anger, which is to be distinguished from earlier phases of more spontaneous hurt and anger . . .
>
> The resolution, . . . forgiveness, appears to come to us in an unexpected context . . . the moment of forgiveness appears to be the moment of recognition that it has already occurred . . .

One experiences a shift in one's understanding of and relationship to the other persons, one's self and the world. The implications of the original situation are cast in a new light: the hurt is no longer merely an injury that another has inflicted and that, therefore, acts as a barrier, but instead becomes appropriated as pain shared with other human beings . . . No longer does one see oneself in a relationship of victim and victimizer . . . After forgiving a family member for sexual abuse, one person stated . . . 'I realise that forgiveness has set me free. Free to continue my life . . . without pain and anger, and free to love again.' The vision of newness is so compelling, so like a gift of grace, one will not choose other than to move gratefully to it . . .

The experience . . . is one of radically opening to the world and others, as well as to the person who hurt oneself. There is a sense of arriving home after a long journey and the world is welcoming, so well remembered and yet transformed . . . There is a movement of transcendence – that is, an unanticipated and yet welcomed opening up to the new, and an experience of being free from burdens and restrictions. (Halling, 2006, pp. 254–260)

Example 11.2 Heuristic research – counselling for midwives when breaking bad news to pregnant women

Anna Roland-Price (writing with Del Loewenthal, 2007) conducted a study exploring the experience of midwives having to break bad news to pregnant women and asking whether counselling/psychotherapy is helpful to these midwives. This research grew out of the researcher's role of running a 'birth reflections' service which offered counselling and support to pre- and postnatal women. As a practising midwife, she was conscious of the special relationship she had with the pregnant women with whom she worked and the challenges she faced when breaking bad news.

She interviewed several of her colleagues, engaging the heuristic method which involved her own personal reflexivity. She found that through engaging in psychotherapy, the nurses acquired a self-awareness which enabled them to 'be with' their patients better and more empathetically. The findings thus demonstrated a valuable role for psychotherapy in the continuing training and support of midwives.

To do the research, Roland-Price applied Moustakas's method in eight analytic-reflexive steps:

1) *Gathering data.* Several colleagues were interviewed with the researcher starting with the question 'Is counselling/psychotherapy helpful in relation to breaking bad news to pregnant women?' Then co-researchers were invited to describe their feelings and experiences of these occasions. After each interview the co-researchers offered feedback on the interview. Later as Roland-Price replayed the audio-tapes she noted down her own experiences and feelings.

2) *Immersion.* After each interview, Roland-Price immersed herself in the transcript of the data – going back over it again and again. She discovered all aspects of her life seemed to be tuned into the process of giving bad news and she got in touch with memories buried in her past.

3) *Incubation.* In this stage of stepping back, and Roland-Price allowed intuition and tacit knowledge to emerge while distancing herself from the data and her own experience.

4) *Individual depiction.* On returning to the data with a re-newed perspective she revised her original depiction of the individual's story.

5) *Completion of individual depictions.* Once she was satisfied that her individual depiction captured key themes, emotions and experiences she repeated the process for the other interviews.

6) *Composite depiction.* The individual depictions were then gathered together to create a composite depiction (including narratives, conversations, illustrations, descriptive passages).

7) *Exemplary portraits.* In this stage, two/three co-researchers were selected as being representative and exemplary portraits created such that both the phenomenon and the individual person emerge in a unified manner.

8) *Creative synthesis.* In this final step, Roland-Price pulled her findings of both her own and co-researchers' experiences together in a poem.

Findings

Overall, the interview data revealed four enduring themes: (i) inner feelings (e.g. anger/pain) and bodily awareness (e.g. 'something inside you swelling'); (ii) sense of detachment when breaking bad news; (iii) the support sought after; and the positive aspects of counselling/psychotherapy where a new awareness and freedom was found. To give a flavour of her findings, selective extracts from the composite depiction and the final poem are offered below:

Composite depiction

A conflict existed between on the one hand, not showing their feelings, putting them away, and on the other, the calling of their inner world to portray all the emotions that come with [giving] bad news – anger, despair, hope, guilt and frustration.

The co-researchers spoke of emotions and said they found them difficult to deal with, learning instead to block them out in order to concentrate on their patient's emotions and the needs of others. After the event, the co-researchers felt totally drained . . . and exhausted . . .

The co-researchers all spoke positively regarding their counselling and psychotherapy. It seemed to give each a greater understanding of the conflicts within their being and, outwardly, give them self-awareness and a greater sense of freedom, allowing them to deal with the external world with confidence. Ultimately, they seemed to 'be there' for their patients. (Roland-Price & Loewenthal, 2007, pp. 76–77)

Creative synthesis

> How hard it's been to hear the pain,
> To hear the other
> And sit in vain.
> Through pain, despair, and all of those things
> I have struggled to be there.
> Anxiety filled my being,
> So gently,
> Like a onion peeled,
> Layer by layer.
> My therapist peeled
> Her words like balm itself.
> Oh, how I've changed.
> Who am I,
> Nurse, midwife, therapist?
> Will freedom come?
> In my desire
> The need to know.
> To hear the Other

The inner feelings experienced by the co-researchers when breaking bad news were deep and meaningful, often reflecting those of the patient receiving the news. In experiencing these feelings, they shared a common sense of inadequacy, almost a sense of fear in showing their own feelings, a sense of not knowing what to do or say and their inability to 'be with' their patient . . . (Roland-Price & Loewenthal, 2007, pp. 79–80)

Example 11.3   Relational-centred research – the experience of mistrust

The example below comes from a group phenomenological study six of us undertook focused on the phenomenon of 'mistrust'(King *et al.*, 2008). We sought to work together to explore different ways of doing phenomenological analysis (rather than to engage dialogal research collaboratively).

We decided to focus on one in-depth interview I had conducted with one of our participants ('Kath') about her experience of mistrust. We analysed the transcript individually, then gathered to discuss our findings as a group. This produced a layered analysis which contained both consensual and individual components. The following extract is taken from my own reflexive account:

> Kath likened her lived experience of mistrust to being 'attacked' by others and then finding herself becoming a different person – a 'ghost' of herself. 'I became a different kind of me, a lesser me'.

> **Kath:** It was this kind of shift and change and the pulling in and the unsafeness of that environment which before had felt secure, clearly wasn't. I was shaky. Lots of the sort of firm things that you believed in were now shaky. Does that make sense?
> **Linda:** Yes, so, when you say 'pulling in' you pulled yourself into yourself
> **Kath:** Yes, I withdrew . . .
> **Linda:** It seems like your very way of being is kind of quite open (mmm, mmm) and direct. And here you've lost even your way of being.
> **Kath:** . . . that really sums it up actually. I felt the person who left that college was not me. Or was a paler shade of me . . . I had to kind of slow down in a sense, not in speed sense but in a kinda closure sense . . . in a protective sense.

> As Kath was speaking I was very aware of her 'big presence'. I had previously known Kath as a 'big personality' and as someone who physically embodied a big, attractive presence. Yet, in the course of our interview, she somehow started to 'fade' in front of my very eyes. I could feel a strange sensation within myself, a sense closing down, closing in, shrinking, trying to become smaller, trying to become a 'paler' version of myself. *Slowly I was disappearing. Then I realised that, strangely enough, this new reality actually felt safer. If I couldn't be seen, I wouldn't be hurt . . .* I dwelt there some more . . . I could understand and accept Kath's need to 'reduce' and close down. At the same time, I began to feel something else. *Losing myself, also felt slightly scary. Who would I be and who would I become if I was to disappear to be replaced by a paler-shade of me? I became aware that I felt somehow sad at the loss of my customary embodied way of being.* I looked at Kath and she too, seemed to me to be sad and a little lost – indeed, vulnerable in her loss. (King *et al.*, 2008, pp. 95–96)

As this excerpt demonstrates, Kath was impacting on me (Linda) emotionally, bodily and empathically but, at the same time, I was impacting on Kath. The illustration shows the way that I checked out her bodily perceptions with Kath in dialogue and her response of 'that sums it up' suggested it was possible I had mirrored something of Kath's experience and in that mirroring there was an intersubjective merging.

However, other group members who analysed the transcript had a different perspective and alternative understandings. Two members of the group, for instance, pointed out that through my form of questioning, I might have fostered an explicit concern with emotionality and engaged a dialogue akin to that found in a therapeutic relationship. They suggested that Kath's narrative initially had a neutral tone but through my therapeutic reflecting back took on the tone of a brave, battling 'victim'. I subsequently reflected on this:

> I may have introduced into the mix something from my own history as a 'caring therapist'. This, in turn, may have triggered something in Kath, encouraging her to edge towards the stance of 'victim'. However, this process is probably even more complicated. While I had several roles which I was inevitably juggling (chief among them in this instance, the roles of therapist and researcher), questions can also be raised about my habitual interactional roles and pattern of operating... If I reflexively probe my motivations, I understand that I have an emotional need to give care to others, perhaps as a result of significant gaps in the care I received as a child. I know that I tend to thrive on the empathy I once longed to receive; my providing of care can be seen as an effective way to deny my own need to be cared for. My child self can be seen as entwined with my adult therapist and researcher selves... What selves were activated in Kath? (Finlay & Evans, 2009, pp. 119–120)

As this example highlights, Kath and I brought different ways of being to the encounter. In this way, researcher and co-researcher bring into the between 'the sum total of who they are in all their complexity and with their own individual histories and ways of organizing their experience [and] their unconscious processes'. Both are then 'faced with the challenge of meeting the other in all his/her complexity' (Evans & Gilbert, 2005, pp. 74–75). Ambiguous and layered inter-subjective dynamics (conscious or unconscious) deserve attention and need to be probed reflexively.

Reflections

Dialogal, heuristic and relational-centred approaches are, in my view, all intriguing methodologies particularly suitable for research by therapy practitioners. They have all been created and developed by psychotherapists or clinical psychologists and have emerged, at least in part, out of therapeutic contexts. The different approaches invite therapists to draw on their relational skills, empathy and reflexive capacity used in practice, and to apply these in the research context.

Generally speaking,[xiii] reflexive-relational approaches have the merit that they foreground researcher impact on the research and actively emphasize the tentative nature of findings. At its best, any focus on the researcher is engaged as part of ensuring an appropriate 'phenomenological attitude' of openness and this should enable deeper penetration into the phenomenon of concern. Their main weakness is that in foregrounding the researcher they invite self-indulgent or skewed findings. Arguably relational-reflexive elaborations are unnecessary when descriptive or hermeneutic methods are applied well.

At a more emotional, intuitive level I can own that I delight and revel in reflexive-relational research, whatever the form. The depth of personal introspection and the dialogical journey involved usually lays the ground, in my view, for research that has deep personal significance and this helps to ensure its evocative resonance and relevance. What I love about these approaches is how they are often transformational whenever they are applied (in either research or psychotherapy).

However, reflexive-relational research is not a straightforward, unproblematic option and it can go wrong. It is all too easy for the researcher to become bogged down in the swamp of self-absorbed, interminable deconstruction and self-analysis such that the phenomenon is lost. Equally, when working in groups, researchers can get derailed by impass and resistance, say, when group dynamics parallel some unconscious process which distorts understandings or potentially disrupts progress. Given these challenges it is important for researchers to take a disciplined but *compassionate* approach (to themselves and others) and to embrace opportunities for supervision.

The scientific status of reflexive-relational research can also be challenged; the nature of the project is open to debate. Inevitably critics challenge its subjective nature. In response, some within the field argue that the intense negotiated dialogue involved (including perhaps involving co-researchers in validating findings) increases the robustness of findings. Moustakas, for example, takes a more essentialist approach claiming that done well, heuristic research results in elucidating essences that 'comprehensively, distinctively, and accurately depict the experience' (1990, p. 32). Others argue that trying to shore up the scientific credentials of an explicitly (inter)subjective project is misguided and that these elements should be celebrated in their own right. Langdridge (2009, p. 222), for instance, owns that his relational-centred research moved the story told in a particular direction and was 'co-constructed in a particular way, emerging out of my intervention and speaking to me as a therapist in this moment'.

My own position leans towards Langdridge's stance. I want to see the research process being conducted systematically, ethically and with self-awareness. But I step back from making grand claims such as asserting co-researchers have verified the 'truth' of the analysis or 'confirmed' interpretations. Surely different researchers are likely to facilitate the telling of different stories and different participants will elicit different interventions from researchers? I believe researchers need to be more humble and travel more hopefully, aspiring merely to make a resonant and reasonably satisfying description of the phenomenon – one that has integrity.

While I celebrate the potential of reflexive-relational research approaches, it is not for everyone. Not every researcher will be motivated to engage in the sustained reflexivity; not every research relationship or research project will demand it. Embracing a relational approach would probably be an unnecessarily complicated elaboration for most phenomenological studies. For this reason, reflexive-relational research should be *applied* selectively according to demands of the research topic, phenomenon and situation . For example, the relational-centred approach discussed above would be most appropriate for case study research into existential topics, particularly when conducted by psychotherapists who are already familiar with reflexive and relational approaches to working. If you already work in reflexive-relational ways generally, then you might consider drawing on your experience and skills to do research.

If you are going to engage a reflexive-relational exploration, try to enjoy going into the unknown and connecting with the other in dialogue. Let yourself go into that mysterious, seductive, evocative, and potentially transformative, realm of the *between* . . .

Notes

[i] I use the term 'co-researcher' instead of participant quite deliberately here. First, it highlights the fact that reflexive-relational research may be collaborative as in the case of the dialogal method and involve co-researchers who may be participants and/or researchers. Secondly, it makes the ethical point that relational-centred researchers often prefer to do research *with*, as opposed to *on*, participants.

[ii] This category is my own convenient construction. In pushing together 'dialogal', 'heuristic' and 'relational-centred' approaches, I do not mean to minimize the significance and contribution of any one approach. I would urge interested readers to recognize the unique form each methodology takes.

[iii] There are other ways of **working relationally**. A significant methodology here for therapists is the co-operative inquiry approach of Heron (1996), stemming from the earlier New Paradigm Research (Reason & Rowan, 1981). Grant's (2005) study on the experience of being in an audience (the 'intentionality of gathering to witness'), to give another example, offers another version of relational research by putting the spotlight on *group phenomenological methods*.

[iv] These kinds of themes reflect the way reflexive-relational approaches lean towards being a **moral science** rather than a more general human/social science. Stevens explains, a moral science psychology is concerned with

> not so much with why we are as we are but with the process of self-creation . . .
> Psychology's role here is not only to raise consciousness about what influences help
> to make us what we are, but also to facilitate reflexiveness or 'mindfulness' through
> stimulating personal reflection about the process of living. (1996, p. 217)

[v] See this article online at: http://www.ipjp.org, volume 5, edition 1.

[vi] See Sayre, Lamb and Navarre (2006) for a good example of using the dialogal method and videotape.

[vii] This practice of identifying prior assumptions at the start of research using sensitizing, self-reflective exercises is commonly used. Colaizzi's method (1973), for instance, recommends engaging 'Individual Phenomenological Reflection' (IPR) as a preparatory stage to data gathering.

[viii] Moustakas (1994) discusses key differences between the descriptive Duquesne method and his own. Briefly, the differences can be summarized as: 1) Duquesne studies focus on particular experiences of participants; heuristic research draws more widely utilizing self-dialogue, art work and other personal documents. 2) Duquesne studies aim towards composite descriptions of essential structures; heuristic research aims to stay close to individual stories and co-researchers remain visible. While Moustakas's version is more reflexive in the way it involves self-search, Moustakas himself never actually uses the term 'reflexivity'.

[ix] In our version, we draw on the relational and developmental components of intersubjectivity and psychoanalytic theories while retaining the gestalt and phenomenological interest in the embodied lived experience in the 'here and now'.

[x] Ken Evans and I (Finlay & Evans, 2009) argue that presence, empathy (or more broadly 'inclusion' in Buber's theory), intersubjectivity and reflexivity are four key dimensions of both relational psychotherapy and relational-centred research.

[xi] Put in Buber's terms, relational-centred researchers aim towards *I-Thou* relating aspiring to be 'free from judgment, narcissism, demand, possessiveness, objectification, greed or anticipation . . . eschewing instrumental and habitual ways of interaction found in *I-It*' (Finlay & Evans, 2009, p. 31).

[xii] The original study was conceived in 1984 when both Halling and Rowe were faculty members at Seattle University. They realized they had a mutual interest in the topic and offered it as an independent study to a group of four graduate students as part of classwork. Halling and Rowe interviewed these four, plus as a group they engaged group discussions concerning the fruits of their literature searching and evolving understandings.

[xiii] To give a more specific evaluation, in my view, the **dialogal approach** offers a collaborative engagement with the phenomenon which respects the breadth of different people's experiences while drawing on the transformative potential of dialogue to deepen findings. The 'empirical variation' engaged ensures a well-balanced range of conclusions providing, that is, the politics of power and negotiation within the work group are sensitively managed. The challenge to this approach is whether 'more' is achieved through dialogue beyond what can be gained through using the descriptive approach with rigorous imaginative variation. **Heuristic research** offers a systematic, structured approach, integrating first-person and descriptive phenomenological approaches while encouraging the possibility of creative exploration and presentations to further deepen understandings. However, the epistemological commitments underpinning the method remain fuzzy, caught between descriptive, hermeneutic and first-person accounts, and this potentially compromises the depth that might be engaged. The **relational-centred** method exploits the special professional skills of therapists (particularly psychotherapists) with its in-depth awareness of the dynamics between self (researcher) and other. A particular value of the method is that it explicitly attends to the possibilities of less conscious parallel processes at work, something that other approaches often ignore. However, the success and rigour of the approach depends largely on the skill/awareness/experience of the researcher which raises questions about the credibility of the research.

Part III
Phenomenological Methods in Practice

Introduction to Part III

Phenomenology has diverse philosophies and manifestations and, as a result, it also has a multiplicity of methodologies (i.e. approaches to research involving a combination of philosophy *and* specific methods of data collection and analysis). There is no one way to *do* phenomenology. Methods have evolved organically depending on the type of phenomenon under investigation, the variety of approach being used and the kind of knowledge the researcher has been seeking.

Some general principles can be specified, however, regarding methods of how data may be gathered or analysed, and about how to produce findings. The following chapters address these principles and focus on the practical *doing* side of research. However, in order to ensure research is coherent our methods (of data collection and analysis) must match up with our methodological approach. It is important therefore to read the following chapters in conjunction with the relevant, approach(es) described in Part II. If you are going to use 'descriptive phenomenology', for instance, guidelines associated with that approach need to drive your specific mode of data collection and analysis.

Chapter 12 on **planning the research** offers practical advice on a range of questions including: how to choose a research topic; how to use supporting literature; which methods to choose; how to find (and gain access to) participants; and how to set up support systems.

Phenomenology for Therapists: Researching the Lived World, First Edition. Linda Finlay.
© 2011 Linda Finlay. Published 2011 by John Wiley & Sons, Ltd.

Chapter 13 examines the process of **gathering data.** Here I discuss the need for the researcher to be attentive, empathetic and curious. Using examples from practice, the chapter focuses on three common sources of data: 'interviews', 'participant observation' and 'written accounts'.

Chapter 14 focuses on **relational ethics.** The ethical challenges researchers face when doing phenomenological research are discussed, including the responsibilities attached to the fact that researchers and co-researchers alike can be profoundly touched by the research process.

In *Chapter 15*, I describe and explain how to engage narrative, thematic, reflexive and creative approaches to the **analysis of data.** I show how each style of analysis highlights different aspects of the phenomenon and so facilitates different insights. The analytic process aims to iteratively engage intuitive possibilities, but I argue that meanings arising will inevitably remain tentative, partial and emergent.

Chapter 16 focuses on how to **produce research**. Five overlapping processes are discussed: pulling it together; marshalling the evidence; developing your argument; writing up; and 're-presenting' the research.

In *Chapter 17* the **evaluation** of research is explored. I argue that 'good' phenomenological research is research that is *r*igorous, *r*esonant, *r*eflexive and *r*elevant (the 4 R's!). Ultimately, the special contribution of phenomenological research is its capacity to capture some flavour of the layered meanings, ambiguity, ambivalence and richness of our experience of our lived world.

Chapter 12

Planning the Research[i]

> Such journeys open vistas to new journeys for uncovering meaning, truth and essence – journeys within journeys . . . this is the beauty of knowledge and discovery. It keeps us forever awake, alive, and connected with what is and with what matters in life. (Moustakas, 1994, p. 65)

Research can be likened to going on a 'voyage of discovery'. As we embark on our research journey we go into unknown territory. We never quite know, in advance, what we will find and what delights or challenges we will face. As an experienced researcher-traveller I am always excited at the start of a voyage because I know I'm embarking on an adventure – one with the potential to open new horizons of understandings.

For novice researchers, the process usually generates more anxiety. Not only are they going into unknown territory, they are likely to feel uncertain, lacking in confidence and confused about how to travel, where to stay and what to explore. They may even feel some resistance to starting. Or they start in a rush, only to find themselves lost en route, going round in circles or passing-by choice beauty spots.

This chapter is geared for those new to research. It offers *practical* guidance on how to plan your voyage of discovery. I take you through the key challenges and critical decisions you will need to make step by step:

- choosing a topic and research question;
- sensitizing to the topic through self-reflection;

Phenomenology for Therapists: Researching the Lived World, First Edition. Linda Finlay.
© 2011 Linda Finlay. Published 2011 by John Wiley & Sons, Ltd.

- locating existing knowledge;
- deciding methods of data collection and analysis;
- gaining ethical approval;
- recruiting and engaging co-researchers;
- setting up appropriate support systems.

Researchers sometimes find this planning stage tedious and, like an impatient traveller eager to enjoy their holiday, they rush into it, often doing interviews without appropriate preparation. There are plans and arrangements that need to be made before embarking on any journey.[ii] It is important to be organized. Planning demands systematic and thoughtful attention, it cannot be approached as though following a recipe. Every piece of research – like every therapy relationship – is unique. It has its own specific demands which need to be planned for in advance and carefully negotiated at every stage of the research. We need to be clear about what we expect and how we hope to deal with it.

However, planning is not sufficient. In phenomenological research it is important to *remain responsive to the phenomenon* and to whatever emerges. In practice the research process is 'messy'. Data needs sensitive collection, our personal baggage intrudes, confusions and ethical dilemmas arise; it is not realistic to imagine that these things can be packaged and tidied neatly away at the planning stage.

Choosing a Topic and a Research Question

The process of deciding what to research can often prove challenging and time-consuming. The challenge is to find a topic and a research question(s) that is *relevant* and *interesting* and is also *do-able* given your time constraints and the other practicalities you may face. The following five tips may help you choose an appropriate topic and question:

1) *Tap into a 'passion'.* Find a topic/research question that excites, or at the very least interests, you. Passion and curiosity will sustain you through some of the more intense or tedious stages of doing research.
2) *Keep grounded and modest in your aims.* Pragmatism needs to balance enthusiasm. Novice researchers (and sometimes the more experienced) can fall into the trap of wanting to make a significant or revolutionary contribution. Grand plans are more suited to life projects rather than single research studies, and are hard to put into practice (Fischer, 2006). You need to remain focused on what you can realistically achieve. Your research should aim to say 'a lot about a little problem' (Silverman, 1993, p. 3), rather than a little about a big one.[iii]

3) *Be specific and precise.* As you work towards defining your research question, try to be as focused, specific and concrete as possible. If you are interested in the broad topic such as 'self-harm', you might re-formulate the research question as '*What* does the act of self-harming mean?' If you're seeking to research phobias, pick a particular angle such as '*What* is the lived experience of confronting a phobia?' Alternatively, instead of investigating the value of therapeutic interventions in general, you might ask, '*What* is the lived experience of having therapy?' Even then it might be more practical to focus more specifically on one aspect; asking, for example, '*How* is a therapist's self-disclosure experienced by the client?'

4) *Let your research question evolve.* Sometimes researchers refine – or even change – their question after they have started on the research. Even a complete change of tack may occasionally be necessary. To give an example, a student started a descriptive phenomenological study on the lived experience of grieving. When she explored her own process of grieving she became intrigued about how she kept 'getting lost'. It was as if her lost-ness was being acted out in her life. With this insight she refocused her research on 'lost-ness' and changed her research design from being a 'descriptive phenomenological' study to 'heuristic research'.

Sensitizing to the Topic Through Self-reflection

To truly question something is to interrogate something from the heart of our existence, from the center of our being . . . We live this question . . . Is this not the meaning of research: to question something by going back again and again? . . . I am indeed animated by this question in the very life I live. (van Manen, 1990, p. 43)

The choice of research topic and question will be driven by personal, professional or academic goals. What is driving you? Are you being required to conduct this research? What expectations have been laid on you and are you laying on yourself? What are the assumptions and presuppositions you already hold about the research topic?

Also, you need to reflect on both the topic for study and on your relationship to that topic as part of engaging the **phenomenological attitude** and bracketing your assumptions/current understandings. This stage is a particularly crucial one in phenomenological research as the researcher prepares to approach the phenomenon to be investigated with 'openness and wonder' – this attitude being fundamental to the method. As can be imagined, it is not easy to enter into this way of being. As van Manen (1990) explains, the problem of phenomenological inquiry is that we know too much.

Our common-sense 'pre-understandings, our suppositions, assumptions, and the existing bodies of scientific knowledge, predispose us to interpret the nature of the phenomenon before we have even come to grips with the significance of the phenomenological question' (1990, p. 46).

Fischer and Wertz (1979) show how they began this process in their report of how they embarked on their study of 'being criminally victimized' (see Example 6.1):

> [We] agreed, as a sensitizing exercise, to jot down notes about our personal experiences of having been the victim of crime. Then we met to discuss, among other issues, what we thought we were likely to find. The recorded anticipations alerted interviewers to possible themes that might require clarification if alluded to by subjects. They also allowed us to become aware of our presuppositions regarding the phenomenon so that we could attempt not to impose them on our subjects. Later we found that some of our notions had been fulfilled (albeit always in special ways), some modified, and some disconfirmed. (cited in Polkinghorne, 1989, p. 46)

In addition to self-reflection, some phenomenologists start by attending to the **etymological** sources of words as a way of getting in touch with meanings. To illustrate this, see how van Manen (1990) unpacks the term 'parenting':

> The etymology of the word 'parenting' refers both to *giving birth* and *bringing forth*; it has connotations of *origin* or *source*. To parent (*parere*) is to originate, to be the source, the origin from which something springs. How is this sense of source maintained in the experience of parenting? I may feel pride at the recognition of having brought this child into the world, [but this] ... is tempered by the strange sense that I much less produced this child than that it came to me as a gift. (1990, p. 59)

Locating Existing Knowledge

A further way to clarify your research and its focus is to explore the existing literature. At some point in your research you will need to search the literature and explore the status of what is currently known about your topic. Partly, this is an orientating exercise to help you to recognize how your topic is currently being framed and to identify key issues and debates. Partly, it offers you the opportunity to identify gaps in the literature and thus provide a rationale for your own research. Being thoroughly conversant with the literature will also enable critical evaluation when you come to look at the contribution of your own research. When writing up your research you will need to discuss your findings in the light of existing research, stating whether your research supports, refutes or extends current evidence (Steward, 2006).

Phenomenologists commonly argue against engaging in a detailed literature review in the early stages of a project. Their point is that ideas might be shaped too much by others before you even get started and that puts a strain on efforts to bracket prior understandings. In any case the researcher needs to focus on lived experience, not theorizing. However, some preliminary reading may help to avoid duplication of effort and a formal literature search may be a required part of gaining ethical approval for the project.

You can access the literature in a number of ways:

1) Specialist **online databases** (such as AMED, Psych-lit, MEDLINE, CINAHL, BIDS) offer lists and descriptions of relevant theoretical and empirical articles. Often the literature cited here involves quantitative studies and may not tap into the qualitative dimensions you are interested in. However, you can narrow your focus to phenomenological studies. One straightforward way to start is to check out *UK PubMed central* (large, free, online life science resource) at http://ukpmc.ac.uk/. How about trying a search of your topic now? I have just searched for 'phenomenology; pain' and it resulted in 433 useful abstracts of research.

2) Articles can also be accessed directly from **journals** which can be searched either online or by hand. Particularly relevant, research (as opposed to philosophically) focused phenomenological journals include: *Journal of Phenomenological Psychology; Phenomenology & Practice; Indo-Pacific Journal of Phenomenology; Existential Analysis.*

3) **Professional websites,** such as the one for the British Association of Counselling and Psychotherapy (www.bacp.co.uk/research/index) or the College of Occupational Therapists (www.cot.co.uk/Homepage/) usually offer information about research and may include databases on systematic reviews, publications and dissertations. Alternatively, try www.healthtalkonline.org which focuses on people's own accounts of their health and illness and includes useful information/videos and references to research findings.

4) **'Google'** or other Internet search engines can also be useful to access references to relevant books and research articles related to particular topics.

Conducting a literature review to explore existing knowledge takes time and effort. It cannot be done quickly, but it is not all hard slog. Playing 'detective' as you track down elusive articles or unfamiliar research projects can be fun and the process of gaining new knowledge is satisfying.

When you have collected your resources together, your next task will be to synthesize and evaluate the knowledge they contain, and to write up. This **literature review** acts as your empirical, theoretical, methodological and/or personal *rationale* for your research. To give an example, Granek (2006) carried out qualitative research on how depression is experienced. In her literature review, she criticized 'objective' measures of depression as embracing medical models which pathologize and do not sufficiently attend to relational dimensions. This point then became her rationale for undertaking a more subjectivist approach to people's stories of depression.

For a research proposal a brief summary of relevant research is usually all that is required. You will want to be similarly selective if you are writing a journal article and limited to around 1000 words for your review. When writing an article reviewing the literature (approximately 5000–6000 words) or a chapter in a thesis, you will need to undertake a more substantial review: one that seeks to be both analytical and critical. The word 'critical' here does not mean have to be negative. A good critical evaluation of the literature aims to draw attention to strengths and limitations of what is out there. Rather than just describing the research, you need to grapple with its value or relevance.

One of the benefits of carrying out a literature review is that it allows you to explore how others have researched your topic area. This should help guide your own choices of methodology and method.

Deciding Methods of Data Collection and Analysis

Before you jump into deciding your tactics for data collection and analysis, you need to be clear about your research strategy in terms of your aim and research **methodology** (see *Chapters 6–11* outlining different approaches). Your choice of methodology has *consequences*, for instance, it will guide how many participants are needed and how to approach the research. Do you want to conduct a descriptive or hermeneutic study? Will you explicitly focus on lifeworld to structure your analysis? To what extent will you want to include yourself and/or relational dimensions as part of what you are researching? Do you want a more structured approach such as using descriptive phenomenology, interpretative phenomenological analysis (IPA) or lifeworld approaches? Or might you want to let your research evolve more organically, intuitively and creatively as fitting first-person, hermeneutic and reflexive-relational approaches?

To help you decide your **methods** you might ask yourself: what sources of data are potentially available and appropriate? Would combining methods offer something more? What can the chosen methods feasibly reveal?

You might also ask which methods would be the most practical given the inevitable constraints of time and competing demands. That said, methods should not be adopted simply because they seem to be the easiest way forward. Instead, you need to be sure that your choice of methods and procedures are consistent with your methodology and appropriate to the research question you are pursuing (Holloway & Todres, 2003).

Having decided your general path, you then need to decide on the specific approach and **procedures** you will use to collect data, and then to analyse it. If you have decided to interview participants, for example, you must next choose between semi-structured or more open approaches. If you are opting for a participant-observation, will you join in as a full participant or will you remain something of an outside observer? You will also need to work out what kind of relationship you are seeking to have with the people you are researching. For instance, are you going to share the research process with them, in essence co-opting them as co-researchers, throughout the analysis phase?

In the following extract, Robbins (2006) describes his rationale for combining methods to allow data *triangulation*[iv] within his descriptive phenomenological study on the experience of joy. He chose Schneier's imagery in movement method as an approach to enable memory to emerge out of a re-created experiencing of the feelings rather than feelings emerging out of memory.

Example 12.1   Choosing a combination of methods

The method involves a step-by-step process that can be understood as a gradual shift from an intuitive 'felt sense' of meaning toward a more fully articulate, explicit, and structural understanding. The technique begins with abstract drawing (image), then proceeds to using role play (movement) to enhance the vividness of an emerging memory, and concludes with a verbal and written description of the experience. Using this approach, I could work with the research participants to assist them in a dynamic movement from an intuitive sense of joy toward the articulation of a vital, lived re-experiencing of an emerging memory of being joyful. By the end, I would have both a verbal and written account of the experience. Even better, I would also have three sources of data: the drawings, gestures, and verbal/written protocols. (Robbins, 2006, p. 194)

When it comes to selecting your **analysis method**, you have a general choice between engaging in thematic, narrative, reflexive or creative forms of analysis. Usually, researchers tend to favour a particular method but they might also combine approaches: for instance, presenting individual narratives which are then synthesized into more general existential themes. In a research paper written by Niall Fitzpatrick and myself (Fitzpatrick & Finlay, 2008), for example, we started by outlining the narratives from five participants and then produced additional, separate existential and lifeworld-focused analyses.

Ultimately, the data collection and analysis options chosen need to fit the research aims and methodology. Procedures need to fit the overall approach taken and the aims of your research. Phenomenologists often *let the phenomenon itself guide* their study of it and sometimes it is not possible to decide methods in advance. Dalhberg *et al.* (2008) for instance suggest researchers adopt an open, bridled attitude while being sensitive to phenomenon and context, and then actively wait for the method(s) to emerge.

Gaining Ethical Approval

Having planned the basic strategy and tactics of the research, the next step is usually to construct a formal *research proposal* or gain formal approval to go ahead with the research. Different institutions offer their own specific guidelines for information that needs to be supplied in the proposal. If you are doing your research to fulfil course requirements, this proposal may involve a relatively straightforward process ending in your supervisor's formal approval. If your research involves clients or work in organizations such as the NHS, you will be required to submit your proposal to a formal Research Ethics Committee[v] (see *Appendix*).

Whatever the required format of the proposal, you will need to address six main areas:

- *Aims/objectives.* What is the purpose of the research and the research question?
- *Literature review.* What is the theoretical, empirical and/or methodological rationale for the study?
- *Research design.* What data collection and analysis methods/procedures are being proposed and who will be the participants/co-researchers?
- *Ethical issues.* What is being done to ensure no harm comes to the participants and to protect their interests?
- *Planning.* What is the envisaged timetable for the research and what resources are required?
- *Support mechanisms.* What arrangements for supervision, support and research training are in place?

Many professional groups and institutions have developed their own codes of conduct for research and research ethics and you will need to follow these.[vi] (If you are a student, you should check whether your own training organization has published a code of ethics). All of these codes attend to core principles of minimizing risk, doing no harm, being competent and treating people fairly and with respect. These principles find expression through practices that ensure *informed consent, due care* and *confidentiality*.

Informed consent

Informed consent means ensuring that participants understand the nature of the project, what the research will involve, the limits to their participation and the risks they may incur (Social Research Association, 2003). If the research is to involve patients/clients then professional bodies will add their voice. For instance, the United Kingdom Council for Psychotherapy (UKCP) states that 'Psychotherapists are required to clarify with clients the nature, purpose and conditions of any research in which the clients are to be involved and to ensure that informed and verifiable consent is given before commencement' (http://www.theburypractice.co.uk/_doc/UKCP-CodeOfEthics.doc).

Three particular challenges arise for researchers when trying to obtain informed consent. First, we often do not know in advance where the research is going to lead. While a participant may agree to be interviewed, it is difficult to predict what is going to happen in the interview. It is likely the interview is going to touch on sensitive issues. The individual needs to know this and understand that personal revelations, and the understandings research can bring, can be unsettling. At the same time the researcher needs to ensure that any such risks are minimized. In this context, Grafanaki (1996) has highlighted the significance of *process consent* as a way of ensuring against unanticipated effects. Instead of simply seeking consent at the start of a study, the researcher needs to build in a series of negotiation points. For example, you could plan to review an interview transcript with the participant before finalizing it, to make sure the participant agrees with the wording.

Secondly, the person being invited into the research needs to be given the right to choose whether or not to participate (or continue to participate) and they need to be given this information in a non-coercive manner. This can pose particular difficulties in practitioner research where patients or clients are being invited to take part in research. Will they feel obliged to say 'yes' to their therapist and do they feel able to refuse? Will they feel used and exploited? If they agree to take part in the research, they also need to be allowed to change their mind and to feel completely free (and within their rights) to withdraw at any time.

Thirdly, if we are offering participants the right to withdraw from the research at any point, it might be worth being more honest about the boundaries here. If research has already been published as an article, the participant would be unable to withdraw. Smith *et al.* (2009) suggest a time-limit such as up to 1 month after the interview with a right to review the transcript.

Due care

It perhaps goes without saying that researchers need to approach their participants with due care, awareness and sensitivity as well as with respect for their well-being. Our studies often touch on significant personal issues and memories and this means that phenomenological research can be evocative and is potentially unsettling. The fact that research can be transformative shows its potential power and so we need to tread carefully. For instance, a colleague recently interviewed someone with a long-standing health care problem. Although the participant had been interviewed many times by professionals over the years, he found this research interview particularly powerful as he felt that he had found his 'voice' and that the researcher had truly witnessed his struggle. While he valued this particular research opportunity, others may not want to be reminded of difficult experiences.

Due care needs to be paid to boundaries and roles. It can be tricky, for example, for the practitioner-researcher to separate their therapist and researcher roles. For research ends we might want to simply hear an individual's story. Wearing our therapist's hat, however, we might be tempted to probe in more challenging ways or to give advice. The participant needs to know what they are signing up for. This process is made even more difficult when you are acting in both capacities when your participant is a client. Here, both the therapeutic and research contracts become muddied and it is possible both will suffer. For example, the participant may feel pressured by the therapist-researcher's 'authority' and feel unable to say 'no'. For these reasons, it is often advisable to avoid research involving your own clients. Working with a colleague's clients is a useful way round this problem.

Confidentiality

In therapy practice, we are well used to ensuring any personal information and records that could identify service users are sensitively managed and carefully restricted. The same process needs to apply in the research situation. Where personal details about participants are open to the public, anonymity should be guaranteed. This is reinforced by the Data Protection Act which requires that information obtained about a participant during an investigation is confidential unless otherwise agreed *in advance*.

It is often hard to guarantee this anonymity in qualitative research. It is quite possible that the level of personal details offered in narratives and case studies will mean individuals can be identified. The anonymity of participants can also be compromised by the fact that others (for example, your colleagues) know that you are doing research with certain people. Extra care needs to be taken here and possible consequences fully discussed. Wise (1987), among others, has even argued the case for including 'misinformation' (such as changing the number, ages and sex of children) and excluding publicly known information which could identify them in order to maintain anonymity.

The process of negotiating informed consent and confidentiality provides an essential foundation for recruiting your participants and engaging them in your research.

Recruiting and Engaging Participants

Not every qualitative research project requires participants. You may decide to draw on other sources of data such as documents or personal reflection and experience. But if your project does involve other people, at some point in your planning you will need to make decisions about whom to recruit and how.

For qualitative researchers in general, and phenomenologists in particular, more is not necessarily better when it comes to sample size as we are not aiming to get a representative range. This is in contrast to quantitative research where samples are supposedly selected in sufficient numbers to act as a microcosm of a particular population (allowing statistical calculations to be made about probabilities that patterns observed in the sample will exist in the wider population).[vii]

The answer to the questions of who should be recruited, and how many, depend largely on the aims of the research and what is appropriate, given the phenomenological methodology adopted. There are no hard and fast rules.[viii] Each researcher needs to justify their strategy in terms of its specific context. In Example 12.2, Sue Morrow (1992, 2006) describes her approach of using a strategic sample in her (phenomenologically orientated, feminist, collaborative) grounded theory research with sexually abused women.

Example 12.2   Strategic sampling for research with sexually abused women

Eleven women in a large . . . metropolitan area were recruited through therapists who specialized in working with adult survivors of child sexual abuse . . . I sent therapists letters explaining the project in detail, along with accompanying letters to be given to appropriate potential participants. Prospective participants called me if they were interested. A particular attraction for participants to participate was a nine-week research support (focus) group that they would attend at no cost . . .

The women ranged in age from 25 to 72 years. One was African-American; one, West Indian; and the remainder, European American. Two identified as lesbian . . . One was mobility impaired, another experienced multiple physical illnesses . . . , a third was hard of hearing, and the remainder were able bodied. Participants came from a variety of socioeconomic classes, educational backgrounds, and religious . . . orientations . . .

Prior to the interviews, I attempted to establish an egalitarian relationship and a context of mutuality with each participant. In my recruitment letter, I informed participants I was an abuse survivor as well as a therapist. (Morrow, 2006, pp. 151–152)

The process of engaging people in the research involves much more than simply deciding sample numbers, characteristics and inclusion/exclusion criteria. Individuals need to feel positively involved, and this means that a relationship has to be developed with them. To some extent the process of negotiating a person's involvement mirrors what happens in therapy. The individual – potentially unwell, vulnerable or damaged – has to take the challenging step of deciding to work actively with the therapist/researcher. The therapist/researcher, in turn, has to gain the person's trust and inspire confidence; they also need to deserve this trust. Together the therapist/researcher and client/participant need to evolve and agree the terms of the therapy/research contract.

Setting up Appropriate Support Systems

Alongside developing relationships with participants, researchers also need to set up appropriate support systems and build relationships with supervisors, mentors or other researchers involved. Practical support systems are also important in relation to IT back-up, library access and peer support.

If you are a student, it is likely that you will be allocated an official supervisor who will help you manage the research process. At the same time you might seek out various mentors to help guide particular aspects of your research. Independent researchers, working alone or in a team of researchers, will similarly want to set up various support networks, be it in the form of peer support or calling on the services of other consultants.

It could even prove beneficial to bring your personal issues about the research into supervision or therapy. We cannot help but be affected ourselves when we engage empathically with others, particularly if a participant shares painful or traumatic experiences. Sometimes we can even become traumatized ourselves as a result of our engagement with survivors and their traumatic stories. Greenall and Marselle (2007) discuss this experience of vicarious traumatization in relation to the research they did with 9/11 survivors:

> Some interviews were so traumatic... that afterwards we experienced feelings of detachment and estrangement... [and] dissociation from the normal world. The trauma we were exposed to made us feel different from others; consequently, one of our team withdrew from social interaction and distanced herself from her partner. (Greenall & Marselle, 2007, p. 545)

How can we cope with such cases of vicarious traumatization? Saakvitne and Pearlman (1996) outline three coping mechanisms: awareness, balance and connection. Awareness involves recognizing signs of vicarious traumatization and employing *self-nurturing* activities. Balance highlights the need to maintain healthy work–life boundaries. Connection with others is then used as an antidote to the isolation and alienation experienced. Both formal supervision (with supervisor or peers) and therapy can be a helpful support to facilitate this awareness, balance and connection.

It is not uncommon these days for research to involve different supervisors, for example, if you are doing research with a client you might have a research supervisor and therapy supervisor.[ix] As another example, PhD research may involve two co-supervisors: one perhaps an expert in the methodology or the research area and the other providing institutional or pastoral support. For these arrangements to work, it is essential that roles are clarified and that there are clear lines of communication between the parties involved. Some boundary setting is usually advisable to decide what is appropriate for each of the supervisors to deal with and how. Equally, if you are taking your research into therapy, it would probably be most helpful if your therapist concentrated on how the research is impacting on you personally, and what is figural for you in the field, rather than getting caught up in the research itself.[x]

In therapy contexts, supervision is seen as a learning process in which a therapist engages with a more experienced practitioner as part of ongoing professional development. This process, in turn, promotes and safeguards clients' well-being. Similarly, in the research context good supervision enhances the researcher's learning and ensures ethical research. In both contexts, supervision provides a 'reflective space where the supervisee can unfold his [sic] own narrative of his work ... reflect on this story with the supervisor as witness and arrive at possible new meanings and insights (Gilbert & Evans, 2000, p. 100).

The phenomenological research journey, like many therapy journeys, can be intriguing, stimulating and enjoyable; it can also prove challenging, painful, stressful and, at times, tedious. Ensuring that you have enough support – whether educational, practical or emotional – is essential.

Reflections

This chapter has discussed a range of decisions and issues that need to be engaged when planning research. Decisions taken, from clarifying the research question to determining methods and procedures, should hang together coherently. Some processes involved when setting up research (such as engaging participants and enabling informed consent) are invariably challenging and require careful reflection.

I have found that qualified therapists can feel ignorant and de-skilled when it comes to research and they may even view it as a distant academic activity done by 'others'. This is precisely why I argue vigorously for phenomenological and relational approaches. I think these approaches offer a way to take our everyday lived experience and human-ness into research. They also offer a way to mirror our therapy practice, concerns, interests and skills. As therapists, we have an advantage, I believe, when it comes to phenomenological research: we can draw on our understandings of the healing quality of the therapeutic relationship and familiar skills, such as interviewing, being empathetic, bodily awareness, taking a holistic approach and being able to use intuitive, inferential thinking systematically (Finlay & Evans, 2009). If you are a therapist currently taking uncertain first steps into the research territory I want to encourage you and reassure you that you already have many of the resources that you will need for your 'voyage'.

With careful, reflective planning at the beginning of research, I would say you stand a better chance of producing sound results. But your plans, just like your research expectations, should remain modest. Research findings can only ever be partial and provisional. They may intrigue, resonate and surprise but they are not going to 'change the world'. Instead of setting out to discover new territory, plan simply to go exploring. Go on a voyage of discovery and see what emerges. Instead of setting up the research with the aim of scaling Himalayan peaks or unveiling new continents, trust that through its respect for individual human stories and experience your research will allow something of real value to emerge. Know that however modest your research it has the transformative potential to open up new horizons.

Notes

[i] Material in this chapter has been drawn from chapter 6 of Finlay and Evans (2009) and has been reproduced here with kind permission of the publishers Wiley-Blackwell.

[ii] Pursuing this metaphor, the process of setting up research is akin to preparing for a journey by going to a travel agent, packing and generally getting organized! First of all, the prospective traveller must decide where they are going (in the case of research, they must choose a topic/research question). Next, they find out more about their destination by getting hold of a travel guide book or searching the Internet (the equivalent, in research, of doing a review of the literature). After that, comes the planning stage when the practicalities of the journey are investigated and sorted out (a process akin to deciding methods of data collection and analysis). For certain destinations, visa applications may have to be made (just as gaining ethical approval is essential for certain fields of research). Then the traveller may organize relevant tour guides or local people to contact if in need (setting up research supervision and support).

[iii] If you are relatively new to research you may be tempted to seek out a topic or question that has never been done before. In fact, your research is likely to be more fruitful if you opt for a topic or area that has already generated literature with which you can critically engage. For example, you might interview podiatrists in a way that mirrors research already done with physiotherapists. Then you can compare responses. For PhD level research you may be required to make an 'original contribution'. But this does not mean you have to find a topic that no one has touched before.

[iv] **Triangulation** involves using different methods, data sources or researchers in the investigation to help increase efficacy or validity of findings. Measuring the same phenomenon from different angles is thought to offer a more accurate reading. However, this implies there is only one objective, knowable social reality – a more positivist, *realist* reading potentially at odds with qualitative and phenomenological approaches (Mason, 2002). Care needs to be taken to evaluate the epistemological status of triangulation. In phenomenology we use it to deepen/broaden and enrich understandings rather than to verify findings. In dialogal approaches for instance, triangulating several researchers' perspectives offers a kind of 'empirical variation' mirroring the process of imaginative variation used in descriptive phenomenology.

[v] Within the United Kingdom, the Research Governance Framework (Department of Health, 2001) has attempted to bring together various statutes and guidelines for research. A key component of this system is the development of Local Research Ethics Committees (LRECs), originally set up in 1968. These committees (comprising relevant people with a broad range of experience and expertise) were set up to review research proposals to ensure ethical research practice. Currently, NHS bodies cannot permit research to go ahead within their organizations unless projects have received formal approval from an LREC (Ballinger & Wiles, 2006).

[vi] See for instance, the various professional guidelines laid down such as the British Association for Counselling and Psychotherapy (BACP) ethical framework (at http://www.bacp.co.uk/ethical_framework/) and the guidelines from the

British Psychological Society (www.bps.org.uk/the-society/code-of-conduct/support-for-researchers_home.cfm). Physiotherapists in the United Kingdom have their own Chartered Society of Physiotherapy whose ethical guidelines are laid down at http://www.csp.org.uk/uploads/documents/csp_effecprac_res07.pdf.

[vii] In qualitative research, the aim is rather to obtain either a 'strategic' or an 'illustrative' sample (Mason, 2002) designed to offer data relevant to the research question. In a **strategic sample**, a range of participants are usually chosen to provide a broad picture of the phenomenon being studied. A researcher may seek to recruit participants who share an experience (such as having a gambling problem) but who differ on demographic variables such as age, sex and ethnicity. An **illustrative sample**, in contrast, seeks to illuminate or be particularly evocative, and tends to be *idiographic* in approach (that is to say, the focus is on individual experience and there is little attempt to generalize beyond this particular sample). Case study research comes into this category. Here a participant may be chosen because their story is particularly interesting and/or powerful.

[viii] While there are no hard rules, some approaches offer guidelines: Giorgi (2009) suggests at least three participants for his descriptive psychological approach; Smith *et al.* (2009) generally recommend three to six participants for an IPA study; my own research is often based on single case studies. Some phenomenologists argue that the number is less important than considering degree of 'variation' between participants. Dalhberg *et al.* (2008) recommend having a relatively heterogeneous sample including participants of different genders and ages in order to get a rich range of experiences. For IPA studies, Smith *et al.* (2009) suggest it might be more appropriate to go for a relatively homogeneous group.

[ix] In the United States and other countries, the system of having a doctoral 'dissertation committee' may be in operation where several chosen advisors direct and support the research.

[x] If you are taking your research process to therapy, you might usefully ask yourself how you are experiencing the meeting with your participants? Are you finding the meeting engaging and are you managing to explore in depth? If not, then what or who is getting in the way? You might consider what unconscious forces may be operating and if the poverty of contact is down to your failure of empathy or the co-researcher not fully engaging. You could also consider what more you could do. Might you be willing, for instance, to experiment with self-disclosure and risk what may appear the 'unspeakable' in the grip of projective identification (Evans, 2007; Finlay & Evans, 2009).

Chapter 13

Gathering Data[i]

The genuine will to know calls for the spirit of generosity rather than for that of economy, for reverence rather than for subjugation, for the lens rather than for the hammer. (Spiegelberg, 1984, p. 680)

The idea of 'data gathering',[ii] with its positivist connotations whereby researchers collect their data based on objective observation and measurement, sits oddly with phenomenological research. To be in tune with the phenomenological spirit it might be better to talk about *generating* data within a research encounter where meanings emerge and are co-created through reflection and dialogue.

Linguistics aside, the purpose of data gathering is to find a way to enable rich description of a phenomenon. How this is done – for instance, whether we use interviews or reflect on a piece of literature – is probably less important than the focus on the description of experience and the way we allow (or perhaps encourage) implicit meanings to emerge.

In the first instance, researchers seek to dwell with the experience as *concretely* as possible. The researcher may ask someone, for instance, to describe an experience in detail: What happened? Can you describe that moment in as much detail and as concretely as possible? Where were you? What did you feel, think and do just before the experience, during and after? The aim is to get into that moment and know how it was or is experienced by the person emotionally/cognitively/bodily and in the context of their life.

Phenomenology for Therapists: Researching the Lived World, First Edition. Linda Finlay.
© 2011 Linda Finlay. Published 2011 by John Wiley & Sons, Ltd.

The researcher then dwells with the knowledge given; dwells in that moment, probing for meanings. The dialogue below illustrates how a researcher might try to empathize and grasp what the experience felt like for the individual concerned. Together, researcher and participant explore and explicate the implicit meanings of a shocking experience. It is at this point of teasing out meanings that the boundaries between data gathering and analysis blend.

> **Interviewer:** What was that like?
> **Participant:** Shocking really.
> **Interviewer:** Shocking?
> **Participant:** I was shaken to the core. It was like a rug being pulled out from under me.
> **Interviewer:** So everything you had taken for granted up till then was. . .
> **Participant:** Exactly! It just disappeared.
> **Interviewer:** I'm getting a sense of you feeling shaky and unbalanced having lost your footing somehow.
> **Participant:** Yes, that's it: Unbalanced. I went into shock. Didn't know how to react.

Data and subsequent descriptions emerge from – blossoms out of – a research context. The challenge is how to open up the space to attune to and nurture this blossoming of meaning. This is the focus of this chapter and I approach the subject from two directions. First, I examine **methods** of gathering data. I offer some pointers about how to engage three different procedures of gathering data: interview, participant observation and written accounts. Secondly, I discuss the data gathering **process** in terms of the need for the researcher to be attentive, empathetic and curious while responding spontaneously and reflexively to the moment. A final section presents a research **encounter**. An extended excerpt from an interview transcript is offered to show some of the processes involved.

Methods for Gathering Data

The process of gathering data in phenomenology cannot be reduced to protocols, procedures and techniques. It is more about engaging the Other (or self) reflectively and being receptive to whatever emerges. Despite that, it is still useful to consider some practical issues arising from the different research procedures available to us. Three of the methods of data collection most commonly used in phenomenological research are briefly explored here: **interview, participant observation** and **written accounts**. (Of course there are other ways to collect data, such as through groupwork and creative media but space does not permit a broader exploration.[iii])

Interview

Interviews can be unstructured conversations or semi-structured with questions loosely prepared in advance as an aide-memoire and to help you focus. Interviews can be informal conversations or involve a more formal approach. Usually, a combination of guiding questions, reflecting back and prompts are used. Haumann's approach to researching psychotherapists' experience of having personal therapy, for instance, was based around asking a few trigger questions, such as:

> Could you describe as fully as possible how your own therapy or analysis influences your work as a therapist? Please try to describe this in terms of your own experience rather than just giving a theoretical explanation of what happens. (Haumann, 2005, p. 23)

She then asked further questions about the participants' own therapy experiences, offering prompts or probes if she sensed the participant needed encouragement to expand.

Whatever the approach, it is often more productive to allow the interview 'conversation' to progress with some fluidity and **spontaneity**. As the researcher, for example, you might suddenly choose to probe an area based on your intuition. Alternatively, your participant could take the interview in unexpected directions. Providing you stay reasonably focused on the research topic being investigated, and your participant is content to proceed, these diversions should probably be allowed. Follow your intuition and yield to whatever feels right in the moment.

> There is a spontaneous quality to a good interview that cannot be completely prescribed ... What one seeks from a research interview in phenomenological research is as complete a description as possible of the experience the participant has lived through. (Giorgi, 2009, p. 122)

As a therapist you have the advantage of being trained to listen and help others express themselves. The downside of this is that you may too easily lead a person into emotional disclosures beyond the terms of the research. Alternatively, you may be so worried about not being a therapist that you become curiously flat, stiff, distanced or disengaged (McLeod, 1999). For this reason, it might help you to conduct one or two pilot interviews before you begin your actual project.

If you are inexperienced in this area here are 10 tips for carrying out research interviews:

1) Do not underestimate the importance of **preparing** your participant in advance. While you do not want your participants to be overly prepared (in the sense of giving you previously rehearsed answers), they need to know what is expected of them.

2) Prepare your **environment** carefully, thinking in terms of your participant's comfort, ease and emotional safety. Also, as part of this preparation, think about how you are going to record the interview. Increasingly, digital equipment is popular and less unwieldy and unobtrusive than traditional tape or video recorders. Recording can be inhibiting initially but most people relax after a few minutes.

3) If you are going to take **notes**, think about how to explain this to your participant. Some people feel that you are taking them more seriously when you write notes; others can react negatively – perhaps because note-taking can seem like a distancing move.

4) Allow a few minutes at the beginning of the interview for your participant to **settle** down. It can help to chat informally at the beginning as part of establishing a rapport and putting the individual at ease.

5) Asking **open, non-directive, singular questions** usually bears more fruit than asking ones that are closed, directive or multiple. Sometimes the participant just needs a place to start. You might, for instance, ask them to *describe in quite concrete terms a typical day or an actual situation in which they had experienced the topic being investigated.* Returning the participant to actual lived events may also steer them away from any tendency to talk in overly intellectual or abstract terms.

6) Try to **listen** carefully. It is all too easy to lose focus, usually by thinking about your own role and planning questions. As you will know from your professional training, the skill of listening actively involves tuning into – really trying to hear with both curiosity and compassion – what the person is saying.

7) Try to be flexible, spontaneous and **responsive** during the interview rather than being fixated on asking set questions. A phenomenological research interview is 'not a situation where a person is passively reporting facts or opinions, but is better seen as an "encounter" where the person is actively engaged in exploring the meaning of events or experiences that have been significant for them' (McLeod, 1999, p. 125).

8) Be mindful of what a **privilege** it is for someone to share their personal experiences with you. You have an ethical responsibility to respect their privacy and dignity and ensure they are not harmed in any way by your interview.

9) Give some time at the end of the interview to **debrief** your participant.
10) Try to leave your participant the **richer for the experience**. The process of being deeply listened to and witnessed can also have powerful impact. As McLeod (1999, p. 125) notes: 'One of the hallmarks of a good qualitative interview lies in the extent to which the informant learns or gains from the experience.'

If you are an experienced therapist, you are likely to feel quite comfortable with these 10 tips for carrying out research interviews. You probably routinely navigate these issues in your practice. Your main challenge may be to avoid falling into the trap of play-acting the role of 'researcher' – perhaps by taking a formal, more distanced approach replete with pre-prepared research-type questions. I suggest that the most productive research encounter is one where the researcher seeks to relate to the participant in a natural, empathic and genuinely human way.

The greater uncertainty or dilemma you will have is to know where the differences lies between the kind of interview you would engage in therapy practice in contrast with that in research. The lines here are blurred. Much depends on the type and number of research interviews involved (influencing the depth of your research relationship) and your own style.

In a one-off research interview, for example, you are less likely to probe and challenge to any significant extent – you will simply want to hear the other's story and through reflecting back and attentive listening you would keep focused on that particular story. However, where deeper research relationships are involved, for instance when engaging dialogal research, the researcher's task may well be akin to that of the psychotherapist's in terms of aiming to facilitate awareness – of both conscious and unconscious aspects – and thus explore shifts in understanding and meaning that can emerge from increased awareness.[iv]

In some research encounters, then, it may be important for the researcher to sense when a participant is *resisting* going deeper into some aspect being explored. While it is important to respect the participant's boundaries, you could reflect on if and how he or she might be supported and nudged to further exploration. One way for you to do this, as a researcher, for example, might be to model the process by disclosing your own uncertainty about pushing further.

Participant observation

Participant observation involves a researcher going into the 'field' and doing naturalistic research *in situ*. For example, Dahlberg (1997, cited in Dahlberg *et al.*, 2008) participated in the activities of a physiotherapy unit aiming to understand how patients with musculoskeletal conditions benefit from the care offered. She both interviewed and observed patients and this included joining in activities in a gym. Dahlberg notes that while the interviews helped to explicate meanings of 'care', it was her participant observation that made it possible to 'grasp the importance of the exercises for their sense of embodiedness and "bodily balance"' (Dahlberg *et al.*, 2008, p. 213). It was in the dressing room after the gym work when she could listen to spontaneous conversations offering further insights about their lived experience of care.

The first decision to take when embarking on a participant observation is to determine beforehand the extent to which you will participate in the group's activities. For example, if you were going to observe an emotional literacy class in action at a school, you would need to decide whether to join in as the 'teacher's assistant' or to observe from a distance. In broad terms you need to choose between taking an insider versus an outsider perspective.

Often, this decision between **participation** and **observation** depends more on the practicalities of the context. The decision can prove especially challenging in covert field studies where you may have to put yourself in potentially risky situations. For example, one researcher, who wishes to remain anonymous, was studying drug use in the British clubbing culture and admits taking drugs in order to be accepted by the group he was researching. While most phenomenological research does not involve such extreme decisions, the degree and manner of participant observation always involves choices with practical and ethical implications attached.

Participant observation also poses other challenges: how to negotiate access to the research field; how to comply with the need to observe naturalistically; and how to approach the difficult task of managing one's emotions in the field.

Negotiating access to the research field can prove problematic as often there are 'gate-keepers'(i.e. people who control access to resources and participants) who need to be satisfied. Studies attempting to explore service users' views and experiences of their treatment, for example, could be derailed by a gatekeeper manager reluctant to have user 'complaints' researched by a stranger. To give another example, Abrahams (2007) discusses the challenges of gaining access to women's groups working in the field of domestic violence. Some of these had, in the past, experienced being insensitively used and exploited by researchers. Abrahams engaged in extensive damage reparation before she could begin her own research.

Once the researcher has gained access, the next question is **how to observe** without unduly changing what is being studied. Care needs to be taken to minimize any intrusion and ensure that observations are naturalistic. For instance, the use of video is gaining popularity as a means of recording details of interactions such as during a counselling session. Here, having the camera in place before recording starts can help participants get used to its presence.

All kinds of pragmatic considerations arise in participant observation research. As part of my PhD research exploring the lifeworld of the occupational therapist, I shadowed and observed three occupational therapists over the course of their working week in a hospital (Finlay, 1998a). I took detailed notes, including both observations and reflections (see Example 13.1). Later I developed my observations into a preliminary analysis of the therapist's lifeworld, while my reflections entered my reflexive analysis chapters (see Example 13.2).

Example 13.1   Example of a participant observation

Negotiating access – I started the participant observations by gaining official permission to observe the therapists concerned . . . My public role as far as all the managers and therapists were concerned was to act as an 'observation student'. This ensured that access to all areas was relatively easy as the system was accustomed to accommodating student observers. Also, my professional qualification acted like a passport; I was accepted as a professional who could be trusted to behave appropriately and keep information confidential. . .

Once inside the field, my professional qualification also eased my passage. I was, by definition, a stranger, an outsider. Yet in a subtle way I was accepted as an insider by the occupational therapists concerned and their occupational therapy colleagues (who knew me or knew of me). I, too, felt on familiar ground. . .

The participant observer role – I adopted different sorts of observer roles (Junker, 1960) depending on the context. When in the presence of patients/clients (for example, on the wards or in their homes), I tended to adopt a 'complete observer' role where I was not expected to participate actively. . .

With staff, I was accepted as a 'participating student/colleague'. This role allowed me to ask questions, write notes and check out impressions generally. . .

Data collection – My means of data collection included unstructured observation, reflection and note writing. In an effort to appear relatively unobtrusive when the therapists worked with patients/clients, I took my lead from the therapists. For example, while observing Jane, I made it a point when we visited clients' homes never to accept a coffee until she did first. I only wrote notes when she did; I spoke only when asked a direct question; I would wait for her to choose her seat and sit down with the client before I sat. With all these behaviours I aimed to have minimum impact on Jane, her work and her clients; I wanted to emphasise her relationship with the clients and maintain my marginal observer status...

Once back in the office ..., I would 'interview' (informally) the therapists about their clinical reasoning and responses. In this way I was able to compare my observations and reflections with theirs...

On returning home after each day, I made notes and expanded them. I then audio-taped my observations and reflections, including my personal responses and some analysis (transcribing the tape in my own time). This daily exercise was time consuming, absorbing around two hours a day, but it enabled me to capture considerable depth of data. (Finlay, 1998a, pp. 124–127)

Example 13.2   Reflexive analysis during participant observation

One aspect of working in the hospital context that I found disturbing (i.e. potentially significant) was that I was required to wear a uniform. Glancing in the mirror on my first morning of work I caught sight of myself in a uniform and panicked. I was aware of my resistance here. The process of writing up my reflexive notes helped me to become aware of how my participants felt in wearing their uniforms each day. An extract is offered here:

1) The uniform is quite nice in that it offers me a sense of being an insider; being accepted and legitimate somehow. This particularly hit me when a doctor entered into a fairly deep personal/professional conversation with Peter and had automatically included me. Clearly the uniform acts as a sort of passport – and I quite like the inclusion.
2) The negative side of my experience ... is that I dislike the restraints, the anonymity, the lack of individuality. If find myself wanting to have the staff I am working with (particularly 'Peter') see me in my usual wear and thus how I 'normally' am...
3) Then there is the feeling of power which I find myself feeling both negative and positive about. People are passing me in the corridor and giving me what I interpret are 'respectful nods'. This uniform clearly has some power and I am feeling it too. I have always known I feel negative about this kind of thing – but my positive response to the feeling of power comes as a horrible surprise...
4) I notice in the changing rooms at the beginning and end of each day how naturally staff wear and take on/off their uniforms in front of each other. It is part of the routine. It has a practical purpose. But I also sense that they too like the identity/status/belonging that it affords them. Their uniforms are always so clean, white and crisply pressed ... It is part of how they 'present' themselves. (Finlay, 1998a, p. 236)

Perhaps the most challenging aspect of participant observation is finding a way to **manage emotions** and the allegiances that inevitably build up as you become immersed in the field. For example, Scott (1997) carried out some (phenomenologically orientated) ethnographic research on child protection practices by intensively shadowing 10 families with 17 allegedly abused children as they moved through the child protection system. She also interviewed and observed the professionals involved. She was shocked by the unexpectedly strong emotional reactions the experience triggered in her. As a social worker with extensive clinical experience in the child protection field, she had not anticipated the intensity of her feelings. It seems the most anguish was caused, not by the abuse, but seeing children and parents suffering at the hands of professionals she herself had taught. She describes how the suffering of the parents and children seemed more visible to her as a researcher than when she was a more desensitized practitioner exposed daily to such distress:

> I felt a sense of helplessness ... which I had no way of alleviating and an unease with the voyeurism inherent in the act of observation ... Most painful ... of all was listening to the intense anguish of a father who had been falsely suspected of sexually abusing his four year old daughter. (Scott, 1997, p. 356)

Written accounts

Data involving written accounts comes in different forms including personal diaries, protocols and/or literature.

Personal diaries   First, we might draw on personal diaries – sometimes a source of rich reflection. The value of this is illustrated in the following extracts taken from the study described in Example 1.1. This 'data' arose in the broader research context where Pat and I sought to explore her lived experience of receiving an implant. She kept a diary of her experience over several months moving through her rehabilitation when she was struggling to adapt and learn to hear.

> I'm feeling *cut off*... Doubts about my ability to pick up my life are again creeping up ... Can I continue working? ... The sounds are not pleasant, it is so confusing. My brain ... needs clearer, better, fuller sounds, almost as if it needs to pop a cork out and let sound in ... I'm tired; *disconnected of conversations*. I really don't like this ...
>
> It scares me that I really like my silence and I miss it and I found it hard to cope with the noise even if it helps and makes me *more part of things* ... What is the hard thing is trying to be part of the hearing, have the expectations of the hearing ... and having to struggle all the time to do what your body is not able to do effortlessly ...

> I am moving on . . . emotionally. I am not comparing and struggling but getting on with both my silence and the noise. The silence reminds me of who I am, the noise increases the contact with the world outside . . . It changed my being in the world for a while. I lost my footing but I think I have taken control. (Finlay & Molano-Fisher, 2008, pp. 159–161)

As this extract shows, personal reflections can be extraordinarily poignant and offer rich revelation. The same applies to protocols.

Protocols   Phenomenological 'protocols' are formal written descriptions or narratives of lived experience used most commonly within descriptive phenomenological method. Participants might be asked to write a description on a side (or few sides) of A4 and this can be used as 'data' in itself or – perhaps more usefully – as a springboard for a more focused, detailed discussion in an interview.

Often people find it challenging, even anxiety provoking, to write a description and prompting questions can help. Van Manen offers some guidelines:

1) You need to describe the experience as you live(d) through it. Avoid as much as possible causal explanations, generalizations, or abstract interpretations. For example, it does not help to state what *caused* your illness, *why* you like swimming so much, or why you feel that children *tend to* like to play outdoors more than indoors.
2) Describe the experience from the inside, as it were; almost like a state of mind: the feelings, the mood, the emotions, etc.
3) Focus on a particular example or incident of the object of experience: describe specific events, an adventure, a happening, a particular experience.
4) Try to focus on an example of the experience which stands out for its vividness, or as it was the first time.
5) Attend to how the body feels, how things smell(ed), how they sound(ed), etc.
6) Avoid trying to beautify your account with fancy phrases or flowery terminology. (1990, pp. 64–65)

Literary accounts   Poetry, art, drama/film and literature (including autobiography, biography and fiction) can be rich, **vicarious** sources of life experience. 'Phenomena such as love, grief, illness, faith, success, fear, death, hope struggle, or loss', notes van Manen (1990, p. 70), 'are the stuff of which novels are made'. We only have to think of classic works such as Proust's *Remembrance of Things Past* or Dostoevsky's *Crime and Punishment* to know how they can vividly evoke aspects of life.

The work of Seamon (1993a) in Example 7.2 is a good example of how a phenomenologist might squeeze meanings out of fiction.[v] Similarly, in Example 13.3 Van der Bruggen and Widdershoven (2004) offer an account of what it is like to have Parkinson's disease by analysing *four novels* about people with the condition. (They also drew on personal accounts from patients and information obtained by searching the literature.) In their analysis they highlight a central theme that 'being a Parkinson's patient is apparently characterized by an existential paradox: life appears simultaneously immobile and unpredictably whimsical' (p. 28).

Example 13.3   Being a Parkinson's patient

This example shows the impact of communication problems. The authors offer an extract from a novel by Harding which describes a family's experience of going on holiday to Malta with Jim – a man in a relatively advanced stage:

'Come on, Dad. What is it?' I'm beginning to lose patience, and I hate myself for it.
  Slowly he raises his good hand, lifts up his spectacles and stares at me. He lowers the glasses and stretches out his hand towards me. (His fingers tremble heavily) . . . They touch my hair and rest there for a second or two. I don't know what's happening . . . He says something, but it comes out all throaty and I don't understand it. I can make out 'Nick', but nothing else . . . His eyes mist over . . . I put my arm around him and without thinking, kiss him lightly on the cheek. His skin is sharp and scratchy to my lips from the permanent residue of stubble because he's so hard to shave. I take my arm from around him, grasp his claw and lead him by it slowly down the steps. (Harding, 2000, pp. 311–312)

Researchers have a choice concerning what method or combinations of method to use. The decision of whether to interview, observe or use textual material is in part determined by the nature of the phenomenon as well as what is practical. The source of the data, however, is probably less significant than the way meanings are accessed. The *process* of gathering data has more impact on the quality of what is revealed than the mechanics of the method.

Processes Involved in Gathering Data

A number of complex, delicate and subtle processes occur when gathering data through reflection and/or dialogue. Openness, empathy and attentive listening are three interlinked processes which characterize, to a greater or lesser extent, the qualities phenomenological researchers bring when in relationship with participants and/or texts.

Openness

A key aim in phenomenological research is to discover new awareness, to find out more about another individual or a specific phenomenon. We hope to be touched, surprised and to have our horizons expanded. This can only happen if we are *open to* our participants (or the phenomenon) and if we start from a relatively '**unknowing**' non-judgemental position characterized by a real **curiosity**. We genuinely want to understand what such and such an experience is like for our participants (or texts); we want to really hear what they are saying. Thus, we need to be prepared to allow things to spontaneously emerge in the intersubjective space between researcher and participant/text and we must have faith that it will. If we are closed to new possibilities and understandings then we will only confirm what we knew already, and the value of our research outcomes will be diminished.

Openness is enabled in phenomenological research through the practice of '**bracketing**': by our attempt to suspend presuppositions (see also *Chapter 5* on the phenomenological attitude). This process is often misunderstood as an attempt to be objective. In fact, what is called for is an especially attentive attitude of openness and receptivity – there is an emptying of the self in order to be filled by the other. Max van Manen (2002) describes this process as 'the unwilled willingness to meet what is utterly strange in what is most familiar'. The aim is 'to see through fresh eyes, to understand through embracing new modes of being' (Finlay, 2008, p. 29). With this openness comes fleeting moments of awe and wonder[vi] – such moments are elusive but can be powerfully transformational (Finlay, 2008):

> When we are struck with wonder, our minds are suddenly cleared of the clutter of everyday concerns that otherwise constantly occupy us. We are confronted by the thing, the phenomenon in all of its strangeness and uniqueness. The wonder of that thing takes us in, and renders us momentarily speechless. (van Manen, 2002)

Empathy

In our empathy, we feel, sense, intuit, attune to and share in the other's experience. There is a *being-with* the other in a relational space (Finlay, 2010a).

A key ingredient in successfully engaging participants in data collection is the researcher's embodied empathic presence. Here the researcher is present as a person meeting the person of the other (Yontef, 1993). This awareness of meeting the other in the present moment lies at the heart of any authentic encounter – be it therapy or research. It is this authentic meeting that provides the other with an experience of being seen, acknowledged and witnessed (Evans & Gilbert, 2005).

If you are a therapist, you will not need reminding of the value of empathy and creating for the client a sense of being understood. Theorists such as Rogers (1951) from the humanistic tradition, and Kohut (1984) from the tradition of self-psychology, underline how essential it is for the therapist to be able to enter into the subjective world of the other in a concerned and empathic manner (Evans & Gilbert, 2005). You already know, from your work as a therapist, that empathy is a relational process, unique to each encounter. Empathy cannot be reduced to mere technique (Myers, 2000).

The value of empathy applies equally to research where it can be understood as a process of seeking ways to allow participants to present themselves to and through oneself as the researcher. It involves an '**intersubjective** process of imaginal self-transposition and mutual identification where self-understanding and Other-understanding is intertwined' (Finlay, 2005, p. 290). Here, empathy is not just about emotional knowing; it is a *felt*, **embodied**, intersubjective experience. We therefore need to talk about 'a research process which involves engaging, **reflexively**, with the participant's lived body, our own body and our embodied intersubjective relationship with the participant' (Finlay, 2005, p. 272).

As researchers we must always remain aware that participants can become stressed and distressed when being observed or talking about difficult subjects and their personal experience. Compassionate, sensitive, attuned care and ethical attention is needed to support them positively. While unduly stressing/distressing a participant is to be avoided, sometimes a level of upset may be unavoidable. However, if such a situation arises it is important to check that the participant is happy to continue. This is one area in which research differs from therapy. It is not within the researcher's remit to push or challenge as a therapist might.

'Attentive listening'

Openness and empathy merge when we engage 'attentive listening'. This is not an appraising, critical listening but a listening where curiosity, contemplation and compassion run free. This kind of listening involves slowing down and dwelling with the other. It involves listening *in silence* to the 'voice' of the other. In that silence something *more* is born. The 'more' goes beyond the words said. And there is always more . . . Phenomenological research rejoices in the product of attentive listening; the product of 'being with' an Other.

From the participant's perspective, the experience of being truly listened to – being **witnessed** and allowed to have a **voice** – can be profound. In addition to knowing one's perspective is appreciated, being listened to opens up space or time to allow a person to **make sense** of their experience and to go beyond previous understandings.

Attentive listening can be likened to Todres' (2007) concept of '*attentive being-with*'. He applies this concept to therapy but, equally, it works for research:

> In this mode of being, the therapist allows his/her attention to be absorbed into the phenomenological world of the other . . . in an attitude of letting-be-ness . . . More and more, therapist and client get a feeling of how it all hangs together. (Todres, 2007, pp. 77–78)

Willis (2010) pushes the notion of attentive, attuned listening further, to encompass the reading of text. He recommends opening one's heart, intuition and imagination in the process.[vii]

> Such 'listening' reading requires a kind of reflective and attentive silence allowing the author to speak to the imagination and the heart. It is not a substitute for a cool and more critical reading but it can be an aesthetic source of precious enrichment. It is the warm flesh on the bones of the human search for wisdom and truth that perhaps for people suitably disposed, might make the quest more desirable as well as more convincing (Willis, 2010, p. 23)

In summary, the data gathering process is one that involves opening oneself in curiosity, being attuned empathetically, listening attentively and responding reflexively. In the next section I attempt to show how these concepts might be applied in practice.

An 'Encounter'. . .

The example below comes from some narrative case study research I undertook on the lived experience of having mental health problems (Finlay, 2004; also see the section on narrative analysis in *Chapter 14* which presents a narrative created out of this dialogue). Kenny was my co-researcher and agreed to be interviewed about his experience. He was a middle-aged man suffering from anxiety and depression – something he had struggled with for over 3 years. He told his story over a cup of coffee in my kitchen. We spoke for approximately an hour and a half.

I started by asking Kenny to describe what it was like living through the early days of his breakdown. The dialogue that emerged was co-constituted; it developed and took shape in that specific context.

The extract below draws upon two sources: the actual interview transcript^{viii} *and* the reflexive notes (in italics) I wrote after the interview. As you read, note how my reflexivity sheds light on Kenny's experience and so forms part of what can be seen as 'data'.

Example 13.4   An interview dialogue

Kenny: The realisation that something was wrong was I was waking up in the morning, praying that there was something wrong with us – anything, just so I didn't have to go to work. I carried on and then suddenly one morning I said 'That's it, I've had enough'. I walked out and never went back. I locked myself in the bedroom. It took weeks and weeks before I would go out. I would read, submerge myself in books, escaped. I wasn't interested in anything. I just wanted to be in my bed. I suppose in some ways it was my little nest. I was safe in my bedroom and nobody could get to us. And I wasn't bothered about anything. The worst part of it was if I was thinking. It seemed to get worse. What's happening? What am I doing? I was scaring myself. It was a dreadful experience that I wouldn't wish on anyone. To be scared is one of the worst things. It is a method of torture.

Linda: It sounds incredibly scary – all the more so because it's being like, that was so different from the way you normally are(?)

Kenny: Yeah, I definitely wasn't me-self.

Linda: Was that the scariest bit, facing someone, facing yourself as someone you didn't know?

Kenny: I was just very fearful – I kept jumping at me own shadow. I wondered 'what am I doing?' But I wouldn't say it was self-inflicted 'cos had I known what was happening I would have done something about it.

Linda: Yes, I guess you wouldn't have got ill in the first place. So what did you do after that initial period?

Kenny: From there we went to see the doctor. He agreed that I should have 2 weeks off and try to relax. I think in some ways it was a huge relief that I didn't have to go back to work. Fortunately the doctor I had was sympathetic. The state I was in – I was shaking, it was visible, the terror in my eyes. I just wanted to get out of the doctor's surgery. I remember trying to relax a bit then, thinking I've got two weeks, I can sort myself out. But it was never going to happen. I had this desperation of what was happening.

As I was listening to Kenny speak, I suddenly realised that I was reacting quite strongly to him and became aware my own bodily responses. I remember noticing how my arms were folded tightly across my stomach. I was protecting myself, but also 'holding myself in' and somehow 'holding myself together'. I then saw that Kenny had adopted the same posture as he recalled his trauma (had I mirrored his posture or had he followed mine?).

[The word 're-member' is significant here. Remembering is not just a cognitive function: it is about reiterating responses in the body: we re-member.]

With us both holding ourselves, it seemed an important moment, one that called for me to tune into what we were both doing. I was a little surprised at the sensations and my reactions. Usually, I would interpret this non-verbal gesture as representing a symbolic wish to protect oneself from others or a way of giving oneself some nurturing/comforting. But here in this situation I was somehow sensing an additional, even different, interpretation . . .

Linda: As you're speaking and remembering, Kenny, I can see you're holding yourself tightly. And I'm doing the same as I'm listening to you. [shared laughter]. It's like you're trying to hold yourself together. Is it like, kinda to stop yourself falling apart. Is that what it was like for you?

Kenny: Yeah, I would go off to bed and just hold myself like that. Sometimes it seemed like for hours. One minute I was alright and the next I could just go into a rage about the simplest thing. And again, it could be a trivial thing and I'd lose it completely. Again I sought the sanctuary of the bedroom. I knew there I wouldn't hurt people. The worse thing was because I was feeling guilty I was getting more angry about it.

I felt his confusion: his rage against himself and this crazy 'alien' it seemed he had become. I felt his fear of losing himself, of losing it in general, and his concern that he might hurt others in his anger and craziness. I felt his guilt about this anger and understood why he might want to lock himself away. It was the only place he could be safe. Perhaps it was the only place he could recover himself to reassure himself that he was still there.

Later, when I was analysing the transcript, I replayed this dialogue over and over as a way of helping me to focus on what it would be like to be Kenny. I adopted that holding posture and 're-membered' the (my? his?) emotions. Again I got that strong sense of 'holding together' that which was falling apart and holding in the craziness and rage so they didn't break out and destroy others.

Linda: From the way you're describing it I can hear how you were just a bundle of different emotions: fear, anger, desperation, frustration, distress. It must have just felt overwhelming(?)

Kenny: Yeah, totally. And then after two weeks, I went back to the doctors and he recommended I see a counsellor. But I didn't think it would help at this stage. It was two months later that he insisted . . . She was nice and got me to start talking.

Linda: Instead of pushing things down and away?

> **Kenny:** Yeah. Saying things out loud is different. I thought suicide might be a way out but I never seriously contemplated it. For all that you were really down there was still something at the back of my mind, clinging on by the fingertips, it was still there – 'We can go on from this'.

The Kenny–Linda example above illustrates the process of co-creating data in dialogue. Kenny shares his personal experience in response to my prompts, questions and reflecting back.[ix] It seems that Kenny felt comfortable enough to share his personal experiences with me. In fact, he had a specific purpose for the story he was telling: he wanted me not only to understand the nightmare of his experience, but also to 'spread the word' that it is possible to claw one's way back to mental health. He was also giving, at some level, a 'performance'.

Does the dialogue set out above parallel interactions you might have with patients/clients in therapy sessions? Perhaps you have asked your client to 'tell their story', then reflected back to check your understanding or asked questions to get them to expand on certain points, as I did? If so, this demonstrates that you already have many of the skills and the experience needed to handle such research encounters. (Even if you are embarking on research for the very first time, remember that your ability to engage with others means you are far from being a novice.)

If you are a therapist, the most challenging thing for you will be to ensure you stay focused on the research project and hold back from making therapeutic interpretations or interventions. This is easier said than done. Not only will your own impulses get in the way, but also your participant, knowing your role, may attempt to elicit that therapist self. Remember that your contract with your participant is to do research, not therapy. Use your research aims to guide your focus and the context to define the lines of inquiry you want to pursue.

Reflections

As therapists, we have a number of advantages when it comes to collecting data. We already have the necessary skills to interview and observe. We know how to use ourselves in relation to others, how to enable the other to feel safe and to speak, and how to share our warmth and empathy. We have the ability to be a presence that is authentic, energized, active and direct. We already know how to be self-aware and how to respond intuitively in the emerging relational context. We realize the importance of being patient when another tells their halting story and we can tolerate that initial sense of chaos without jumping in to clarify too soon. These are the qualities to draw upon (and perhaps nurture) when engaging phenomenological research with others. Just as therapists use themselves as tools in therapy, researchers use themselves as research tools in phenomenological research.

I am frequently puzzled by the limited attention the phenomenological literature pays to data gathering compared with the analytic process. While the importance of having an open, non-judgemental, empathetic, ethical phenomenological attitude is usually acknowledged – and rightly so – rarely is anything said about the relational processes we might engage.[x] I have tried in this chapter to claim back some space for the process of 'being-with'. In this mysterious space *between* anything can, and often does, emerge. Let yourself go, be open and unknowing.

The data gathering process is less about applying techniques and more about encountering and dialoguing with the other (or oneself), be it in person-to-person contact or through text. Churchill (1990, p. 63) says that 'research praxis is a fundamentally human endeavour'. I agree.

Notes

[i] Some of the material in this chapter has been drawn from chapter 7 of Finlay and Evans (2009) and has been reproduced here with kind permission of the publishers Wiley-Blackwell.

[ii] I am making a distinction in this chapter between 'gathering' and 'analysing' data. However, these two processes often merge in practice. For instance, during interviews descriptions of lived experience are gathered but may also be simultaneously reflected upon more analytically. Where phenomenological research involves a reflection on texts the data is already gathered in one sense but further data is gathered in terms of the reflective-analytical dialogue engaged in with oneself.

[iii] If you are an occupational therapist, art therapist or drama therapist you might like to consider how you could utilize your own modes of therapeutic activity as a way to gain information about people's lived experience. For instance, instead of interviewing someone about their experience of an illness, why not ask them to paint or sculpt what the illness means to them? Also, if you commonly work with groups, you might prefer to work with a 'focus group' rather than conducting individual interviews.

[iv] If a participant, in coming into deep relational contact with a researcher, becomes aware of previously unconscious material, some anxiety is likely to be generated. With this anxiety comes a natural self-protective desire to defend against new and potentially disturbing awareness. Some 'resistance' may ensue. This process of resistance is usually out of awareness and, if challenged, creates ambivalence such as feeling confused and torn between conflicting desires to hide or to let repressed material into consciousness. This ambivalence about whether to maintain the status quo versus thinking/behaving differently affects the relationship with oneself (for example, denial and depression shown possibly as unexpressed anger) and with others (for example, gaps in memory or displacement of anger onto someone else). With ethical considerations to the fore, the researcher will need to tread sensitively and respect the choices made by the participant about what they want to share.

[v] See also Seamon (2010c) and how he offers a post-modern phenomenological account of 'home' and 'becoming-at-home' via the example of the TV comedy/drama *Six Feet Under*.

[vi] Hansen offers an explication of '**wonder**':

> Only when we authentically are moved by 'something', which we experience as very important and meaningful and at the same time experience the limitation and infinitude of the written and spoken word, and when we openly expose our vulnerability, struggle and longing, *then*... there are signs of wonder in our faces and thoughts. (Hansen, 2010, p. 171)

[vii] Willis (personal communication) suggests that aesthetically attuned reading is fostered by sharing with kindred spirits who act as attentive companions and through a dogged, hard-won kind of connoisseurship dedicated to its cultivation while rejecting cheap substitutes.

[viii] The interview questions and answers have been transcribed largely word for word, except for some grammatical confusions, 'ums', 'ers' and hesitations which have been edited out to aid clarity. Similarly, I have not included the kinds of pauses and notes on intonation here which other transcription methods highlight.

[ix] The focus of the dialogue was on Kenny's mental health struggles. By mutual consent, neither Kenny nor I talked about other personal issues such as Kenny's relationship with his wife and family. His domestic circumstances could well have been a source of tension and problems but I respected these boundaries. Kenny had not consented to talk at that level and I tried to stay with what Kenny was bringing to our encounter. I sought instead to show my empathy while also trying to make it easy and comfortable for him to tell his story. By my manner (verbal and non-verbal), I tried to help Kenny to feel safe enough to share. I also followed my intuitions and drew on my bodily felt sense in the 'here and now' to possibly shed light on Kenny's 'then and there'. I also attempted to empathically reflect back. I played a part in negotiating the intimacy-distance of the moment – at times, encouraging more disclosure; at other times gently protecting Kenny and containing his disclosures.

[x] There are notable exceptions such as the work of Churchill (2010b) on empathy and the second-person perspective.

Chapter 14

Relational Ethics[i]

Relational ethics requires researchers to act from our hearts and minds, acknowledge our interpersonal bonds to others, and take responsibility for actions and their consequences. (Ellis, 2007, p. 3)

Professional guidelines for the ethical conduct of research tend to emphasize certain key principles: participants should be respected, protected and never deceived; their informed consent should be gained beforehand; they should be debriefed afterwards; confidentiality should be maintained; and so on.

These guidelines sound reasonably straightforward. In practice, however, every research encounter brings up context-specific ethical uncertainties and challenges (Finlay, 2009c). With phenomenological research in particular the challenge may be felt more acutely as our research topics can involve personal and sensitive material and they may even be considered 'invasive' (Usher & Holmes, 1997). No matter how strictly and carefully various ethical procedures and protocols are followed, situations arise in the field which make our heads spin and hearts ache (Ellis, 2007). The process of negotiating an ethical path can be tricky, and compromises usually need to be made.

This chapter focuses on the relational ethical challenges which arise at different **stages** of any research project involving participants. During every stage researchers confront the tricky task of minimizing the impact of likely (inevitable?) power imbalances between ourselves and our co-researcher(s).

Phenomenology for Therapists: Researching the Lived World, First Edition. Linda Finlay.
© 2011 Linda Finlay. Published 2011 by John Wiley & Sons, Ltd.

How do we move towards more collaborative, egalitarian, open relationships (as opposed to exploitative, instrumental ones) as suited to our humanistic values? For many phenomenological researchers, understandings of the other are found in the fullness of our open relation where 'dialogue, parity and reciprocity' are threaded through all phases of research (Heron, 1996, p. 11).

Pre-research Phase

If you are a practising therapist, you will be familiar with the tensions generated when negotiating an initial therapy contract. Often, a delicate balancing act is involved as you seek to set boundaries and establish trust. Similar tensions arise in the research context, except that the research you are proposing is not something that potential participants have asked for and, furthermore, it may not offer them any direct benefits (although sometimes a small fee or expenses are given). Thus, a different sort of contract needs to be negotiated.

It also may be necessary, depending on the type of research you are planning to do, to negotiate a broader contract for entering the 'field'. If, for instance, you are intending to do a participant observation study, then you may need to negotiate the contract and boundaries with a number of people at various organizational levels.

All this means that a great deal of ground work needs to be done before a project gets underway – ground work that reaches beyond purely procedural concerns such as obtaining informed consent and ensuring confidentiality/anonymity. Ethical permission needs to be obtained from relevant parties, then the **research contract** as a whole needs to negotiated and a level of trust and/or consent established with all involved (see *Appendix*).

In addition to formalities, the pre-research stage requires the foundations of mutual trust within the research relationship being put in place and the research aims and process generally agreed upon. In Buber's terms, we are called on to move beyond a functional, instrumental 'I-it' relationship, in which we see the other in terms of their use to us, towards an 'I-Thou' relationship – one of openness to their personhood. This process is easier said than done. In a situation where the researcher initiates and controls contact and holds professional knowledge, the relationship is inevitably an uneven one.

The significant step demanded of the phenomenological researcher is to release control, or rather take 'control in a new humanistic sense by being clearly conscious of the choice' of ensuring co-researchers have both choice and voice themselves (Krüger, 2007, p. 19). Such an impulse fits the recommendations of the phenomenological philosopher Levinas (1961/ 1969) who puts concern for the Other at the centre of his ethics. He argues that ethical human relating involves an ongoing effort to constrain one's own freedom and spontaneity (or allow oneself to be constrained) as part of a project of being 'open' to the Other.

Data Gathering Phase

During the data gathering stage researchers face ethical challenges relating to the use (and misuse) of power, concerning their duty of care to keep participants safe. This power comes from researchers' professional authority and the way they control the research. Researchers must work hard to relinquish their '**power**' and yield to whatever might emerge in the relational moment.

Inevitably, researchers will sometimes find themselves being instrumental. Alert to opportunities to obtain data from the other, they may push hungrily ahead. This is inevitable, even at a simple level when, during interviews, we are selective about which questions/answers to follow up. At a more subtle level, the researcher is the one who uses 'expert' knowledge (such as using empathetic responses and reflecting back techniques) to both 'open up' a participant's expressions and close them down again. There are no clear-cut answers here about what level of disclosure or degree of restraint is desirable. The negotiation can only take place within the dialogical relationship and the key is to remain aware of ethical responsibilities as Example 14.1 illustrates.

Example 14.1   Co-researcher distress

In a tape-recorded interview, Maria, the informant, becomes excited and emotionally involved with the story of her life as a mother of her handicapped child. Suddenly, and to her own surprise, she bursts out in tears – but continues with her story. At this point, the researcher becomes particularly alert and tempted because behind the tears and a sad destiny, he detects that the informant actually reveals something which is right to the point of the theme he wants to explore in his research.

So, how should the researcher in this example handle the dilemma . . . Should, in the name of science, the tape recorder be stopped and the interview cancelled in order to take care of the informant's personal process? (Kruger, 2007, p. 20)

How should we manage our power as researchers while protecting (and perhaps even empowering) our participants? Ideally, the research process is at once strategic *and* respectful. As in therapy, we attempt a balancing act: we seek to use our professional skills to enable and facilitate disclosure while at the same time intervening to protect our co-researcher from too much exposure. Such 'dialectical oppositions' (Ellis, 2007, pp. 20–21) involve moving back and forth between expression and protection, between disclosure and restraint (Bochner, 1984).

As in therapy, the researcher endeavours to enable participants to feel they have control over what they are sharing; they consent to whatever is going to constitute the 'data' to be worked with. At the same time researchers need to be reflexively aware of the **power** (and lack of power) they wield. Power, of course, comes in different guises, inhabiting structural dimensions such as class, race/ethnicity and gender. Researchers need to be alert to how these different types of power cross-cut one another. It is too simplistic to suggest power is exerted in one direction only. Participants control the agenda too and they can claim power, for instance, acting in a passive aggressive way. Consider the trepidation you might feel if you were a woman interviewing a violent male sex offender; or if you were a phenomenological researcher interviewing a doctor who was hostile to 'unscientific' qualitative research.

Beyond questions of power, researchers have a **duty of care** to ensure the safety (emotional and physical) of their participants. Phenomenological research often taps sensitive material and can be emotionally intense to experience (for the researcher as well as co-researcher). Participants may feel exposed and vulnerable while the experience of re-telling their stories has the potential to re-traumatize them. Example 14.2 illustrates ways in which the research challenged one participant. Here, Pat (participant) explains to me (researcher) in an email why she had wanted to disengage from our research to do with exploring her experience of receiving a cochlear implant. (Example 1.1 offers background information about this research.)

Example 14.2   Research and emotional intensity

Pat: Hi Linda. I am ready again, sorry about [being out of touch for such a] long time, thanks for the space . . . couldn't handle the analysis. Felt I wanted to move on, not to dwell in the past . . . Even if I have progressed, I feel I will never feel 'normal' as I felt before because my bubble has been burst!! . . . I am scared about what else I don't know will come in the analysis and I rather hide it and don't face it! (Finlay & Molano-Fisher, 2009)

In this example, both Pat and I needed to balance the potential harm of our focus on Pat's emotional world against the potential benefit of telling her story. We made the decision to carry on. Pat felt she wanted to share her experience as there were lessons to be learned by professionals as well other deaf individuals considering the possibility of implants. As Cutcliffe and Ramcharan (2002) acknowledge, emotionally charged research may be distressing for some but it can also often be therapeutic and validating.

Example 14.3 highlights how what arises needs to be sensitively handled and managed.

Example 14.3   Collaborating with while protecting co-researchers

In the following quotation Ellis describes the relational ethical process she engaged when collaborating with two other researchers on studying their experience of bulimia nervosa. She was mindful of the personal and emotional nature of the project, and this was intensified by the fact that ethical concerns arose as her co-researchers were her PhD students. They decided to write privately and hold any disclosures as confidential until they all agreed to disclose more publically. As a group they also had to continually process how they were feeling and whether or not to stay with the project.

> I emphasized that Christine and Lisa not reveal anything to me they might regret later because they might be concerned with how I, their professor, saw them . . . . In each meeting, we created opportunities to change our minds, and to add to or delete from the stories we had told. (Ellis, 2007, pp. 20–21)

As Ellis shows here, a number of steps can be taken by researchers to protect their participants. In the research by Ellis and her students, they agreed to use mild discomfort as a cue to explore further while they were also committed to protecting one another from distress. As she notes: 'We tried to develop trust by openly sharing our lives; however, we also had to respect each other's needs for privacy and restraint' (Ellis, 2007, p. 21).

Phenomenological researchers need to recognize the potential for the research to be intense and possibly even painful. Even research that seems apparently straightforward may deeply touch participants. We need to appreciate the gift they are giving us by sharing and to be prepared to handle whatever comes up.

While being supportive of research participants, however, we need to take care to not transgress boundaries between research and therapy and that means trying to stay within the terms of what you have negotiated in your research contract. Also, unlike the therapy context, we might negotiate terms where certain personal or sensitive material is ring fenced as 'no go areas' or the material may later be deliberately excluded from the research. Towards the end of the research, a separate post-research discussion may prove fruitful to help the participant integrate their experience. It may also be necessary to arrange for some external counselling to be offered if extra support is needed.

The above discussion and examples highlight how the data gathering phase of research involves much more than simply collecting data. Ethical and relational negotiations, concerned with power, protection, respect and the safety of the participants, are similarly intertwined when it comes to analysing the data.

Data Analysis Phase

In this phase, phenomenological researchers confront the question of the extent to which they could, or should, involve participants in the analytical process. The outcome depends, in part, on the type of research involved. Many phenomenologists would not involve participants in the analysis as it is too much to expect them to bracket their natural attitude. Dialogal and relationally oriented research, in contrast, seeks to involve co-researchers.

In Example 14.4, I discuss the ethics of my collaboration with Ann in a phenomenological study on Ann's lived experience of multiple sclerosis (see Example 3.1).

Example 14.4   Participant validation?

Ann and I collaborated in this research in a number of ways. First of all she agreed to share her experience with me as she was keen that I 'spread the word' to therapists about what it was 'really like to have MS'. Together, we embarked on a project whose findings, we both understood, would eventually be made public. Ann was content for me to share the findings with therapists. . .

Ann was a physiotherapist and had a reasonable understanding of the aims, process and intended outcomes of my case study research. This was important as it meant that her consent to take part in the research was properly informed. It also meant that Ann could take on a more collaborative role in the research *to the extent that she wanted to.* . .

Ann . . . affirmed certain themes, suggesting I had captured her experience 'nicely'. At other points she suggested my analysis (particularly my metaphorical flourishes) needed to be 'toned down' as she didn't feel they adequately represented her ordinary, everyday experience. One notable example here was my initial use of an analogy: that of Ann situation being akin to 'living with an alien monster'... I therefore deleted all references to the monster while retaining (I ruefully acknowledge) some sense of the notion of alien infiltration...

While Ann gave me some feedback, I retained control of my analysis and writing... I could have involved Ann much more collaboratively, but chose not to.' (Finlay, 2006b, pp. 194–195)

Some phenomenologists embrace the idea of **participant validation** or member checking as a way to 'prove' the validity of their research. Here, researchers refer their evolving analysis back to their participants for confirmation: when the participant agrees with the researcher's assessment, it is seen as strengthening the researcher's argument. But such confidence may be misplaced. It needs to be remembered that participants have their own motives, needs and interests. They also have varying degrees of insight. Moreover, what may have been 'true' for them at the time of the interview may no longer be the case. Their ability to put themselves back into the specific research context may well be limited. For all these reasons, processes of participant validation need to be engaged in carefully and with awareness of the complex conscious, unconscious and contingent dimensions which may lead a co-researcher to support or refute any one analysis. (The researcher is, of course, subject to their own complex conscious, unconscious and contingent elements: hence my insistence on some researcher reflexivity.)

In his evaluation of participant validation, Ashworth (1993) supports it on moral-political grounds but warns against taking participants' responses too seriously as it may be in their interests to protect their 'socially presented selves'. As he notes:

Participant validation is flawed... since the 'atmosphere of safety' that would allow the individual to lower his or her defences... and act in open candour... is hardly likely to be achieved in the research encounter. (Ashworth, 1993, p. 15)

In the case of the research with Ann above, it could be argued that Ann's involvement in the co-production of the findings strengthens the trustworthiness and ethical basis of this research. That is not the same as saying that Ann has validated this study thereby ensuring its veracity. As phenomenological researchers we do not claim to seek a 'truth' which can be validated in this way. Instead we acknowledge that findings are produced in a specific context. Rather than seeing the process of involving participants in analysis as being about validating the 'correctness' of findings, we should emphasize that it is about empowering them to share in meaning-making processes (Haumann, 2005).

Concluding the Research

The final phase of research involves tying things up with participants, writing up and disseminating the research. While the first process may be conducted within the relational context, the second usually occurs away from participants. However, in all these stages the issue of reciprocity comes to the fore. Is there an opportunity to give something back?

Tying up the research with participants usually involves some sort of debrief towards closure of the research relationship. When and how this is achieved varies enormously depending on the type of research involved. For some research, it may occur at the end of the interview/observation stage with researcher and participant perhaps sharing their experiences of doing the research in an interactive summing up. Certainly, in whatever methodology is adopted, participants should be given time to reflect on their experience and the space to discuss further issues.

In more collaborative types of research, closure may come with seeing a tangible, jointly produced end product. Participants may, for instance, get a real 'kick' out of seeing their story in print. Others may appreciate the fact that the researcher is going on to write official reports which can 'make a difference' or they are planning to share the findings in some productive, constructive way.

After achieving some degree of closure of the research relationship, researchers will present their findings to the wider professional and academic community and here fresh ethical questions emerge. To begin with, there is the issue of how others may react to experiences that co-researchers have been willing to share. For example, in the Ellis, Kiesinger and Tillmann-Healy (1997) research on the experience of bulimia described above, the co-researchers needed to think very carefully about how they would be seen by others after telling their stories – particularly as they were about to apply for academic jobs. The research article they collaboratively wrote was to become part of their job application packets and clearly identified them as women with eating disorders if not other emotional vulnerabilities (Ellis, 2007).

Also pertinent is the impact of the research on the participants themselves. In the following passage, Haumann (2005) discusses her discomfort that her participants had little say or power over her interpretations. In this research she was exploring psychodynamic psychotherapists' own experiences of personal therapy. Haumann was particularly concerned about her analysis of the issue of power and unresolved conflicts between her participants and their therapists. She describes herself as feeling on a 'slippery slope':

> On the one hand the participants were also therapists and should be able to know that my interpretations were not 'truths', but only *my* interpretations, and could be useful comments on their therapies. On the other hand, these interpretations could also invade the space of therapy, do real damage there and also undermine the participant's ability 'to interpret his experience in his own way'. (Haumann, 2005, p. 22)

Haumann's comments suggest that a pernicious ethical challenge of writing up research is the sense of discomfort researchers may feel about treating participants as *objects* to 'talk about' rather than as persons to 'talk with'. Put in Levinas' (1961/1969) terms, the power we can misuse is a function of the way we objectify others in relation and that we should choose to act to reduce such dominance. Josselson nicely expresses this discomfort of exploring the guilt and shame that go with writing about others in an objectifying way:

> My guilt, I think, comes from my knowing that I have taken myself out of relationship with my participants (with whom, during the interview, I was in intimate relationship) to be in relationship with my readers. I have, in a sense, been talking about them behind their backs and doing so publicly . . . I am guilty about being an intruder and then, to some extent, a betrayer . . . I am using them as extensions of my own narcissism and fear being caught, seen in this process. (Josselson, 1996, cited in McLeod, 2001, p. 198)

There are no easy ways to preclude such feelings of discomfort. However, being reflexively aware both of the nature of our research enterprise and of our ethical responsibilities is a good place to start. Just as in life, we have to make choices in difficult, uncertain circumstances, and cope with competing demands and responsibilities.

It also helps if you believe your research has the potential to benefit, at some level, your co-researchers even if your initial intention was to benefit a wider community. In the following extract a participant in Morrow's study of the experience of sexual abuse shares her positive response to the experience of being a co-analyst:

> The participant co-researcher analytic process was a shared voice . . . That creates the experience of being understood. The amount of, just, honor and respect – it's just not like anything I've ever experienced . . . You have done something really extraordinary. It's so much more than a dissertation . . . It's the place that believes I'm honourable, worth knowing. (Morrow, 2006, p. 165)

Reflections

Ethical research practice involves much more than following rules and procedures. Instead, it is a process that begins with an idea and does not end until the research is no longer being disseminated. Issues arise in interactions within research relationships and compromises may need to be made. Every research encounter brings up ethical challenges which, because context specific, need to be individually negotiated. Rather than rely on professional ethical codes to guide us through this process, I argue that it is essential that researchers grapple *reflexively* with the ethical problems and uncertainties that arise (Finlay, 2009c).

As ethical phenomenological researchers we celebrate efforts to embrace research that listens to, and values, the other's 'voice' while we also acknowledge the complexities involved. The process of gaining informed consent and maintaining co-researchers trust and goodwill, particularly when the research involves sensitive subjects and/or vulnerable people, invariably challenges.

I appreciate, too, the complexity of the power relations involved where power is never one-way and always enacted in subtle and multilayered ways. However, I believe that by giving up some of our control as researchers, we open ourselves to new possibilities.

It behoves us to use our researcher power wisely and ethically while acknowledging both the limits of our research and its potential to broaden understanding and add to the sum of human knowledge. As Krüger (2007, p. 21) says, 'To live with this inherent power is to enter the realm of ethics. The only way of surviving as a true professional is to . . . live with the paradox: to behave ethically and exert power – simultaneously.'

Note

[i] Material in this chapter has been drawn from chapter 10 of Finlay and Evans (2009) and has been reproduced here with kind permission of the publishers Wiley-Blackwell.

Chapter 15

The Process of Analysing Data

Something new has entered us, something unknown; our feelings grow
mute in shy embarrassment, everything in us withdraws, a silence arises.
(Rilke, 1904)

Novice researchers can fall into the trap of spending huge amounts of
time and energy on data collection – for example carrying out the interviews as though that is the real research. In fact, the most significant
part of the research comes with the labour-intensive phase of process-
ing data and analysing meanings. Too often novice researchers skip su-
perficially over data; for instance, simply reporting what was said in the
interview. This misses a potentially wondrous opportunity to engage a
phenomenon deeply.

From the chapters in Part II, you will have seen that there is no one way to
do phenomenological analysis: analysis varies according to the phenomenological approach embraced. It also varies with the type of data collected,
the researcher's own predilections and what is required of them by others. Some analytic approaches emphasize scientific rigour and a careful,
systematic working through of the data; others emphasize fluid, intuitive,
evolving, dynamic presentations. Some approaches try to represent and
stay as close to the data as possible; others prefer to pursue more explicitly
interpretive versions.

Phenomenology for Therapists: Researching the Lived World, First Edition. Linda Finlay.
© 2011 Linda Finlay. Published 2011 by John Wiley & Sons, Ltd.

Whatever the approach taken the phenomenological researcher must make sense of the data and synthesize it in such a way that participants' voices (or other data) are adequately re-presented and the phenomenon is opened up for the reader. With all phenomenological analysis, the focus is on pulling out explicit and hidden meanings through iteratively examining the data. Engaging this process involves researchers 'dwelling' with the data, examining it and then progressively deepening understandings as meanings come to light. The analysis process is often a messy one, involving both imaginative leaps of **intuition** as well as systematic working through of many **iterative** versions. Early versions often bear little resemblance to the neatly packaged themes we see outlined eventually in research papers.[i]

In the first section of this chapter, I offer some general tips for 'engaging analysis' (in both senses of the phrase). Then I outline the four general types of analytic forms that phenomenologists tend to employ: narrative, thematic, reflexive and creative. We have a choice about how to present (re-present) our analysis and so I offer some brief critical reflections on each analytic form.

In practice, analyses may not be so cleanly delineated and several types might be usefully combined. (In my own work I frequently combine narrative, thematic and reflexive analysis, for instance.) As you study the examples offered, you will see that the different types of analysis highlight different aspects of the data and enable different insights. Each method reveals certain aspects or dimensions while concealing or de-emphasizing others. Different interpretations assume figural significance against a ground of possible meanings; choice of analysis can be seen to shape emergent understandings. Any one analysis, says Churchill (2000, p. 164), can only be presented as a 'tentative statement opening upon a limitless field of possible interpretations'.

Engaging Analysis

The good and the bad news is that there are no clear-cut recipes explaining how to engage phenomenological analysis, although guidelines are available (see *Chapters 6–11*). It is reassuring to know there is no one right way (good news) even while it can be more daunting to start the analysis (bad news). You have permission to evolve the approach that works for you. That said, I offer below some general statements about what makes for better, richer, deeper analyses. Dwelling, wonder, evidencing and ambivalence are key watch words both for 'engaging in analysis' and for ensuring the 'analysis is engaging'.

Dwelling

It is important with phenomenological analysis to take time to dwell with the raw data such that *implicit*, layered meanings come to the fore. The process involves a focused act of discovering sedimented meanings, nuance and texture out of silence. The more you stop and linger, the more you will feel yourself engaging the phenomenon, perhaps re-experiencing the sense of it. 'When we stop and linger with something, it secretes its sense and it's full significance becomes... amplified' (Wertz, 1985, p. 174).

At its best, the process of doing the analysis becomes an *embodied lived experience* in itself. It is not just a cognitive, intellectual exercise. When I am well immersed in an analysis I am there sensing, moving, empathizing, responding and resonating with my whole body-self. In a sense I am re-living the experiential accounts and 're-membering' (re-embodying) what was said.

The process of engaging the data is similar to the way psychotherapists nurture their awareness and understanding of a client. Moustakas even suggests his heuristic research methodology can be used in psychotherapy:

> To truly know this person in the stirrings and deepenings of heart and mind, the therapist must not pressure, direct, or control, but rather must wait and permit awarenesses and meanings to generate in their own time. (1990, pp. 109–110)

One practical and immediate way to dwell with the data is to consider **transcribing** interviews oneself (or take time with transcribing reflective field notes). Too often researchers seek to save time and outsource this job. It is a laborious process but I suggest that it provides an opportunity to hear the interview again and to remind oneself of tone and other non-verbal noises or silences which are so useful when grappling with implicit meanings.

Apart from doing the transcription, take the analysis slowly, expecting to take many passes at it. It can help to engage analytical steps, for instance those recommended by Wertz in *Chapter 6*. My particular approach is to start by aiming to **empathize** through repeatedly listening to the participant's description of their world and trying to get a feel for their situation. Then I linger over **selected passages** or chunks of data (for example, focusing on powerful or puzzling passages) in order to begin to divine what certain aspects mean to the participant. I would suggest that it is easier if you are selective here – feel free to ignore portions of the interview or observation that are not particularly relevant to your project focus. At the same time it is important to stay with the data, and even the literal words, rather than jump too quickly into premature analysis and interpretation. It is particularly important to avoid importing theoretical ideas in at this early stage.

From there, I take a **step back** and begin to think, with real interest, about where the participant is, how he/she got there, what it means to be there, and so on. Here you are trying to focus on the way the situation appears to the participant. Sometimes it helps to interrogate the analysis using lifeworld orientated questions such as:

- What does it mean to be this person? Who does s/he think s/he is? What does s/he think about? (self-identity)
- What is his/her subjective sense of embodiment? (embodiment)
- Where does he/she experience his/her day? Are some places safer than others? Does he/she feel closed in? Is there a feeling of 'insidedness'/'outsidedness'? (spatiality)
- How does s/he experience his/her day? Is it pressured, rushed and speeding by? Boringly slow and endless? Discontinuous? (temporality)
- How does s/he experience relating to others? Who are the significant people involved and how are their relationships impacted? (relationships)
- What drives the person? What motivates them? What gives their life meaning? (project)
- Is there any discourse/language being used that seems significant and reveals either personal or shared cultural meanings? (discourse)
- Is there a mood/tone attached to the phenomenon? What background 'existential feelings' are being expressed such as 'feeling distant', 'fretful', 'fulfilled', 'cynical' or 'yearning'? ('mood as atmosphere')

Embracing an attitude of wonder

Rather than plodding through transcripts in the hope of accounting for every last word said, seek out the parts that resonate for you; where something said seems particularly significant or is interesting, surprising, quirky, poignant, special or paradoxical in some way. It is easy to lose the gestalt, the wood for the trees, and in the process be swamped by the data. When this happens, it can help to stand back and think, 'What are the three most pertinent issues emerging about this experience?' or 'Were there any particularly powerful moments in the encounter?' As you follow the data where do you get touched or hooked or puzzled or surprised? Then wonder about these experiences in awe, curiosity and focused reflection.

Van Manen describes the process of adopting wonder as part of the phenomenological attitude so that it shatters our taken-for-granted views of our world.

> Wonder is the unwilling willingness to meet what is utterly strange in what is most familiar . . . We are confronted by the thing, the phenomenon, in all of its strangeness and uniqueness. (van Manen, 2002)

Embracing an attitude of wonder can involve a kind of 'epistemological earthquake' where we 'arrive at the world as if for the first time . . . The more we reflect and wonder – the deeper the wonder seems to grow and the more enigmatic the world and life seem to be' (Hansen, 2010, p. 172).

Evidencing the analysis

While phenomenological writings can sometimes take flight into literary prose, when we do phenomenological *research* we usually need to ground our analysis empirically in data. Here we might utilize participants' words from interviews or we might simply focus on a concrete example of lived, everyday experience.

Smith offers advice for IPA researchers when he cautions that the analysis needs to be 'plausible and persuasive' in terms of the evidence presented to support the claims made:

> Extracts should be selected to give some indication of convergence and divergence, representativeness and variability. This way the reader gets to see the breadth and depth of the theme. (Smith, in press)

He goes on to recommend that for papers with small sample sizes (1–3 participants) each theme is supported with extracts from each participant. For papers with sample sizes of 4–8, he suggests extracts from half the participants is considered appropriate evidence. While this advice relates specifically to interpretative phenomenological analysis (IPA), the idea of evidencing claims in some way holds for all qualitative research approaches.

The following is an example of how a phenomenological description might be 'evidenced' using the voices of participants. This extract comes from a study I collaboratively embarked on with Virginia Eatough on the 'experience of connecting with a kindred spirit' (Eatough & Finlay, 2009). Example 15.1 describes kindred spirits' feelings related to *falling in love*.

Example 15.1   Falling in love

With love, there is a palpable embodied response to the connection and attraction – a sense of the heart being captured (hooked). The other stands out from the crowd and may evoke sexual fantasies and/or feelings of falling in love. As the *heart flips* there is a sense of feeling alive and one feels a change in surroundings/ambience as the world feels brighter, more beautiful. As one person expressed:

> I felt my heart flip when he smiled at me. To be fair he was probably smiling at everyone that way. But it felt special as if to me alone; as if my soul was being warmed. (participant no. 10)

There is a flowering in the presence of the other; of being enhanced by the other. The other makes one feel special. There is a sense of 'glow' and opening of body/mind/soul, being warmed by the other as a flower is warmed by sun and rain. There is a sense of fittingness with the other, a sense of the 'rightness' of the connection. The other is both comfortably safe and feels the same as one while being exciting and challenging in their difference.

> I felt so 'whole'. . . each time I spoke I felt heard and met and honoured by S . . . I so enjoyed my sense of myself growing fuller in her presence . . . And in our sharing there was a sense of profound togetherness, perhaps like two figures, side by side, looking into a deep wondrous pool of water, and seeing their reflections merging in the ripples into one . . . each knowing they are separate, but at the same time feeling profound 'togetherness' in a place beyond. (participant no. 11)

And, there is a yearning to be replenished by the other; a need to somehow maintain the connection and/or contact in whatever way or means possible, along with a sense of loss when the other is absent.

> I met what I want, who I want. She is not for the having. But now met I ache for the loss. (participant no. 2)

Capturing ambivalence

The best phenomenological accounts capture the ambiguity, ambivalences and paradoxes of human experience. Rarely, if ever, is an experience simple or clear-cut; our emotions are invariably mixed, our experience layered. It is precisely this complexity that we need to try to tap in our analysis. It is here that poignancy and resonance is found.

An example of how phenomenology can capture ambiguity is offered by Dahlberg in her account of 'loneliness' when she says:

> Loneliness is the figure against a background of commonality; being-alone is the other side of being-with; loneliness is intertwined with togetherness. This understanding of existence gives us a more ambiguous picture. (2007, p. 206)

Dahlberg explains that a person can be lonely in the presence of others yet not feel lonely when alone. She suggests fostering a secret place of loneliness where we can let go of stressful human relationships and welcome dialogues with ourselves and nature, going beyond ourselves. Such a space may have the power to enable better health and well-being.

Palaian (1993, cited in Moustakas, 1994, p. 151) offers another example of how ambivalence can be embraced within an analysis. The extract in Example 15.2 comes from her study of the 'experience of longing'.

Example 15.2   The experience of longing

The experience of longing is a paradoxical experience . . . Longing turns in on itself. One reaches out across an expanse toward fulfilment in trust and hope. In the reaching out pain and loss are experienced as an imminent yearning for fulfilment. Longing is the grief of the unattainable . . . It is the hope toward possibility and infinite entrancement. Both despair and promise exist together in longing, rhythms of death and birth . . . Longing is at the interface of the losses of yesterday, the open wounds of separation, and the joyful creations of tomorrow. Longing hurts so desperately and still it continues; still the hunger, and the itch arises within.

After you have dwelt with the data with an open, wondering attitude and then developed some idea of the important issues and textured nuances at stake, it is time to turn to consider how best to shape and re-present your analysis. Here you might use thematic, narrative, creative or reflexive analytic forms.

Thematic Analysis

Thematic analysis is a method for analysing and describing important patterns (themes) within data (Braun & Clarke, 2006). Most qualitative methodologies, phenomenology included, incorporate elements of thematic analysis. For some methodologies this is just the initial step in finding sequences for in-depth analysis. Other methods specify their own sophisticated procedures for identifying and working with themes. Braun and Clarke (2006) provide a step-by-step guide to typical phases:

- Familiarizing yourself with your data;
- Generating initial codes;
- Searching for themes;
- Reviewing themes;
- Defining and naming themes;
- Producing the report.

It is often said that themes 'emerge from data'. While it is true that themes need to be grounded in and reflect the data, the idea that they somehow pop out and are self-evident is not true. It does not do to sit waiting passively for themes to arrive. Mostly, meanings have to be searched for as they are implicit and themes have to be painstakingly shaped up in successive iterations.

Haumann (2005) makes this point when she describes the way she interrogated her data on psychotherapists' experiences of their personal journey in her phenomenologically inspired study. In the initial phase of textual analysis she used *intersubjectivity* theory to generate a conceptual framework. This underscored the shifting power distributions and identification processes. The Jungian notion of the *wounded healer* was used as a key theme to draw attention to the way therapists relate to patients as objects rather than subjects. The effects of personal therapy were then understood in terms of enhanced abilities to relate person to person and for reflective thinking. The final stage of analysis involved generating an intersubjective *model* of personal therapy and development.

While Haumann used psychotherapy theories as her lens through which to analyse data, other pre-set frameworks can similarly be used to interrogate data and structure an analysis. An analysis might, for instance, be effected using **lifeworld concepts** as themes of embodiment, self-identity, sense of time/space, relations with others and so on (Ashworth, 2003). Take, for example, my collaborative research with Pat Molano-Fisher (Finlay & Molano-Fisher, 2008) about her experience of receiving a cochlear implant after 50 years of being profoundly deaf. We analysed her story in terms of three themes: (i) **embodiment**: disrupted body–world interconnection; (ii) **sociality**: disconnection and a sense of shame; (iii) **mood as atmosphere**: feeling 'alien' and 'alienated'. (See Example 1.1 for a summary of the overall research findings.)

Example 15.3 is part of the 'mood-as-atmosphere' theme. Of particular interest is Pat's sense of being an 'outsider' – her *not-at-home* feeling (Heidegger's notion of *unheimlich*). Note how the analysis implicitly intertwines with other lifeworld fractions of disrupted selfhood, embodiment, self–other relations and spatiality.

Example 15.3   Mood-as-atmosphere: feeling alienated

Assaulted by the surreal noisiness of the world and finding her relations with others disrupted, Pat feels a disconnection from her world. People's voices – including those of her husband and children, the individuals with whom she is most intimate – sound alien to her. At the same time she is fearful of her own alien-ness – a state which she associates with losing control.

> When I saw films where the aliens abducted people and then put a switch on them I was even more affected because I tried to envisage the switch on me ... I laughed at the jokes friends did about getting sucked by the magnet into a high lamppost ... In between the jokes there was the fear of changing so much and being under a control of a computer, of hospitals and audiologists and the country itself.

Sensing the strangeness, weirdness even, of both herself and of others, Pat experiences anxiety, fear and a desire to withdraw. Slowly she works through her mixed emotions. However, she never fully recaptures the openness to others she had experienced previously. As she puts it, 'Now, except for work, family and few very close friends I have withdrawn quite a bit from social contact.'

While Pat is not suffering from any illness, she feels 'ill at ease' with her new implant ... At the same time, her new experiences allow her the opportunity to question her existence and open up the possibility for new authentic Being. (Finlay & Molano-Fisher, 2008, p. 264)

The eventual form taken by themes can vary, but a good thematic analysis is one that does more than string together extracts from the research. Instead, it will seek to identify and synthesize themes that are **coherent**, convincing and grounded in the data (Braun & Clarke, 2006). Ideally, themes should be more than ordinary category headings: they should also be interesting, written in a lively style or they should **resonate** in some way.

Consider, for example, Avis' (2010) use of metaphors when she describes the process of being and becoming a client as part of training to be a counselling psychologist. One theme of 'being and becoming a trainee client' included several sub-themes:

A)   Peforming – being the 'good client' and 'good therapist';
B)   Masked self – awareness of therapeutic rules could impede process;
C)   Forced self – being a reluctant client;
D)   Lifting the mask – from 'inhibited trainee' to 'letting go'.

Themes that capture layers or **polarities** are also evocative. For instance, Ken Evans and I collaborated on research exploring psychotherapists' perspectives on statutory regulation (Evans & Finlay, 2009). Four emergent, interlinked themes were found: 'feeling proud–feeling shame'; 'belonging–isolation'; 'credibility–ineligibility'; 'fight–flight'.

More than just naming themes, however, the skill lies in describing and explicating (i.e. explaining meanings). Example 15.4 offers a brief demonstration of how this might be done. Here, Fitzpatrick and Finlay (2008) explored the lived experience of the rehabilitation phase following flexor tendon surgery. In this rehabilitation, participants were required to complete an hourly exercise regime and wear a splint constantly for 4–6 weeks. Three themes were identified overall: 'battling–retreating', 'denying–accepting' and 'struggling–adapting'. The first of our themes is reproduced here as a taster. Note how both individual examples and outside theoretical references are woven into the description.

Example 15.4   The lived experience of the rehabilitation phase following surgery: 'retreating–battling'

'Illness', says Toombs (1993, p. 96), 'is a state of disharmony, disequilibrium, dis-ability and dis-ease which incorporates *a loss of the familiar world*'. The trauma of the original injury and surgery is followed by the dawning awareness of multiple losses; despair and anxiety accompany the realization of dis-ability. The loss of function, of confidence and motivation, of daily roles and activities, and of taken-for-granted physical safety, all push the individual to retreat from the life they once lived.

The result is a diminishment, a shrinking of life. Without everyday roles and activities, life's landscape feels barren and boring . . . John retreats from socializing with his family and playing his sports. Jane abandons the final term of her college, putting her life and her future on hold . . .

At some point, the retreat must be halted if rehabilitation is to be successful. So, the battle begins. The individual takes a stand to fight, to get through, to subdue the enemy (the injury, the pain, the disability). The injured person moves forward, determinedly and positively re-engaging with life. Helped by his wife 'out of love' to do his exercises, John finds that this support fuels his determination to 'beat the injury'. (Fitzpatrick & Finlay, 2008, p. 149)

Thematic analysis offers the opportunity to highlight important conceptual features or nuances of lived experience. Yet, as themes open up possibilities, other avenues are closed. Researchers need to be cautious about offering an account of 'general themes' and asserting that they fit all their participants. The particular voices and experiences of the individuals studied can blur or retreat into the background, with some individuals' experiences being more strongly reflected in the themes than others. The themes can also become somewhat inflexible and may not sufficiently reflect the evolving nature of participants' experiences. To help balance these limitations it can help to supplement thematic analysis with narrative accounts. (When I do case study research, for example, I will often start with the narrative and then home in on significant lifeworldly themes.)

Narrative Analysis

Narratives can be presented in different ways. Commonly, the researcher tells a participant's 'story' about particular life events or experiences, following the participant's own **chronology**. This chronology may extend over years or just recognize the person's experience *before, during* and *after* an event. Researchers then have the option to engage in some form of **secondary analysis**: for instance, employing theoretical frames or examining the narrative genre or type of story (for example, a 'heroic quest story'[ii]) and identifying relevant themes, scripts and metaphors. In other words, the narrative involves both a person's story and a method of inquiry where the researcher reconstructs that story.

The precise tenor and tone of the narrative analysis varies considerably across different qualitative methodologies (Reissman, 1993). Example 15.5 offers a taste of what a phenomenologically orientated narrative analysis might encompass. This extract has been taken from a fuller published account of Kenny's *occupational narrative*[iii] (Finlay & McKay, 2004). It is based on my interview with Kenny and described in *Chapter 13* showing how researchers might move from data collection to analysis phases.

Example 15.5   Kenny's story

Rock bottom: Five years ago Kenny was a 'gibbering idiot' – he had hit 'rock bottom': 'I was absolutely terrified. I was jumping at me own shadow . . . I was just shaking the whole time, having panic attacks. I locked myself in the bedroom. It took weeks and weeks before I would go out. I would read, submerge myself in books, escape. I wasn't interested in anything. I just wanted to be in my bed.'

Doing something: Suddenly one morning, something in his head shifted . . . He recognized how destructive it had been to have 'done nothing' for so long. 'I was beginning to feel useless', he admitted. He made the decision that day that he was going to get back into work somehow. That was the beginning of his recovery. (Finlay & McKay, 2004, pp. 30–31)

Narrative analysis

Kenny's story is a chronological account of his illness and journey back to health and work. This progressive occupational narrative (Braverman *et al.*, 2003) is a simple story – not particularly dramatic or unusual. Kenny tells of everyday experiences and ordinary events. He speaks of the value of occupation and a special relationship with an understanding employer. His story can also be understood as a quest story (Frank, 1998) in that Kenny seems to have framed his illness as a condition from which something can be learned and passed on to others. His quest was to find meaning and purpose in his mental health problems and to re-emerge stronger with new qualities and insights: with a new identity in fact. The life Kenny has re-claimed has involved compromise and sacrifice. He shares his victory while recognizing its provisional status . . .

Primarily Kenny's story is one of survival and self-discovery (Davies, 2001). In such narratives individuals heroically emerge from difficult experiences to share their story . . . We hear something of Kenny's fight to regain control and how he progressed from being a 'gibbering idiot' to becoming an 'iceman' who can master stressful situations without getting ruffled . . . Being able to successfully 'kick down' each new hurdle empowers Kenny and gives him more confidence. (Finlay, 2004, p. 478)

Narratives offer a way into individuals' life stories in all their particularity and richness. Through hearing individuals' voices we are reminded to honour and witness their experience – to truly listen. Through the story we hear how experience unfolds over time rather than being presented as a static theme.

While research narratives are usually grounded in participants' words and may be presented as reflecting the individuals' reality, their constructed nature needs to be emphasized. Researchers need to take care to distinguish between a life story that is lived and one that is told and then re-told by a researcher. Individuals present what they want to be known about themselves (Reissman, 2003) and then via the co-created dialogue between participant and researcher, the narrative is re-versioned. The story heard, interpreted, analysed and re-told by one researcher is likely to be different from one by another.

Reflexive Analysis

The aim of reflexive analysis is to examine, critically and in a self-aware way, how the researcher, the context and the relationship between researcher and participants have influenced the data gathered and findings.

The examples below show how we have a choice as researchers about the extent we engage reflexivity. Do we just offer a paragraph or two contextualizing the research process or is there value in engaging reflexivity in a sustained way? Equally, it is possible to turn an entire piece of writing/presentation into a reflexive piece. The autobiographical examples in *Chapter 10* are a case in point. See also Etherington (2004) who devotes a book to reflexive writing (her own and others).

In Example 15.6, Virginia Eatough (2009) offers a hermeneutic analysis of the embodied experience of being angry. In a study firmly anchored in phenomenological philosophy, she brings her reflections back to her own horizons of experience showing that the exercise of being reflexive can, itself, enable or reveal insights about the phenomenon being focused on.

Example 15.6   A hermeneutic account of the embodied experience of being angry

The women's descriptions of what it is like to be angry brought to the fore the body's involvement in our emotional experiences. They conveyed this through compelling images of heat, explosiveness and internal turmoil . . .

When Marilyn said of her mother 'she petrified me just with a dirty look' my immersion in that experience enabled me to recall times when my mother gave me such looks, experiences which live with me to this day. Reliving and re-imagining those experiences brought me closer to Marilyn's and gave rise to a better understanding of how she felt. Retreating from both our experiences I reflected upon Marilyn's use of the word 'petrify' with its implications of being stunned or paralysed with terror. I thought about this in the context of the stormy relationships we had with our mothers. I theorized that Marilyn's sense of self was threatened with potential obliteration. This tentative interpretation might be something Marilyn would be unable or unwilling to consider. It is a result of my reflections from a distance, yet it was borne out of my empathic engagement with Marilyn's words. (Eatough, 2009, p. 195)

In Example 15.7, Puig (2010) examines some of her own process and responses when conducting her study on counselling psychologists' experience of working with refugees and asylum seekers. Through her re-flections she gained some insights into her participants' experience of pain, trauma and helplessness and how they coped with their work.

Example 15.7   Researcher reflections on a study exploring counselling psychologists' experiences of working with refugees and asylum seekers

On reflection I chose the research topic with some naivety, not really knowing what to expect from the interviews . . . Participants' accounts were heavily laden with pain, trauma and helplessness and it was some-times hard to stay with the transcripts. I found myself cutting off at points and skipping words and phrases as my own defence, often having to return to sections again. It was as though a parallel process was oc-curring and I was experiencing the pain of my participants as they spoke of their overwhelming feelings. Upon analysing the transcripts I realised this also occurred during the interviews. I sometimes asked more head level questions such as: 'Which model do you work with?' which yielded more cognitive answers rather than emotional material . . . Even so, par-ticipants still gave rich accounts and this was interesting to reflect upon as it seemed this avoidance is often what participants experienced with their clients. (Puig, 2010, p. 119)

Example 15.8 is taken from the research by Ken Evans and myself (Evans & Finlay, 2009) on psychotherapists' experience of professional statutory regulation. It combines both critical evaluation of the research process and personal reflection on the topic. We express our surprise at the power of unconscious processes which seemed to be enacted during our data col-lection. Specifically, we noted how the shame experiences being talked about in our focus group seemed to parallel the shame in the wider professional field.

Example 15.8   A reflexive account of investments in research

When Ken had initially suggested, rather apologetically, that the focus group convene in the lunch hour, so as to limit any disruption of the per-sonal and professional development remit of the group. All other partic-ipants expressed their preference to include the focus group exploration in the scheduled work time. Subsequently, while sharing two historical experiences of feeling marginalised Ken expressed shock, amazement and anger as he realised that he had internalised the oppression of these historical experiences. He had been trapped within a parallel process whereby he mirrored his own sense of marginalisation by unwittingly marginalising the focus group by suggesting that it be subsumed within a lunch break, outside the main agenda! This was a . . . dramatic example of the influence of unconscious forces on the research endeavour. (Evans & Finlay, 2009, p. 11

As the examples above show, reflexive analysis needs to be done in such a way that it contributes to the understanding of lived experience or provides a critical framework through which to evaluate the research. Importantly, reflexivity is not 'an opportunity to wallow in subjectivity nor permission to engage in legitimised emoting' (Finlay, 1998b, p. 455). The best reflexive analysis uses personal revelation not as an end in itself but as a springboard for interpretations and more general insight.[iv]

Thinking about the value of reflexivity, I agree with 'Peter' (cited in Etherington, 2004, p. 231) when he says:

I suppose the greatest gift I have gained from reflexivity is a healing of the split between research and practice. I am the same person, with the same mind and the same heart wherever I am. The discipline of research is just that. It can help me to be rigorous but it doesn't need to privatize my brain or to sequester my heart.

Creative Analysis

Creative forms of analysis – like reflexive forms – challenge the goals and format of traditional academic, scientific research. Creative analysis includes the use of poetry, prose, drama, visual arts and dance to express or represent the voice of researcher and/or co-researchers and to illustrate the lived experience being studied. In this sense, creative analysis can be a way of 'giving voice' to participants, as well as a way of handling data and presenting research findings about the phenomenon itself. Researchers may set out explicitly to use alternative forms to juxtapose, disrupt or challenge taken-for-granted assumptions. The aim underlying the use of creative media – mirroring the processes used in the arts generally – is to evoke and resonate; possibly even to unsettle or shock. At the same time, a heart-felt, soul-full creative process may itself inspire new expressions and insights.

Unsurprisingly with such creative approaches, the lines between 'fiction' and 'fact' may be fuzzy. Similarly, the process of data gathering, analysis and writing up (or publicly sharing one's work) is often blurred. There are no 'rules' in this genre.

In Example 15.9, Shields (1998) offers an account of her personal research inquiry into beauty, body image and the feminine; blending heuristic, feminist, first-person phenomenological, transpersonal and organic approaches.

Example 15.9   Integrated feminist creativity

Shields describes how she had felt negatively about her appearance all her life. Coming from a long line of beautiful women, she felt she was the 'ugly duckling' who had not met family expectations. She wanted to gain a deeper understanding of what physical attractiveness meant to her and so chose beauty and body image as a topic of inquiry. She followed her intuitions arising in her *dreams* about how to proceed with the research. She eventually collected 15 hours of *dialogue* with her mother and grandmother.

When writing up her dissertation, she eschewed standard report formats and, instead, presented the dialogues in their original forms and gave accounts of her dreams using different kinds of fonts. She also included photographs of her female lineage. Looking back, she describes how her relationships with her mother and grandmother have been significantly deepened. For her, the research had been a *transformational* experience which continues today. She writes, 'It has been gratifying to hear that many women have been moved to tears when reading my dissertation.' (Shields, 1998, p. 198)

In Example 15.10, Galvin and Todres (2009) offer a poem to capture an 'alive' sense of the experience of caring for a partner with Alzheimer's. They call their approach 'embodied interpretation' – a poetic, hermeneutic way of re-representing other peoples' experiences based on Gendlin's practice of drawing on 'felt sense'. Galvin and Todres note the short step from phenomenology to poetry:

> The eros of poetry spoke to a certain aesthetic motive that we found had been excessively left out in the research world to which we were socialised . . . We want to do the kind of qualitative research that communicates human experiences in ways that people can really feel and relate to . . . Such entry into alive meanings is not something that can be actively constructed by effort, but rather requires the kind of receptivity of the lived body that 'lets be,' in a bodily participative way. (Galvin & Todres, 2009, pp. 309, 311)

Example 15.10   The experience of caring for a partner with Alzheimer's

To see one loved so much,
change in this way? . . . No!
It is so natural to refuse that this is happening; her memory can function
as before.
How deep is the urge to want to stop it?
It deserves at least an angry 'No'
a great refusal
A denial in any way that is possible.
At times
it is also a sinking feeling
A 'nausea'of awareness that relentlessly breaks through.
His being sickened by her saying something over
and over
and over again
He needs to temper this: her memory loss can't be stopped
anger towards self, her, professionals.
but his is not enough
Helplessness dawns.
Saying 'no' to her memory loss heightens their struggle.
She feels pressurized
Upset
He feels remorse, such deep remorse carries a dawning
trying to deny that her memory . . .
that she is seeping away
Just does not work. (Galvin & Todres, 2009, p. 307)

Creative analysis – in whatever form – can evoke, resonate and offer new ways of looking at a topic. Potentially powerful art forms they may be, but what is their status? What relation do they bear, if any, to rigorous scientific methods of inquiry? Is there a danger that researchers (and participants) may get caught up in the artistic endeavour, with its soaring flights of metaphoric imagination, while in the process losing sight of the phenomenon being researched? Alternatively, might amateurish attempts at artistic expression lose something in the telling? Such questions continue to dog this intriguing, if controversial, approach to analysis.

Reflections

My personal advice for novice researchers embarking on phenomenological analysis is to seek – in whatever way works – richness in complexity, depth in ambivalence and poignancy in paradox. Also, I would encourage you to model on good examples of analysis while having faith in your own hunches and embracing your own preferences.

Phenomenological analysis is always challenging. It is easy to feel overwhelmed with the quantity and complexity of data that needs to be analysed. In my PhD research, for instance, I had a 12-inch pile of transcripts and reflective field notes to tackle! One way to handle such quantities of data is to analyse small chunks at a time; for instance, do some analysis after each interview. It might also help to know that you can return to your data at a later time to re-analyse, taking a different slant.

Whichever analytic approach or approaches we choose to use, we need to remember that it will only offer a selective glimpse. However powerful, comprehensive and nuanced, our findings must remain tentative, partial and emergent. It is always possible to see more in data at a different point in time, and another researcher will usually unfold a different story. Modesty, rather than grand claims to 'truth' or 'self-evident' findings, lies at the heart of qualitative research. Further explication is always possible.

Given the complex, opaque, ambivalent and ambiguous nature of human experience, it is challenging to make sense of our social world or of an individual's confused expressions and experiences. Analysis, in my view, should be judged not on its ability to present 'answers' but rather on its capacity to capture something of this 'mess'. The key question is: does the analysis bring the phenomenon to life?

Notes

[i] For more detailed guidance on how to do particular types of analysis I recommend going to specific articles, chapters and books which highlight and work through particular methods. I particularly recommend Wertz (in press), Smith *et al.* (2009) and Langdridge (2008).

[ii] Frank (1995) classifies illness narratives into three main types: 'chaos narratives'; 'restitution narratives'; and 'quest narratives'. He cautions against using these mechanically, however: 'stories are not material to be analysed; they are relationships to be entered' (p. 200). For further information on these and other types of narratives see, for instance: http://www.dulwichcentre.com.au/illness-narratives.html.

[iii] Kielhofner *et al.* (2002) discuss the relevance of **occupational narratives** for occupational therapy. These narratives are the stories told and enacted which integrate 'unfolding volition, habituation, performance capacity, and environments through plots and metaphors that sum up and assign meaning to these elements. Both our identity and our competence are reflected and enacted in the stories which we make sense of and go about doing in our occupational lives' (2002, p. 127).

[iv] Often the greatest challenge of engaging in reflexive analysis is finding the space to display it in published articles where there are severe word count constraints and the

attention (rightly) has to be kept on the phenomenon being researched rather than the process. However, it is possible for researchers to embrace reflexivity fully at all stages of the research – without necessarily displaying the whole process in any one article. Researchers might simply choose to acknowledge their presence and position in a paragraph under the 'methodology' section or alternatively, researchers might be reflexive in their 'discussion' or 'evaluation' sections to demonstrate rigour or trustworthiness. These strategies of using reflexivity as method and in evaluation can be accommodated in most journal articles. And, sometimes, it is possible – even desirable – to go further.

Chapter 16

Producing the Research[i]

The wonder of that thing takes us in, and renders us momentarily speechless ... It ... should challenge the researcher to write in such a way that the reader of the phenomenological text is similarly stirred to the same sense of wondering attentiveness to the topic under investigation. (van Manen, 2002)

The end is nigh – or is it? The analysis is done; themes, narratives and findings are in place ... You have reflected deeply on your research ... What next? How do you form and shape your research into something meaningful, something digestible by others?

'Birthing a baby' comes to mind ... You are feeling full, heavy, clumsy, nervous, blocked up, unsure and waiting ... the gestation is virtually complete and labour pains have started ... Just how are you going to produce this 'baby' – this *voice* – that has been so hard to conceive and grow?

Birth brings with it a radical transition between two worlds. The by now cramped and completely filled space of the uterus narrows even more ... and the baby is squeezed and pushed through the birth canal ... the walls of the birth canal close up around the baby and mould skull and limbs into the shape of the passage ... This must be the first time that the human being experiences the encroachment of the world, the push of forces against the boundary of the skin that was there but heretofore never felt. And then, after the crowning, the infant emerges into the coolness, brightness, clearness, and expansiveness of [the world] ... The first breath draws inward, and the voice emerges in a cry. (Simms, 2008a, p. 33)

Phenomenology for Therapists: Researching the Lived World, First Edition. Linda Finlay.
© 2011 Linda Finlay. Published 2011 by John Wiley & Sons, Ltd.

Perhaps the biggest challenge for a phenomenological researcher is how to produce the findings in a way that portrays participants' experience in all their complexity. How are we to develop descriptions that are faithful to the phenomenon and can evoke the embodied lived world? How are we to express our findings in ways that are graceful, poignant and elegant (Polkinghorne, 1983) yet achieve communicative resonance? How are we to going to offer relevant arguments to convince a wider audience of the value and interest of our work? Alternatively, what is a 'good enough' piece of work or, if you are a student, what constitutes a 'pass'?

Qualitative human science research in general – and phenomenological research in particular – presents a range of problems and choices which have to be worked with if the complex nature of the findings and their implications are to be expressed, to say nothing of demonstrating the rigour and trustworthiness of the research. These issues provide the focus for this and the next chapter which is concerned with evaluating the quality of research. This chapter discusses the process of 'producing research' in terms of five overlapping processes:

- Pulling it together;
- Marshalling your evidence;
- Developing your argument;
- Writing up;
- 'Re-presenting' the research.

Pulling it Together

This stage of pulling our findings (and perhaps ourselves!) together is often the most challenging. With no easy map or clear-cut route to follow it is easy to lose sense of direction. Surrounded by transcripts and piles of paper it is easy to feel overwhelmed. Is it possible to adequately re-present our research and journey? 'Shame' can kick in at this moment, telling us we are not up to the task or that we have nothing of value to say. If writing itself is a problem we can become blocked, perhaps with old 'scripts' giving us cause to doubt ourselves.

> My Creativity . . . is cat-like, not your domestic moggy, but pre-human, prowl-ing, tearing at flesh with long sharp teeth. It feeds on everything and anything, alive or dead. It devours, voracious in its appetite. No secret or embarrass-ment or ill-loved tendency can escape its notice. So it grows and grows on tender sweet meats and blood pudding.
>
> Sometimes it can look beautiful, sleek, clever as it weaves between oaks and elders and copper birches. But on closer examination, the muck sticks to its tangled fur . . . it stinks, of fear, terror that it will be shot down by a

flaming arrow shot by those who, in turn, fear its coming. The arrows are tipped with poison: 'Is that it?' or 'Why can't you write like X? I hear she had difficulty getting a publisher at first too' or 'That's very nice dear'. Worse are the taunts that come from the inside: what's the point, this is no good anyway and no-one appreciates me!

The arrows and derision cannot kill – not entirely – but once wounded the creature retires to its stinking lair and sulks, sometimes only coming out during the inconveniently early hours of the morning. (Personal communication with Kate Evans)

Fischer offers some valuable advice when feeling this shame and getting 'lost':

Phenomenology is the method that makes the apparent obvious . . . Our findings often will . . . seem quite mundane . . . the 'Oh, I knew that' variety. But in fact, before our research, we did not comprehend them in a full way nor in a way that was useful for other people . . . It is . . . a good idea to track formally surprises, revisions, and discoveries of your misassumptions as you go. This record reminds you that you are not making up what you find. (Fischer, 2006, pp. xxxiv–xxxv)

At this stage it can help to take a step back and ask, 'What are the key findings, surprises and/or points of interest that have emerged?' You have permission now to be **selective**. Focus on, say, three key ideas and themes or a handful of particularly suitable or powerful quotes. You do not have to report everything. Just give your readers/examiners/audience a *sense* of what that experience is like – what the lived world feels like.

Find a **story-line**. For instance, when doing my research with Pat on her lived experience of having a cochlear implant (Finlay & Molano Fisher, 2008), the story that stood out for us – the one that 'emerged' out of the data – was the trauma and ups and downs of her rehabilitation. Pat did not simply move from deaf to hearing; she was catapulted onto a 'roller-coaster ride'. It seemed that the best way to encompass this experience was to construct a narrative showing this.

If you are still stuck, you could *talk* to someone: explain your work to them; discover what you tell them first and what engages them. Perhaps, *brainstorm* ideas and write a paragraph or two about one theme emerging in your research. It can help to engage in spontaneous '*free writing*',[ii] giving yourself permission to play with your own words; just fly and discover landscapes and landing grounds. It can also help to practise by using a writing habit, say making daily entries in a *journal* (Evans, 2009).

Marshalling Your Evidence

Once you have a sense of where you are going and you have started writing up, your next challenge is to marshal your 'evidence': what *examples* illustrate your point? Are there particularly powerful *quotes* from the interview or other data which you might offer? What other academic *references* could you cite to substantiate your argument?

Example 16.1 offers an example of how such examples, quotes and references might be marshalled. The extract comes from a broader research study where I theorized[iii] the nature of the therapeutic relationship in psychotherapy. I argued for **six dimensions of '*being-with*'** which, I proposed, are present at every stage of, and in every moment of therapy:

- Embodied *being-with* (i.e. focus on physical and non-verbal aspects);
- Person-to-person *being-with* (i.e. focus on cognition and emotions);
- Inter-personal *being-with* (i.e. focus on multiple selves/subjectivities);
- Intra-personal, transferential *being-with* (i.e. focus on unconscious);
- Structural, cultural *being-with* (i.e. focus on social aspects);
- Transpersonal *being-with* (i.e. focus on spiritual aspects).

In my argument I suggested that while psychotherapists are likely to be familiar with each of these intersubjective dimensions, the complex way in which they interlink and shape each other needs greater emphasis. My research was an attempt to integrate awareness of processes occurring at different levels in psychotherapy practice. It helped me to articulate tacit dimensions of my practice. I also hoped it might inform other psychotherapists and offer a way for them to view their own work.

To substantiate and evidence this argument, I turned to the data plus wider academic references. My data was the dialogue between myself and my client 'Lisa' taken from one psychotherapy session, together with my subsequent reflexive notes. In Example 16.1 I explore the spiritual or 'transpersonal' dimension occurring within the session. In the dialogue with 'Lisa' I find myself sharing my maternal counter-transferential feelings (i.e. I step into a reparative transference as I attempt to ease, rightly or wrongly, some of the guilt she is feeling about her temptation to have an extramarital affair).

Example 16.1   '*Being-with*': a phenomenology of relational dimensions within a psychotherapy session[iv]

Hycner (1991) explains that the very recognition that there is something more to *being-with* than the sum total of the individuals physically present; he acknowledges a transpersonal element. The transpersonal (beyond personal) or spiritual dimension of *being-with* is the hardest to pinpoint. For some individuals, relationships may involve a mystical, religious, mysterious connection; for others, a spirit of love, compassion, empathy, intuition, healing, or delight-in-the-other; humanity may animate the relationship. For some, transcendence resides in a Divine other or sacred moment where one is taken beyond oneself; for others transcendence is located within the person and refers to our capacity to be moved and to move forward.

The following excerpt of dialogue shows how Lisa and I began to embrace [Buber's] *I-Thou* relating:

[The pull of the maternal transference feels particularly powerful. I take the opportunity to share in the spirit of I-Thou. Committing to the 'between' I allow myself to raise what seems figural. I hope Lisa will receive this and reciprocate in I-Thou.]

Linda: Suddenly I'm feeling maternal . . . I just want to say to you, 'Its okay,' [Lisa: hm] you know that every woman, probably every person . . . we all have these feelings when we're in a long-term relationship. It's inevitable. [Lisa laughs]. So I kinda want to say 'don't feel too guilty [Lisa: yeah]'.

Lisa: But that's not maternal is it?

[I am astounded that Lisa has made this link and challenge to me. She is acknowledging, I believe, a juxtaposition between her experience of her mother and me.]

Lisa: My mother would be saying 'Don't mess everything up! You've got this you've got that. Look at all the good things you've got. Don't screw it up. Just forget him. Aarararargh.'

[She beautifully articulates her introjects here! That I may model for her a non-judgmental acceptance of her behaviour and give her permission to be who she wants to be – possibly unlike her mother – is hugely significant. I'm impressed that it is no longer entirely out of her awareness . . .]

Linda: . . . I do 'mother' a little differently than your mother [Lisa: yeah]. It's like, maybe with me and therapy you can, kind of, get some of your unmet needs from your mum. Maybe that's what therapy offers(?) Cos we kinda re-do it again. I mean, not really, but in spirit. [Lisa: yeah]. .. [Lisa laughs and we pause for several seconds] . . .

Lisa: Yeah, I've gone from him trying to kiss me last week, and now I'm talking about going away for the night and having sex with him now. In just one week. What the bloody hell will I have done by next week?! [she laughs]

[I seek to end the session with my last bit of reaching out to the Lisa who has shyly, slowly, emerged out of the 'cave'.]

> **Linda:** I look forward to hearing about it! [Lisa laughs] But in the meantime, I just want to say 'hello' to this Lisa that has not come out before. [Lisa laughs again warmly]
>
> **Lisa:** Hiya!

*[She says this in a shy sweet voice and gives me a shy wave. I give a shy sweet wave back and we share a precious moment. It feels a **true meeting** ...]*
(Finlay, 2010a, pp. 44–45)

Developing Your Argument

Having marshalled your evidence it is time to pull together your argument so that it convinces and enables others to understand better. Consider, for example, Simms' (2008b) phenomenologically inspired biographical study of children's lived spaces in the inner city from the 1930s to 2000:

> Urban places are not just bricks and mortar for providing shelter. The place we call home is inscribed into our bodies; the street we call ours is the setting for our communal longing and belonging; our neighbourhood is the first world that we know as a child. The bulldozing of the inner city for urban renewal projects . . . devastated the emotional landscape of the African American community of The Hill District. Root shock, the experience of trauma after having been displaced . . . undermined trust, destabilized relationships, created anxiety, depleted social, emotional, and financial resources . . . It dispersed the community and destroyed the web of familiarity and connection that was part of a healthy community (Simms, 2008b, p. 87).

Demonstrating the way places create clearings for, and foreclose on, community activities, Simms critiques The Hill's urban renewal programme. She argues the value of listening to the voices and needs of child citizens which call for the development of safe, child-friendly urban neighbourhoods which allow freedom and encourage neighbourly exchange in close proximity to adult daily activities.

Mason (2002) provides some useful advice for arguing the case for one's research:[v]

- *Arguing evidentially* ('I can make this argument because I can show you the relevant evidence.') . . .

- *Arguing interpretively or narratively* ('I can make this argument because I can show you that my interpretation or my narrative is meaningful or reasonable.') ...
- *Arguing evocatively or illustratively* ('I can make this argument because I can evoke understanding or empathy in you, or because I can provide meaningful illustration.') ...
- *Arguing reflexively or multivocally* ('I can make this argument because I can make you aware of a meaningful range of perspectives, experiences and standpoints, including my own.) (Mason, 2002, pp. 176–177)

Preferences about type of argument rest largely on our chosen methodology and approach. When arguing evidentially, our challenge as phenomenologists is to demonstrate that we have marshalled our evidence systematically[vi]. While this is the particular concern of descriptive phenomenology, lifeworld approaches and interpretative phenomenological analysis (IPA), most phenomenological researchers will try to show how the data constitutes evidence, for instance, by using illustrative quotes and examples. As Halling (2002, p. 30) notes:

> Without well-chosen examples and quotes, the analyses of phenomena and people, however insightful, will fail to bring the reader into a close relationship with the subject matter.

Mason (2002) goes on to suggest three steps towards making a good argument (and I expand her steps to reflect our specific phenomenological interests):

1) *Select the data to include in your argument carefully.* Are you seeking to use data in a realist or interpretivist way? Is it illustrative or constitutive of your argument?

2) *Use that data imaginatively.* With phenomenology, we have permission to engage in creative modes of presentation. A special 'haiku' with all its layered evocations may well be worth a thousand words. Thus, creative experiential forms or polyvocal experimental ones or may be used to evoke and provoke more powerfully than straightforward traditional presentations. Such forms nudge us to recognize how all texts are constructed problematizing notions of 'truth' and 'validity' (Richardson, 1994).

3) *Check that you are convinced by your argument.* This step involves putting your assumptions and analysis to the test, making sure they have been transparently and systematically constructed. In phenomenological terms it is important to demonstrate the application of an appropriately phenomenological attitude in terms of approaching the

phenomenon with openness and bracketing previous understandings. Can you highlight some finding that has come as a surprise?

It is also important to both show and argue for potential value, relevance or significance of findings. I find it constructive to try to explicitly answer the '*So what?*' question. How do the findings help us in our practice? What value is there in understanding the phenomenon more deeply? Has something new or different been learned that was unexpected? Do the findings deepen or deviate from existing research?

You probably will not be surprised to hear that I believe our phenomenological findings matter a great deal and that our research has the potential to offer much. In my own phenomenological research practice I have seen its relevance and impact time and again: I have seen how potentially **transformational** the phenomenological process can be for the individual participants concerned. Often they will say they have learned something more about their experience – the research process has helped them to *make sense of* their own experience. They have also valued the opportunity to give '*voice*' to their experience and to have it *witnessed*. The process of doing the research has often helped participants make fuller sense of their experience. How wonderful if we simply manage this.

Then there is potential for transformation in those who read or hear about the research. I have seen the way that members of an audience can be visibly moved, perhaps even to the extent of becoming tearful, when I have presented research findings, for example, of what it is like to live with disability. Therapists in the audience say they have gained deeper awareness and appreciation of their clients' experience, helping them to 'listen' better. It is to be hoped such learning will positively inform their practice.

To give a concrete example, I have received a number of communications from around the world from doctors and audiologists who have expressed an interest about the research Pat and I conducted (Finlay & Molano Fisher, 2008) described in *Chapter 1*. But perhaps even more thrilling was Pat's own response. She has continued to be inspired by our research experience and she speaks of the research as being a bit like going on a therapeutic journey. As she said in an email communication as we were writing up the research:

> Use the experience we had together as much as you can. It is interesting and valuable. Remember it requires readiness and painful honesty: also respect for each other's skills. Not many people can handle this well. You could have roller-coasted me and you didn't, I respect you for that . . . Without you my story might not have been told . . . What we did was fascinatingly difficult believe me, and we not only ended up with the end product but many other things as well.

Writing up

How do words come?
As appetite, fatigue, like the rhythms of the seasons
awaiting an unfolding
from the calling of the 'more'
the flesh of the world
the interwoven body
Here I am
flickering sense
wells in me
just enough...

The body knows
delicate murmuring
sensing of some gentle form
and then it goes
Unformed yet felt... there is much more than this
much more than this
fleetingly,
vague stirrings echo words, each felt whisper,
an opening to what is known
The body knows
More than this. (Galvin & Todres, 2009, pp. 312–313)

Our challenge, says Halling (2002), is how to communicate effectively with one's readers at both an intellectual and personal level. More than this, phenomenological writing needs to describe well. Perhaps more than any other qualitative research approach, phenomenologists are required to be attentive to the way we express our findings. A phenomenological text is most successful, van Manen declares, when readers feel directly addressed by it:

> Textual emotion, textual understanding can bring an otherwise sober-minded person (the reader but also the author) to tears and to a more deeply understood worldy engagement... To write phenomenologically is the untiring effort to author a sensitive grasp of being itself. (van Manen, 1990, pp. 129, 132)

Unfortunately, most of us are not gifted professional writers and artists; attempting to 'stir the sensibilities' can be a struggle too far. I personally find it helpful to express myself in terms of metaphors as a way of giving my writing a literary edge. Another useful technique is to draw explicitly on the different senses of taste, smell, sight, touch, sound and the way they co-mingle in order to bring words alive. Thus, we might see colours when we hear wonderful music; a sound can have a sour taste. 'Visual and auditory experiences', says Merleau-Ponty (1945/1962, p. 235), 'are pregnant with each other'. Our senses intertwine and open onto the structure of things. In using such metaphoric and sensory techniques, we draw upon an embodied appreciation of the lived world.

In his book *Embodied Enquiry*, Todres follows Heidegger and explores the mysterious relation between language and Being: 'The shape of understanding is first "wet through" by the insight of intimate participation and this can come to language in tentative ways' (2007, p. 19). While some truth about our lived experience can be captured by our language, he wants to assert that the lived body is intimate to understanding. Todres argues that the lived body is the messenger of the unsaid. First, a vaguely experienced felt-sense arises. Then, dipping between the felt sense and language, meanings unfold. Out of a waiting silence, the body resonates with the 'more' of moment-to-moment experiencing. 'There is always a "more" in living,' argues Todres, 'and we cannot say this all at once and finally' (2007, p. 27).

Todres' project, then, is to restore a poetic heart to academic writing. Balancing a concern with 'texture' and 'structure' in our qualitative enquiry into human experience allows us, Todres says, to retain more holistic, embodied, resonant forms of knowing which are not fixed. He argues for an inner poetry to the qualitative research undertaking.

Researchers can facilitate an embodied understanding by making it 'habitable' for others and by evoking lived experience through words in a lively, engaged way. We need to write our descriptions in such a way as to communicate a bodily sense of *being-there*. At the same time readers, too, need to participate to ensure the possibility of an aesthetically rich understanding. This is Todres' project of **embodied enquiry**. As he says, a qualitative research endeavour informed by embodied enquiry would find ways to evoke the presence and aliveness of human phenomena such that we are lead to a palpable and humanized empathic understanding.

Many of the quotations from research write-ups offered throughout this book demonstrate 'good' evocative writing. Just one short example should suffice here. In the following quotation, Todres (2007) describes our existential vulnerability as a 'wound' of human longing and need:

> In living a human life we come with the seasons, with dryness and wetness, with the rhythms of darkness and light, of going away and coming back, of continuities and great discontinuities, with its janus-face of both potential anguish and renewal. Framing and permeating all this is finitude; there, in the possibility of not being, and there, in the fragility of flowers, in the beauty of a sunset, and in the passing of a smile (p. 116).

As I read passages like the one above in Todres' work *Embodied Enquiry*, I am inspired. An image comes to mind:

A gently flowing, gloriously meandering river, one which purifies, irrigates, quenches the thirst and inspires with its scenic beauty. In geological ('structure') terms, I see the river – one called 'Embodied Enquiry' – being carved over time and out of a philosophical landscape. I see it fed by mountain streams and tributaries (the ideas of key existential philosophers). As 'texture', I feel the poetically fluid words of the river, 'wet through' with meaning. The water invites intimate participation and adventure; it calls me to dive into the unknown and bathe in its sensuous depths. (Finlay, 2010b, p. 381)

'Re-presenting' Your Research

It is all too easy to fall into the trap of thinking that once you have written up your research (or submitted your thesis, presented it at a conference or had it accepted as an article) you are done. Really, you are at the beginning. Now is a new journey – one where your understanding and message continues to evolve as you re-present your research in different ways, contexts and for different audiences. For instance, I have re-presented my research with Ann on her experience of multiple sclerosis (Finlay, 2003a) in many forums: primarily I have spoken of it at different conferences plus offered a comprehensive account in the *Journal of Phenomenological Psychology*. But extracts, quotations and messages from that research and from my reflexive diary have appeared in many other articles and chapters. Each time I work with the material my understandings shifts and I see *more*.

I personally find it tragic that so many dissertations languish in university library bookshelves gathering figurative dust. The researchers – most likely exhausted by old efforts and new priorities – somehow turn their backs on their own work. What a waste of labour and new discovery! Richardson throws down the gauntlet:

> Qualitative work could be reaching wide and diverse audiences, not just devotees of the topic or the author. It seems foolish at best, and narcissistic and wholly self-absorbed at worst, to spend months or years doing research that ends up not being read and not making a difference to anything but the author's career. (1994, p. 517)

Surely, as therapists, we have a professional obligation to transform our research into practice and share it more widely? Do we not want to use or apply the research in some way? Do we not want our colleagues to learn from our work? In addition to career advancement, should not research carried out by therapists offer something to enhance practice or to inform professional education? It can only do these things if the research is taken forward and disseminated. Unfortunately, the process of sharing research widely is easier said than done.

The challenge of working out how to disseminate our research comes back to who we are and where/how we seek to have impact. If you are a practising therapist doing applied research, you will especially want to communicate with colleagues or service users. Peer presentations, conferences, research forums and local interest groups will probably be your first port of call. If you are in the academic world, 'publish or perish' is a spectre that looms large for academics in the increasingly competitive university world and you will be working to publish articles in journals.[vii]

The key to presenting and *re*-presenting research well is to be mindful of the audience and their needs and concerns. Can you find a format for your message that communicates? If you are writing for a particular journal, for instance, it helps to be familiar with the level and type of articles readers expect. If you are presenting at a conference, you need to have a sense of audience knowledge and interests.

Newcomers seeking to disseminate their research more widely might model on others. It can be illuminating to watch experienced presenters at work. Alternatively, might it be possible to collaborate with more experienced colleagues? At the very least, find a mentor/supervisor who can guide and support your venture and give you constructive feedback after patiently listening to or reading your work.

Finlay and Steward (2006) offer six tips for (re-)presenting research (written or performed):

1) **Find a specific focus** – Here, you want to find a 'story-line' which will hook the reader/listener in.
2) **Be selective** – Home in on specific aspects of your research which might be particularly relevant and significant. It can be useful, for instance, to limit yourself to just three key points.
3) **Keep your audience in sight** – Who are you writing for or speaking to and what are they interested to learn?
4) **Write/speak in an interesting way** – Aim to make some impact. The best presentations seem to highlight the unexpected, humorous, poignant or particularly intriguing findings.
5) **Adopt an appropriate style and tone** – Ask yourself if you are principally out to inform, debate, impress or instruct.
6) **Be creative** – Might there be more creative, fresher ways of presenting your research? Look on your research as 'wet clay' (Richardson, 1994, p. 523) there to be shaped! (Finlay & Steward, 2006, pp. 253–254)

Reflections

What makes for a good phenomenological presentation or article? For me, clarity and accessibility are important criteria. Academic presentations of research can all too easily appear confusing, daunting, boring and of little relevance to our actual practice. Perhaps you yourself have picked up a research article with good intentions, only to toss it aside after battling to make sense of impenetrable language and jargon?

Phenomenological research is 'animated by the desire to do justice to human existence' (Halling, 2002, p. 20). Yet it has a particular problem as it can often be difficult to grasp, steeped as it often is in dense philosophical ideas (Giorgi, 1997; Halling, 2002). Some writers versed in writing for academic audiences become enmeshed in jargon; their writing corrupted by obfuscating concepts, they have lost sight of the need to *communicate*. Coles (1961, cited in Halling, 2002, p. 29), for instance, was critical of way technical language had come to dominate discourse in his field:

> As the words grow longer and the concepts more intricate and tedious, human sorrows and temptations disappear, loves move away, envies, jealousies, revenge and terror dissolve. Gone are strong, sensible words with good meaning and the flavor of the real.

We confront many challenges when producing our research and it is all too easy to feel overwhelmed and daunted by the task. However, in the spirit of promoting small scale practice-based research evidence that is 'good enough', I would like to encourage budding phenomenological writers to take a risk and give it a go. By sharing your phenomenological insights – in whatever form – know you will be sharing *something* of worth and value. I agree with Halling (2002) when he advises:

> Given the shortage of phenomenological exploration of so many areas, it is likely that even modest or limited studies could make a useful contribution to the understanding of specific human experiences. If we ourselves are honest and forthright about the limitations of such studies, then there is no reason to hold back . . . Let us not be too reticent to speak truth as we find it. (2002, p. 36)

Richardson (1994) suggests that learning to write (and I would add learning to present research) can be seen as part of a process of inquiry. She argues that researcher's self-knowledge and understanding of their topic develops *through* writing. She seeks to 'encourage individuals to accept and nurture their own voices' (1994, p. 523). Ultimately, producing and disseminating your research is a new journey in itself – a process of discovery of ourselves and of knowledge. I hope that, as you take up opportunities to share your research more widely, you too will value and nurture your own individual voice.

Notes

[i] Some of the material in this section has been adapted from Finlay and Steward (2006) and has been reproduced here with kind permission of the publishers Wiley-Blackwell.
[ii] In her seminal work, *Writing Down the Bones*, Goldberg gives the following 'rules' for free writing:

> Keep to a time limit.
> Keep your hand moving.
> Don't cross out.
> Don't worry about spelling, punctuation, grammar.
> Lose control.
> Don't think. Don't get logical.
> Go for the jugular (if something comes up in your writing that is scary or naked, dive right into it. It probably has lots of energy). (Goldberg, 1986, p. 8)

[iii] This kind of theorizing approach offers an alternative route into doing research and is an example of research in its broadest sense as '*scholarly activity*'. In other words, research does not just mean scientific empirical activity where a researcher formally studies the behaviour and experience of participants.
[iv] This extract has been reproduced from Finlay (2010a) in the *British Journal of Psychotherapy Integration* with the kind permission of its editor, Maria Gilbert.
[v] These differences in approach imply different understandings of what constitutes 'data and analysis', 'description', 'truth' and theory-building and so on. The differences go to the heart of what we are trying to do in our human science research. Is our purpose to follow the model of *natural science* or do we wish to support a more *moral science* (concerned with human potential) or *political science* (i.e. having a critical edge seeing our work as part of the process of social change) (Wetherell, 1996)? Our project in phenomenology is most commonly concerned with supporting a moral science concerned with human potential and existence though, depending on our methodology, we may also go in other directions.
[vi] To argue **interpretively or narratively**, the aim is to show that our interpretations are both reasonable and suitably nuanced. The examples in *Chapter 7* and *Chapter 10* particularly illustrate this approach where researchers aim to produce findings that capture the messy, ambivalent richness of experience. Arguing **evocatively or illustratively** involves getting readers/the audience to understand experientially – to 'feel' the power of our research. This is similarly the particular concern of both hermeneutic and first-person phenomenologists. Finally, in arguing **reflexively or multivocally**, our aim is to show sensitivity to the co-created nature of our research. The examples in *Chapter 11* stand out as prizing this approach.
[vii] Of course, getting work published is easier said than done. It is beyond the scope of this chapter to address this but there are helpful books on writing up and getting published; for instance, Wolcott (1990) and Richardson (1994).

Chapter 17

Evaluating Research[i]

An excess of the Apollonian tendency to make everything controlled and explicit, and the inquiry will lose depth, range and richness . . . An excess of the Dionysian propensity to allow for improvisation, creative spontaneity, synchronicity, situational responsiveness and tacit diffusion, and the inquiry will lose its focus. (Heron, 1996, p. 47)

Good phenomenological research evokes the lived world. It challenges or deepens our understandings of the lived experience being studied. It helps us grow and enriches our work as practitioners. Good phenomenological research is also likely to be rigorous and transparently trustworthy. These are the qualities we try to bring into our own phenomenological research and they are what we look for when evaluating other people's work.

Of course, what is considered 'evocative', 'enriching' or 'trustworthy' research partly depends on the beholder – whatever works for you. It also depends on the type of methodology involved. If you are evaluating a piece of research, it helps to do so within the frame of its own terms and values. For example, there are the approaches that prioritize scientific rigour and with these you would want to look for evidence that research has been systematically, coherently and conscientiously conducted. Giorgi's descriptive phenomenology, Dahlberg's reflective lifeworld approach and Smith's interpretative phenomenological analysis (IPA) fall into this category. Other phenomenological approaches are characterized by more artful, resonant,

Phenomenology for Therapists: Researching the Lived World, First Edition. Linda Finlay.
© 2011 Linda Finlay. Published 2011 by John Wiley & Sons, Ltd.

aesthetic forms exemplified in the work of hermeneutic writers such as Jager, van Manen, Todres, Galvin and Willis.

I start this chapter by discussing some established **criteria** that qualitative researchers and phenomenologists commonly use to evaluate research. Then, I offer my own criteria developed with Ken Evans (Finlay & Evans, 2009). In our view the best qualitative research shows evidence of *rigour, resonance, reflexivity* and *relevance* (the **4 R's**). Depending on the type of research, one or other of these criteria might be specifically fore-grounded and valued. By way of illustration, I present **extracts** from research projects that I believe fall into the category of good phenomenological research.

Evaluation criteria

It would be nice if knowledge claims stemming from therapy research were 'so powerful and convincing that they ... carry the validation with them, like a strong piece of art' (Kvale, 1996, p. 252). Unfortunately, this rarely happens. More commonly the value of qualitative research needs to be demonstrated, argued for and justified. Without this, researchers lay themselves open to the criticism from quantitatively orientated colleagues who regard qualitative research as 'merely subjective assertion supported by unscientific method' (Ballinger, 2006, p. 235).

Qualitative researchers require evaluation criteria quite distinct from those of quantitative investigators: criteria that are responsive to our particular values and goals. (For instance, quantitative researchers value consistent, reliable use of measures to allow for studies to be replicated. By definition, qualitative researchers do not believe situations can be replicated and that what emerges as 'data' is the product of that specific interpersonal and social context.) Our criteria need to acknowledge that 'trust and truths are fragile' and that good research is that which engages 'with the messiness and complexity of data interpretation in ways that ... reflect the lives of ... participants' (Savin-Baden & Fisher, 2002, p. 191).

Lincoln and Guba (1985) propose the four criteria of credibility, transferability, dependability and confirmability as a way of formalizing the rigour and trustworthiness of qualitative research.[ii] *Credibility* replaces the conventional quantitative criterion of 'internal validity' by focusing on the degree to which findings make sense. *Transferability* replaces the concepts of 'external validity' and 'generalizability' by seeking to give readers enough information to judge the applicability of the findings to other settings. *Dependability* and *confirmability* replace 'reliability' and 'objectivity'. They encourage researchers to provide a transparent and self-critical reflexive analysis to act as an audit trail about their research processes which can be laid open to external scrutiny.[iii]

In the phenomenological field a number of researchers suggest ways to ensure good quality qualitative research. For instance, Smith *et al.* (2009) – drawing on Yardley (2000) – present four broad principles for assessing quality: *sensitivity to context; commitment and rigour; transparency and coherence; and impact and importance.*[iv] These are all useful categories to bear in mind when appraising your own or others' research. **Rigour** in IPA, for example, is shown by the quality of analysis:

> The analysis must . . . be sufficiently interpretative, moving beyond a simple description of what is there to an interpretation of what it means. Good IPA studies tell the reader something important about the particular individual participants as well as something important about the themes they share. (Smith *et al.*, 2008, p. 181)

Smith *et al.* go on to recommend extracts from participants' interviews need to be offered to illustrate each theme. (For smaller sample sizes extracts from all the participants would usually be presented.) (See Smith (in press) for an extended discussion on what makes a good IPA study.)

Dahlberg *et al.* (2008) similarly argue the case for rigour in phenomenology but their focus is more concerned with coherence and twinning epistemological concerns with method:

> Too little attention is paid to the coherence among the epistemological assumptions, research questions, methods, and results of investigations and their values. Weak philosophical and epistemological insights easily end up in a mish-mash of methods. Phenomenology, hermeneutics and the reflective lifeworld research approach offer a consistent epistemology that form a solid basis for research, a firm foundation that prevents the researcher from scientific malpractice at the same time as it preserves the richness and beauty of the lifeworld. (p. 350)

Like Dahlberg *et al.*, Todres and Galvin (2006) argue the case for *both* scientific concern which foregrounds the '**structure**' of the phenomenon, and a communicative concern which highlights '**texture**'. Put in other words, they value both rigour and resonance.

In their study of the experience of caring for a partner with Alzheimer's disease, Todres and Galvin persuasively combine both descriptive *and* hermeneutic methodology. They highlight the structures of six key themes which they call phenomenon. Then, having described the experience in detail, they offer an embodied interpretation of that theme. Example 17.1, taken from the description of the phenomenon/theme of 'learning to live with L's memory loss', shows this process (see also p. 255 where the findings are presented in poetic form).

Example 17.1   Caring for a loved one with Alzheimer's: structural description *and* textural interpretation

Through numerous experiences of L's memory loss, M first learned that he could not control or stop its exacerbation. Initially he found this extremely irritating and used the term 'nauseous' to express his visceral, angry, emotional reaction to what was, to him, the repetitiveness of her saying or doing something over and over again.

His initial angry response to her forgetfulness manifested itself in an attempt to control her into being less forgetful. This was part of his caring burden and at times, he needed respite from it as his own health was suffering.

Coming to terms with L's increasing memory loss involved a complex process of learning to be patient with her behaviour . . . He became aware that his impatience produced a downward spiral in which L would become further unsettled and confused; M would then feel remorse and wanted to avoid this in future . . .

Embodied interpretation

To see a loved one change in this way. No . . . How deep is the urge to want to stop the exacerbation of memory loss in the loved one? It deserves at least an angry 'No,' a great refusal, a denial in any way that is possible. At times, it is also a sinking feeling, the 'nausea' of an awareness that relentlessly breaks through. We need psychological strategies to temper the awareness that the memory loss cannot be stopped: anger towards self, loved one, professional . . . He feels remorse and such remorse carries a dawning awareness that this way of trying to deny the memory loss does not work. It is ironic that the passionate 'no' to the memory loss is a care that can be experienced as a lack of care. As the intimate carer is able to 'let in,' and accept to some degree, that the change is happening; care begins to take the form of patience. (Todres & Galvin, 2006, p. 53)

The 4 R's

Research can be evaluated in terms of what Ken Evans and I call the 4 R's: *rigour, relevance, resonance* and the extent that *reflexivity* is demonstrated (Finlay, 2006d; Finlay & Evans, 2009).

Rigour asks: has the research been competently managed and systematically worked through? Is the research coherent and does the report clearly describe it? Has the structure of the phenomenon been well described? Is the evidence marshalled well and is it open to external audit? Are the researcher's interpretations both plausible and justified? To what extent do the findings match the evidence and are they convincing? Have the knowledge claims been 'tested', validated and argued in dialogue with others (including participants, supervisors or colleagues)?

Relevance concerns the value of the research in terms of its applicability and contribution. Does the research add to the body of knowledge relating to an issue or aspect of social life? Does it enrich our understanding of the human condition or of the therapy process? Is it empowering and/or growth-enhancing for either the participants involved and/or the readers? Does it offer therapists any guidance and will it help to improve their practice in some way?

Resonance taps into emotional, artistic and/or spiritual dimensions which can probably only be judged in the eye of the beholder. To what extent are *you* 'touched' by the findings? Are they sufficiently vivid or powerful to draw readers in? Can readers enter the research account emotionally? Are the findings textured and do they resonate with readers' own experiences and understandings? Or do they disturb, unsettle and push the boundaries of the taken-for-granted? Are the findings presented in a particularly powerful, graceful or poignant way? Polkinghorne (1983) alludes to this idea of resonance in his recommended criteria of 'vividness', 'accuracy', 'richness' and 'elegance' as ways of judging the trustworthiness of phenomenological research.[v]

Finally, **reflexivity** is a broad category which refers to the researcher's self-awareness and openness about the research process. To what extent has the researcher taken into account their own subjectivity and positioning and the possible impact of these on the research? Have they explored how meanings were elicited in an interpersonal, intersubjective context? Has the researcher monitored the potential for the abuse of power in the research relationship? Does the researcher demonstrate ethical integrity and concern for the wider impact of the research? At the same time, does the researcher display an appropriate level of humility in acknowledging the limitations of any findings and in the knowledge claimed?

Figure 17.1 presents these four criteria in the shape of a pie whose pieces are a moveable feast. Each of the quadrants can be enlarged or reduced depending on the researcher's aims and values and the research context. The best research *communicates* and is presented in a way that *fits the audience's or readers' interests*.

The quandrant sizes may also shift according to the stage of research. For instance, more attention might be paid to rigour and reflexivity during data collection and analysis, while resonance and relevance might come to the fore at the writing up stage.

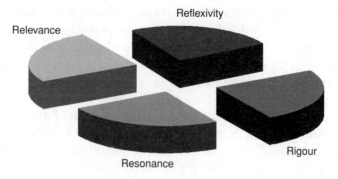

Figure 17.1   Evaluating research using the 4 R's.

Examples of 'good' phenomenological studies

The sections that follow present extracts from three separate pieces of research. I recommend you go to the published sources to appreciate the research in its fullness. However, the extracts are offered here to exemplify what a 'rigorous', 'resonant' or 'reflexive' piece of research *might* look like. (As they each relate to some aspect of health/illness I am already assuming they are all 'relevant', so I do not give a separate example of 'relevance'.) Of course, the selection of these examples reflects my view of good research. Do you agree with me?

Example 17.2   Rigorous research? The experience of chronic back pain

Osborn and Smith (1998) report an *IPA study* of nine women's experience of chronic lower back pain. They highlight the way that experience of pain – the distress it causes and the disability resulting – is mediated by its sufferer's meanings. They conclude that:

> Participants shared an inability to explain the persistent presence of their pain or to reconstruct any contemporary self-regard. While they used social comparisons to try and help them make sense of their situation, these comparisons proved equivocal in their outcome. Participants were unable to establish the legitimacy of the chronic nature of their pain and in certain situations felt obliged to appear ill to conform to the expectations of others. By default, participants treated their own pain as a stigma and tended to withdraw from social contact. They felt confused, afraid for their future and vulnerable to shame. (p. 65)

To go into more detail, here is an extract from one theme – 'withdrawing from others':

> To the participants, their chronic pain was problematic as it was an invisible and private experience but had profound social consequences . . . They were required to reconcile the restrictions of their pain with the demands of their social network, and more often than not this resulted in their withdrawal from social contact . . .
>
> The accounts of the participants in this study highlighted how their experience of chronic pain was closely linked to a sense of stigma, shame and apologism. Chronic pain left them anticipating and fearing misunderstanding and rejection and while the lack of social contact was mourned, the personal costs associated with engagement with others meant that they preferred to withdraw from that social world. (1998, p. 78)

In the fuller article, Osborn and Smith demonstrate their rigour by offering a layered analysis. The numerous quotes (from 8/9 of the women) provide some transparency about how the researchers reached their conclusion. Themes concerning the lived experience are unpacked in detail and systematically, and then helpfully related to other literature. Ideas such as 'social comparison' and 'shame' are interesting and nicely extend understandings of lived experience.

In Example 17.3, Rameshera Rao uses *descriptive phenomenology* to explicate the experience of self-harming by cutting. Through her powerful description she shows her empathy for the self-cutter and tries to elicit a direct emotional response in the reader. She gives a phenomenological description of the self-cutter's experience of cutting as 'wounding to heal'.

Example 17.3   Resonant research? The experience of self-cutting

This passage has been taken from the broader study in which Rao demonstrates the care and rigour taken with her phenomenology. In this passage, Rao summarizes her research findings on the basis of a composite account of several cutters' descriptions. Her intent is as much literary as it is scientific.[vi]

> Self-cutting occurs in the context of a painful interpersonal event which calls into question the individual's already tenuous competence and worthiness . . . when she experiences the pain of rejection, disappointment, or distrust, her body is . . . attended to in terms of its limitations . . .
>
> For the cutter, conventional expressions of pain are difficult to articulate and/or remain unheard. Prior to cutting, she may have tried other actions to gain a handle on herself, but these do not diminish her pain. Unable

to take effective action against the painful and unexpected event, she falls .
helplessly into despair. She feels trapped, unable to free herself from the
intolerable situation and accompanying bodily discomfort . . .

The cutter opens lacerations and feels "a high." The act of cutting dimin-
ishes the rising pressure, racing thoughts, and overwhelming emotions.
She is assured by the ability to create, localize, and regulate cutting. This
is the one action she can take in a time of helpless desperation. Cutting
is always a comforting movement that momentarily frees her from the
"stuckness" of suffering. It is healing to recover a sense of calm, mastery,
and agency when she feels helpless, out of control, and stuck in despair. It
is healing to reveal and release hidden emotional pain. Wounding herself
makes the invisible, palpably visible and tangible. Hers is a language of
pain; her lacerations, efforts to make sense of that pain . . .

Amid her overwhelm, she is relieved to focus and "get it together" . . . Following cutting, she has a reason to engage in nurturing
self-care. Physical healing may parallel emotional healing. She may cut
for attention to the deeper wound, namely her distress . . . The act of self-
cutting pulls her together only to tear her apart with its self-destructive,
shaming, and addictive consequences. Nevertheless, "wounding to heal"
is the cutter's way of coping . . . and surviving. (Rao, 2006, p. 56)

In her research account, Rao (2006) offers detailed quotations from her
women participants to substantiate her composite description establishing
rigour and ensuring resonance. What she does not do is to reveal herself and
to discuss her own role within the research: in other words, show evidence of
reflexivity. This style is in keeping with her descriptive phenomenological
methodology following Giorgi (1985) which aims to remain focused on
participants' descriptions and reflexivity is downplayed in pursuit of rigour
(for instance, in systematically applying imaginative variation). However,
in this version of phenomenology, reflexivity is enacted in other ways, such
as by showing evidence of careful bracketing and sensitive reflection.

The extract in Example 17.4, taken from McGreevy's (2010) broader
hermeneutic doctoral (DNursing) research exploring overweight nurses'
experience of interacting with overweight patients, foregrounds reflexivity
more explicitly.

**Example 17.4   Reflexive research? Being an overweight
nurse/researcher**

While her thesis as a whole also demonstrates her broader concern with
rigour, relevance and resonance, here she engages reflexivity as a way
of understanding her participants more deeply as well as to provide
a more transparent, ethically sensitive account. She includes herself in
the research and acknowledges her own positioning as an overweight

nurse/researcher. She does this as part of questioning the extent this may have made a difference to the research – a good illustration of sound reflexive practice. In addition, she uses this and other examples to explicate a new concept: what she calls '**embodied empathy-in-action**'. She found that her own experience of bodily empathy with this participant was paralleled in the accounts nurses offered of their interactions with overweight patients.

> Embodied empathy was a significant feature when I offered participants an opportunity to ask me questions in a relatively naive attempt to balance the researcher-participant power base . . . This extract is taken from the second interview with Frances and comes quite late in the conversation when it seemed even more relaxed:
>
> > **Researcher:** Is there anything you would like to ask me about my own experiences of weight and being an overweight nurse? . . .
> > **Frances:** *How do you feel about being overweight then and doing this [study]?* . . .
> > **Researcher:** I've put on three stone since Christmas. Actually what's really interesting was when I thought about doing this I'd actually lost an awful lot of weight and, I don't know, I could actually play the psychology card and say 'of course I couldn't do this research unless I had empathy with my participants, therefore the only reason I've put all this weight on is so that I can do this research', which, of course, is absolute nonsense, but actually I do wonder how comfortable I would have felt, because I hadn't met a lot of my participants ever before, if I'd have sat here being $9^1/_2$–10 stone, whether I would have had the same responses from . . .
> > **Frances:** *Mmm. That's a good point.*
> > **Researcher:** Because I think I'm the same age as most of my participants and I'm a similar weight to most of my participants
> > **Frances:** The thing is, I can sort of talk to you because you are the same as me. You understand about the "crunch pangs!" . . .
>
> It was at this point that we laughed in unison as we mimicked eating crunchy food and I felt that my own bodily experiences were merging with those of Frances (McGreevey, 2010, p.186).

Reflections

Rigour, resonance, relevance or reflexivity. Which are the most important dimensions for *you*? Thinking about the pie quandrants, what sizes would the four pieces be?

Behar once said, 'Call it sentimental . . . but I say that anthropology that doesn't break your heart just isn't worth doing' (1966, cited in Bochner, 2001, p.143). Substitute anthropology for phenomenology. I personally believe that the best articles are **resonant**, textured and wield emotional power. For me, research that sets itself up mainly to establish its scientific credentials is less appealing and shows a loss of faith in the richness of what human experience and human science research can offer. I believe that the special contribution and strength of phenomenological research is precisely the way it can capture the ambiguity, ambivalence and richness of lived experience while touching the diversity and complexity of the social world. I value the communicative power of research (and research writing) that challenges, unsettles and disturbs normal taken-for-granted complacency. I like the way phenomenological research draws the reader into the researcher's discoveries and allows new and deeper views into the worlds of others.

There is, of course, a place for different sorts of research and writing depending on the audience/readership. Both science and art are important. A research article destined for a medically orientated journal would need to engage much more with scientific credibility than with artistic flair. A presentation to a user group would probably need to have more emotional and practical credibility. For therapy journals, both elements could be valued and perhaps Todres and Galvin's (2006) approach of combining structure and texture – head and heart – offers a useful model.

In the future when you are considering a piece of research (be it your own or another's) ask yourself: does it express lived experience? Are you impacted by the research in some way? Does this research demonstrate something of the value, interest and integrity of practice? Is this research that therapists want to do and read about? Would this kind of research build a case that will convince sceptical audiences, funding bodies and ethical panels that the research is worthwhile? If the answer to any of these questions is 'yes', then you can be confident you have found some good quality research.

Notes

[i] Material in this chapter has been drawn from chapter 5 of Finlay and Evans (2009) and has been reproduced here with kind permission of the publishers Wiley-Blackwell.
[ii] Lincoln and Guba (1986) later reworked their ideas to incorporate a fifth criterion of 'authenticity' which tapped into themes related to ethics and empowering action.
[iii] Other researchers have challenged what they see as Lincoln and Guba's preoccupation with scientific rigour by arguing for a greater focus on artistic and ethical dimensions. Bochner (2000, 2001), for instance, encourages sociological and narrative researchers to engage an: 'Ethical, political, and personal sociology that listens to the voices of ill,

disabled, and other silenced persons . . . to . . . empower . . . engage emotionality . . . and give . . . sociology a moral and ethical centre' (Bochner, 2001, p. 152).

[iv] **Sensitivity to context** relates to the extent the researcher shows awareness and skill in the research process. **Commitment and rigour** concerns the researcher's investment and the effectiveness of research conducted. **Transparency and coherence** refers to how clearly the different stages of the research are presented in any write-up and if the argument hangs together. The criteria of **impact and importance** point to the test of research being whether or not it says something useful or interesting.

[v] I am grateful to Kate Galvin and Les Todres who remind me that writings striving for resonance might need to be presented more softly to protect others, to avoid doing violence to emotions of readers (be they members of the public and/or of vulnerable patients/clients). Equally, the 'resonance volume' might have to be turned up in a re-sensitizing exercise to ensure practitioners can 'hear' what their patients/clients may be experiencing.

[vi] This research illustrates how research in the descriptive tradition following Giorgi, Wertz and others, can still be resonant and evocative. Resonance is not the sole province of hermeneutic phenomenology.

Appendix

The following offers a model of how to provide an account of ethical dimensions. Here McGreevy (2010) states her case for her doctoral (DNursing) research (on overweight nurses' experiences of their relationship with overweight patients):

> I sought access to enter the research field from the Brighton East Research Ethics Committee branch of the National Research Ethics Committee and a favourable ethical opinion was granted to my study on 4th August 2007: REC reference number: 06/Q1907/76 (Appendix 1). I had to demonstrate that I had considered the potential for harm to participants, which included the time required to participate in the study. The interviews took on average 60 minutes each and participants were also sent their own transcripts as an opportunity for any further comment, reflections or clarification.
>
> There was an additional concern regarding the sensitive nature of the research study that some participants may find the sensitive questions emotionally painful which may surface psychological issues and problems for them. I had arranged free confidential counselling if any participant felt that they would benefit from this.
>
> Participants were all provided with a full explanation of the research study prior to each of the interviews by using a Participant Information Sheet (Appendix 2). Signed informed consent was obtained (Appendix 3) and the participants were advised of the possible risks of participating and the support mechanisms in place should they require them. The participants were advised that they could withdraw from the interview process at any

time without providing an explanation and without invoking any penalty or repercussions. Participant consent was renegotiated at each stage of data generation until the transcripts received their final review by participants.

Participants were reassured that they were anonymised at the point of data generation and all documentary notes, tape recordings and transcripts had no identifying information. They were advised that only I would have access to the data identification material and that this would be kept in locked storage in compliance with the Data Protection Act and Information Governance Protocols until after the study and a time prescribed by law, when it would be destroyed.

The Ethics Committee required some further clarification prior to granting approval for this research study and there was a need for me to offer reassurance regarding the research rigour of phenomenological methods of inquiry . . . It was necessary to emphasise that issues of reflexivity are imperative, as is the necessity to be self-critical, in order to maintain high standards of professional investigation. (McGreevy, 2010, pp. 57–59)

References

Aanstoos, C.M. (1987). A descriptive phenomenology of the experience of being left out. In F.J. van Zuuren, F.J. Wertz and B. Book (Eds), *Advances in Qualitative Psychology: Themes and Variations* (pp. 137–155). Berwyn, PA: Swets North America.

Aanstoos, C.M. (1991). Embodiment as ecstatic intertwining. In C.M. Aanstoos (Ed), *Studies in Humanistic Psychology*. Carrollton, GA: West Georgia College Studies in the Social Sciences, Volume XXIX.

Ablamowicz, H. (1992). Shame as an interpersonal dimension of communication among doctoral students: An empirical phenomenological study, *Journal of Phenomenological Psychology, 23*, 30–49.

Abrahams, H. (2007). Ethics in counselling research fieldwork, *Counselling and Psychotherapy Research, 7*, 240–244.

Abram, D. (1996). *The Spell of the Sensuous: Perception and Language in a More-than-Human World*. New York: Vintage Books.

Allen, C. (2004). Merleau-Ponty's phenomenology and the body-in-space encounters of visually impaired children, *Environment and Planning D: Society and Space, 22*, 719–735.

Angus, L.E. and McLeod, J. (Eds) (2003). *The Handbook of Narrative and Psychotherapy: Practice, Theory and Research*. London: Sage.

Ashworth, P.D. (1993). Participant agreement in the justification of qualitative findings, *Journal of Phenomenological Psychology, 24*, 3–16.

Ashworth, P.D. (1996). Presuppose nothing! The suspension of assumptions in phenomenological psychological methodology, *Journal of Phenomenological Psychology, 27*, 1–25.

Phenomenology for Therapists: Researching the Lived World, First Edition. Linda Finlay.
© 2011 Linda Finlay. Published 2011 by John Wiley & Sons, Ltd.

Ashworth, P. (1997). The meaning of participation, *Journal of Phenomenological Psychology, 28*, 82–103.

Ashworth, P.D. (2003). An approach to phenomenological psychology: The contingencies of the lifeworld, *Journal of Phenomenological Psychology, 34*, 145–156.

Ashworth, P.D. (2006). Introduction to the place of phenomenological thinking in the history of psychology. In P. Ashworth and M.C. Chung (Eds), *Phenomenology and Psychological Science: Historical and Philosophical Perspectives.* New York: Springer.

Ashworth, P. and Ashworth, A. (2003). The lifeworld as phenomenon and as research heuristic, exemplified by a study of the lifeworld of a person suffering Alzheimer's Disease, *Journal of Phenomenological Psychology, 34*, 179–206.

Avis, T. (2010). *The Elephant in the Room': a study exploring how trainee counselling psychologists experience mandatory personal therapy and how counselling psychologists experience having trainee counselling psychologists as clients.* Dissertation, City University, London.

Bains, S. (2007). Transforming the wounds of racism: an autoethnographic exploration and implications for psychotherapy. Accessed May 2010 from: http://www.psychotherapy.net/article/Transforming-the-Wounds-of-Racism

Ballinger, C. (2006). Demonstrating rigour and quality? In L. Finlay and C. Ballinger (Eds), *Qualitative Research for Allied Health Professionals: Challenging Choices.* Chichester, West Sussex: John Wiley & Sons, Ltd.

Ballinger, C. and Wiles, R. (2006). Ethical and governance issues in qualitative research. In L. Finlay and C. Ballinger (Eds), *Qualitative Research for Allied Health Professionals: Challenging Choices.* Chichester, West Sussex: John Wiley & Sons, Ltd.

Banister, P., Burman, E., Parker, I., Taylor, M. and Tindall, C. (1994). *Qualitative Methods in Psychology: A Research Guide.* Buckingham: Open University Press.

Barber, M. (2010). Alfred Schutz. Accessed October 2010 from: http://plato.stanford.edu/entries/schutz/

Blouin, P. (2009). *Pornography and eroticism.* Paper given at the International Human Science Research Conference, June 2009, Molde, Norway.

Bochner, A.P. (1984). The functions of communication in interpersonal bonding. In C. Arnold and J. Bowers (Eds), *The Handbook of Rhetoric and Communication* (pp. 544–621). Thousand Oaks, CA: Sage.

Bochner, A.P. (2000). Criteria against ourselves, *Qualitative Inquiry, 6*, 266–272.

Bochner, A.P. (2001). Narrative's virtues, *Qualitative Inquiry, 7*, 131–156.

Bramley, N. & Eatough, V. (2005). The experience of living with Parkinson's disease: An interpretative phenomenological analysis case study, *Psychology and Health, 20*, 223–235.

Braud, W.G. and Anderson, R. (Eds) (1998). *Transpersonal Research Methods for the Social Sciences: Honoring Human Experience.* Thousand Oaks, CA: Sage.

Braun, V. and Clarke, V. (2006). Using thematic analysis in psychology, *Qualitative Research in Psychology, 3*, 77–101.

Braverman, B., Helfrich, C., Kielhofner, G. and Albrecht, G. (2003). The narratives of 12 men with AIDS: Exploring return to work, *Journal of Occupational Rehabilitation, 3*, 143–157.

Bremer, A., Dahlberg, K. and Sandman, L. (2009). To survive out-of-hospital cardiac arrest: a search for meaning and coherence, *Qualitative Health Research, 19,* 323–338.

Broyard, A. (1992). *Intoxicated by my Illness: And Other Writings on Life and Death.* New York: Fawcett Columbine.

Buber, M. (1923/2004). *I and Thou* [Trans. W. Kaufman]. London: Continuum.

Buber, M. (1937/1958). *I and Thou* [Trans. R.G. Smith]. New York: Charles Scribner's Sons.

Buber, M. (1965). *The Knowledge of Man: Selected Essays* (Edited with an introductory essay by Maurice Friedman. Trans. M. Friedman & G. Smith). New York: Harper and Row.

Carel, H. (2008). *Illness.* Stocksfield: Acumen.

Casey, E.S. (1993). *Getting Back into Place.* Bloomington: Indiana University Press.

Chang, H.V. (2008). *Autoethnography as Method: Developing Qualitative Inquiry.* Walnut Creek, CA: Left Coast Press.

Channine, C. (2009). An introduction to Interpretative Phenomenological Analysis: A useful approach for occupational therapy research, *British Journal of Occupational Therapy, 7,* 37–39.

Churchill, S.D. (1990). Considerations for teaching a phenomenological approach to psychological research, *Journal of Phenomenological Psychology, 21,* 46–67.

Churchill, S.D. (2000). Phenomenological psychology. In A.D. Kazdin (Ed), *Encyclopedia of Psychology.* Oxford: Oxford University Press.

Churchill, S.D. (2003). Gestural communication with a bonobo: Empathy, alterity, and carnal intersubjectivity, *Constructivism and the Human Sciences, 8,* 19–36.

Churchill, S.D. (2006). Encountering the animal other: reflections on moments of empathic seeing, *Indo-Pacific Journal of Phenomenology, 6* (special edition), 1–13.

Churchill, S.D. (2007). Experiencing the other within the we: Phenomenology with a bonobo. In L. Embree and T. Nenon (Eds), *Phenomenology 2005* Vol. IV, *Selected Essays from North America* (pp. 147–170). Bucharest: Zeta E-Books.

Churchill, S.D. (2010a). *Second person perspectivity: Towards a depth phenomenology for understanding others.* Paper presented at the Annual convention of the American Psychological Association, San Diego, August 12–15, 2010.

Churchill, S.D. (2010b). Methodological considerations for human science research in the wake of postmodernism: Remembering our ground while envisioning our future. In M. Tarozzi and L. Mortari (Eds), *Phenomenology and Human Science Research Today.* Bucharest: Zeta E-Books.

Churchill, S.D., Lowery, J.E., McNally, O. and Rao, A. (1998). The question of reliability in interpretive psychological research: a comparison of three phenomenologically based protocol analyses. In R. Valle (Ed), *Phenomenological Inquiry in Psychology: Existential and Transpersonal Dimensions.* New York: Plenum Press.

Colaizzi, P.F. (1973). *Reflection and Research in Psychology: A Phenomenological Study of Learning.* Dubuque, IA; Kendall Hunt.

Cronin-Davis, J. (2010). *Occupational therapy practice with male patients diagnosed with personality disorder in forensic settings: A qualitative study of the views and perceptions of patients, managers and occupational therapists.* Dissertation, St John University, York.

Csíkszentmihályi, M. (1992). *Flow: The Psychology of Happiness.* Sydney: Random House.

Cutcliffe, J.R. and Ramcharan, P. (2002). Leveling the playing field? Exploring the merits of the ethics-as-process approach for judging qualitative research proposals, *Qualitative Health Research, 12,* 1000–1010.

Dahlberg, K. (1997). Kroppen: vår tillgång till världen [The body as the access to a world]. *Nordisk Fysioterapi, 1,* 10–14.

Dahlberg, K. (2006). The essence of essences/the search for meaning structures in phenomenological analysis of lifeworld phenomena, *International Journal of Qualitative Studies on Health and Well-being, 1,* 11–19.

Dahlberg, K. (2007). The enigmatic phenomenon of loneliness, *International Journal of Qualitative Studies on Health and Well-being, 2,* 195–207.

Dahlberg, K., Dahlberg, H. and Nystrom, M. (2008). *Reflective Lifeworld Research* (2nd edn). Lund, Sweden: Studentliteratur.

Dahlberg, K., Todres, L. and Galvin, K.T. (2009). lifeworld-led healthcare is more than patient-led care: An existential view of well-being, *Medicine, Health Care and Philosophy, 12,* 265–271.

Davies, K. (2001). Silent and censured travellers? Patients' narratives and patients' voices: Perspectives on the history of mental illness since 1948, *Social History of Medicine, 14,* 267–292.

De Beauvoir, S. (1947). *Pour Une Morale de L'ambiguïté.* Accessed August 2010 from: http://www.marxists.org/reference/subject/ethics/de-beauvoir/ambiguity/index.htm.

De Beauvoir, S. (1949/1984). *The Second Sex* (Trans. H.M. Parshley). Harmondsworth: Penguin.

De Beauvoir, S. (2010). *The Second Sex* (Trans. C. Borde and S. Malovany-Chevallier). New York: Alfred A. Knopf.

Department of Health (2001). *Research Governance Framework for England.* London: Department of Health.

Dreyfus, H.L. (1993) Heidegger on the connection between nihilism, art, technology, and politics. In C. Guignon (Ed), *The Cambridge Companion to Heidegger.* Cambridge: Cambridge University Press.

Eatough, V. (2009). 'My heart was killing me': A hermeneutic phenomenological study of the lived experience of anger. In L. Finlay and K. Evans (Eds), *Relational-centred Research for Psychotherapists: Exploring Meanings and Experience.* Chichester, West Sussex: Wiley-Blackwell.

Eatough, V. and Finlay, L. (2009). *Discovering a kindred spirit connection.* Paper presented at the International Human Science Research Conference, Molde, Norway, June.

Eatough, V. and Smith, J. (2006a). 'I was like a wild wild person': Understanding feelings of anger using interpretative phenomenological analysis, *British Journal of Psychology, 97,* 483–498.

Eatough, V. and Smith, J.A. (2006b). I feel like a scrambled egg in my head: An idiographic case study of meaning making and anger using interpretative phenomenological analysis, *Psychology and Psychotherapy, 79,* 115–135.

Ellis, C. (2007). Telling secrets, revealing lives: Relational ethics in research with intimate others, *Qualitative Inquiry, 13,* 3–29.

Ellis, C. (2008). *Revision: Autoethnographic Reflections on Life and Work.* Walnut Creek, CA: Left Coast Press.

Ellis, C., Kiesinger, C.E. and Tillmann-Healy, L.M. (1997). Interactive interviewing: Talking about emotional experience. In R. Hertz (Ed), *Reflexivity and Voice.* Thousand Oaks, CA: Sage.

Etherington, K. (2004). *Becoming a Reflexive Researcher: Using Our Selves in Research.* London: Jessica Kingsley.

Evans, Kate (2009). 'Rhythm 'n' Blues': Bringing poetry into group work, *Group-work, 19,* 27–38.

Evans, Ken (2007). Relational-centred research: A work in progress, *European Journal for Qualitative Research in Psychotherapy, 2,* 42–44.

Evans, Ken and Finlay, L. (2009). *To be, or not to be ...* registered: A relational phenomenological exploration of what State Registration means to psychotherapists, *European Journal for Qualitative Research in Psychotherapy, 4,* 4–12.

Evans, K.R. and Gilbert, M. (2005). *An Introduction to Integrative Psychotherapy.* Basingstoke, Hampshire: Palgrave Macmillan.

Finlay, L. (1998a). *The life world of the occupational therapist: Meaning and motive in an uncertain world.* Unpublished PhD thesis. Milton Keynes: The Open University.

Finlay, L. (1998b) Reflexivity: an essential component for all research? *British Journal of Occupational Therapy, 61,* 453–456.

Finlay, L. (2002a). 'Outing' the researcher: The provenance, principles and practice of reflexivity, *Qualitative Health Research, 12,* 531–545.

Finlay, L. (2002b). Negotiating the swamp: The opportunity and challenge of reflexivity in research practice, *Qualitative Research, 2,* 209–230.

Finlay, L. (2003a). The intertwining of body, self and world: A phenomenological study of living with recently diagnosed multiple sclerosis, *Journal of Phenomenological Psychology, 34,* 157–178.

Finlay, L. (2003b). Through the looking glass: Intersubjectivity and hermeneutic reflection. In L. Finlay and B. Gough (Eds), *Reflexivity: A Practical Guide for Researchers in Health and Social Sciences.* Oxford: Blackwell Publishing.

Finlay, L. (2004). From 'gibbering idiot' to 'iceman' – Kenny's story: A critical analysis of an occupational narrative, *British Journal of Occupational Therapy, 67,* 474–480.

Finlay, L. (2005). Reflexive embodied reflexivity: A phenomenology of participant researcher intersubjectivity, *The Humanistic Psychologist, 33,* 271–292.

Finlay, L. (2006a). 'Going exploring': The nature of qualitative research. In L. Finlay and C. Ballinger (Eds), *Qualitative Research for Allied Health Professionals: Challenging Choices.* Chichester, West Sussex: John Wiley & Sons, Ltd.

Finlay, L. (2006b). The embodied experience of multiple sclerosis: An existential phenomenological analysis. In L. Finlay and C. Ballinger (Eds), *Qualitative Research for Allied Health Professionals: Challenging Choices.* Chichester, West Sussex: John Wiley & Sons, Ltd.

Finlay, L. (2006c). Dancing between embodied empathy and phenomenological reflection, *Indo-Pacific Journal of Phenomenology, 6,* 1–11.

Finlay, L. (2006d). 'Rigour', 'Ethical integrity' or 'Artistry': Reflexively reviewing criteria for evaluating qualitative research, *British Journal of Occupational Therapy*, 69, 319–326.

Finlay, L. (2008). A dance between the reduction and reflexivity: Explicating the 'phenomenological psychological attitude', *Journal of Phenomenological Psychology*, 39, 1–32.

Finlay, L. (2009a). Debating phenomenological research methods, *Phenomenology and Practice*, 3, 6–25.

Finlay, L. (2009b). Ambiguous encounters: A relational approach to phenomenological research, *Indo-Pacific Journal of Phenomenology*, 9, 1–17.

Finlay, L. (2010c). Reflexively probing relational ethical challenges, *Qualitative Methods in Psychology*, 7, 30–34.

Finlay, L. (2010a). 'Being-with': A phenomenology of relational dimensions within a psychotherapy session, *British Journal of Psychotherapy Integration*, 7, 33–48.

Finlay, L. (2010b). A review of: 'Todres, L. (2007). Embodied enquiry: Phenomenological touchstones for research, psychotherapy and spirituality,' *The Humanistic Psychologist*, 38, 375–381.

Finlay, L. (in press). Five lenses for the reflexive interviewer. In J. Gubrium, J. Holstein, A. Marvasti and K. McKinney (Eds), *Handbook of Interview Research*. Thousand Oaks, CA: Sage.

Finlay, L. and Ballinger, C. (Eds) (2006). *Qualitative Research for Allied Health Professionals: Challenging Choices*. Chichester, West Sussex: John Wiley & Sons, Ltd.

Finlay, L. and Evans, K. (Eds) (2009). *Relational-centred Research for Psychotherapists: Exploring Meanings and Experience*. Chichester, Sussex: Wiley-Blackwell.

Finlay, L. and Gough, B. (Eds) (2003). *Reflexivity: A Practical Guide for Researchers in Health and Social Sciences*. Oxford: Blackwell Publishing.

Finlay, L. and McKay, E. (2004). Mental illness: listening to users' experience. In L. Finlay (Ed), *The Practice of Psychosocial Occupational Therapy*. Cheltenham: Nelson Thornes.

Finlay, L. and Molano-Fisher, P. (2008). 'Transforming' self and world: a phenomenological study of a changing lifeworld following a cochlear implant, *Medicine, Health Care and Philosophy*, 11, 255–267.

Finlay, L. and Molano-Fisher, P. (2009). Reflexively probing relational ethical challenges, *Qualitative Methods in Psychology Newsletter*, 7 May, 30–34.

Finlay, L. and Steward, B. (2006). Disseminating the research: Towards knowledge. In L. Finlay and C. Ballinger (Eds), *Qualitative Research for Allied Health Professionals: Challenging Choices*. Chichester, West Sussex: John Wiley & Sons, Ltd.

Fischer, C.T. (1984). A phenomenological study of being criminally victimized: Contributions and constraints of qualitative research, *Journal of Social Issues*, 40, 161–177.

Fischer, C.T. (Ed.) (2006). Introduction. In: C.T. Fischer (Ed), *Qualitative Research Methods for Psychologists: Introduction through Empirical Studies*. Amsterdam: Elsevier.

Fischer, C. & Wertz, F. (1979). Empirical phenomenological analyses of being criminally victimized. In A. Giorgi, R. Knowles & D. Smith (Eds), *Duquesne Studies in*

Phenomenological Psychology: Volume III. Pittsburgh, PA: Duquesne University Press.

Fischer, W.F. (1974). On the phenomenological mode of researching 'being anxious', *Journal of Phenomenological Psychology*, 4, 405–423.

Fitzpatrick, N. and Finlay, L. (2008). 'Frustrating disability': The lived experience of coping with the rehabilitation phase following flexor tendon surgery, *International Journal of Qualitative Studies on Health and Well-being*, 3, 143–154.

Fonow, M. and Cook, J.A. (Eds) (1991). *Beyond Methodology: Feminist Scholarship as Lived Research*. Bloomington, IN: Indiana University Press.

Frank, A.W. (1995). *The Wounded Story Teller: Body, Illness, and Ethics*. Chicago, IL: University of Chicago Press.

Frank, A.W. (1998). Just listening: Narrative and deep illness, *Families, Systems and Health*, 16, 197–212.

Gadamer, H.-G. (1975/1996). *Truth and Method*. London: Sheed and Ward. (Second revised edition, originally published in German in 1965.)

Gallegos, N. (2005). Client perspectives on what contributes to symptom relief in psychotherapy: a qualitative outcome study, *Journal of Humanistic Psychology*, 45, 355–382.

Galvin, K. and Todres, L. (2009). Poetic inquiry and phenomenological research: The practice of embodied interpretation. In: M Prendergast, C. Leggo and P. Sameshima (Eds), *Poetic Inquiry: Vibrant Voices in the Social Sciences* (pp. 307–316). Rotterdam: Sense Publishers.

Garza, G. (2007). Varieties of phenomenological research at the University of Dallas: An emerging typology, *Qualitative Research in Psychology*, 4, 313–342.

Gendlin, E.T. (1962/1970). *Experiencing and the Creation of Meaning. A Philosophical and Psychological Approach to the Subjective*. New York: Free Press of Glencoe. (Reprinted by Macmillan, 1970. Also available at The Focusing Institute, 34 East Lane, Spring Valley, New York 10977; http://www.focusing.org.)

Gendlin, E.T. (1992). The wider role of bodily sense in thought and language. In M. Sheets-Johnstone (Ed), *Giving the Body its Due* (pp. 192–207). Albany, NY: State University of New York Press.

Gendlin, E.T. (1996). *Focusing-oriented Psychotherapy: A Manual of Experiential Method*. London: Guilford Press.

Gendlin, E.T. (1997). *Experiencing and the Creation of Meaning*. Evanston, IL: Northwestern University Press.

Gilbert, A. (2006). A phenomenological exploration of the impact of a traumatic incident (death of a child) on Social Services staff, *European Journal for Qualitative Research in Psychotherapy*, 1, 1–9.

Gilbert, M.C. and Evans, K. (2000). *Psychotherapy Supervision: An Integrative Relational Approach*. Buckingham: Open University Press.

Giorgi, A. (1975). An application of phenomenological method in psychology. In A. Giorgi, C. Fischer and E. Murray (Eds), *Duquesne Studies in Phenomenological Psychology* (Vol. 2, pp. 82–103). Pittsburgh, PA: Duquesne University Press.

Giorgi, A. (Ed) (1985). *Phenomenological and Psychological Research*. Pittsburgh, PA: Duquesne University Press.

Giorgi, A. (1986). Theoretical justification for the use of descriptions in psychological research. In P. Ashworth, A. Giorgi and A.J.J. de Koning (Eds), *Qualitative*

Research in Psychology: Proceedings of the International Association for Qualitative Research. Pittsburgh, PA: Duquesne University Press.

Giorgi, A. (1989). One type of analysis of descriptive data: Procedures involved in following a phenomenological psychological method, *Methods, 1,* 39–61.

Giorgi, A. (1994). A phenomenological perspective on certain qualitative research methods, *Journal of Phenomenological Psychology, 25,* 190–220.

Giorgi, A. (1997). The theory, practice, and evalution of the phenomenological method as a qualitative research procedure, *Journal of Phenomenological Psychology, 28,* 235–260.

Gallegos, N. (2005). Client perspectives on what contributes tosymptom relief in psychotherapy: A qualitative outocme study, *Journal of Humanistic Psychology, 45,* 355–382.

Giorgi, A. (2006). Concerning variations in the application of the phenomenological method, *Humanistic Psychologist, 34,* 305–319.

Giorgi, A. (2008a). Difficulties encountered in the application of the phenomenological method in the social sciences, *Indo-Pacific Journal of Phenomenology, 8,* 1–9.

Giorgi, A. (2008b). Concerning a serious misunderstanding of the essence of the phenomenological method in psychology, *Journal of Phenomenological Psychology, 39,* 33–58.

Giorgi, A. (2009). *The Descriptive Phenomenological Method in Psychology: A modified Husserlian approach.* Pittsburgh: Duquesne University Press.

Giorgi, A. (2010). A history of the International Human Science Research Conference on the occasion of its 25th Annual Meeting, *The Humanistic Psychologist, 38,* 57–66.

Giorgi, A. and Gallegos, N. (2005). Living through some positive experiences of psychotherapy, *Journal of Phenomenological Psychology, 36,* 195–218.

Giorgi, A. and Giorgi, B. (2003). The descriptive phenomenological psychological method. In P.M. Camic, J.E. Rhodes and L. Yardley (Eds), *Qualitative Research in Psychology: Expanding Perspectives in Methodology and Design* (pp. 243–273). Washington, D.C.: American Psychological Association.

Goldberg, N. (1986). *Writing Down the Bones: Freeing the Writer Within.* Boston: Shambhala.

Goodman, D. and Becker, B. (2009). *The psyche awakened: Trauma, violence, and the other.* Paper presented at the Psychology for the Other seminar, 2009, Seattle, WA.

Grafanaki, S. (1996). How research can change the researcher: The need for sensitivity, flexibility and ethical boundaries in conducting qualitative research in counselling/psychotherapy, *British Journal of Guidance and Counselling, 24,* 329–338.

Granek, L. (2006). What's love got to do with it? The relational nature of depressive experiences, *Journal of Humanistic Psychology, 46,* 191–208.

Grant, S. (2005). Practical intersubjectivity, *Janus Head, 8,* 560–580.

Greenall, P.V. and Marselle, M. (2007). Traumatic research: Interviewing survivors of 9/11, *The Psychologist, 20,* 544–546.

Halling, S. (2002). Making phenomenology accessible to a wider audience, *Journal of Phenomenological Psychology, 33,* 19–39.

Halling, S. (2005). When intimacy and companionship are at the core of the phenomenological research process, *Indo-Pacific Journal of Phenomenology*, 5, 1–11. Accessed February 2010 from: http://www.ipjp.org/index.php?option=com_jdownloads&Itemid=25&task=summary&cid=81&catid=18&m=0

Halling, S. (2008). *Intimacy, Transcendence, and Psychology: Closeness and Openness in Everyday Life.* New York: Palgrave Macmillan.

Halling, S. and Leifer, M. (1991). The theory and practice of dialogal research, *Journal of Phenomenological Psychology*, 22, 1–15.

Halling, S., Leifer, M. and Rowe, J.O. (2006). Emergence of the dialogal approach: Forgiving another. In C.T. Fischer (Ed), *Qualitative Research Methods for Psychologists: Introduction through Empirical Studies.* Amsterdam: Elsevier.

Hansen, F.T. (2010). The phenomenology of wonder in higher education. In M. Brinkmann (Ed), *Erziehung: Phänomenologische Perspektiven* (pp. 161–177). Würzburg: Verlag Königshausen & Neumann.

Harding, J. (2000). *What We Did on Our Holiday.* Black Swan.

Haumann, H.J. (2005). *An intersubjective perspective on the role of personal therapy in being a psychotherapist.* PhD thesis, Rhodes University, Rhodes, South Africa.

Heidegger, M. (1927/1962). *Being and Time* (Trans. J. Macquarrie and E. Robinson). Oxford: Blackwell.

Heidegger, M. (1987/2001). *Zollikon Seminars: Protocols-Conversations-Letters.* M. Boss (Ed), Evanston, IL: Northwestern University Press. (Originally published in German in 1987.)

Heron, J. (1996). *Co-operative Inquiry: Research into the Human Condition.* London: Sage.

Hertz, R. (Ed) (1997). *Reflexivity and Voice.* Thousand Oaks: Sage Publications.

Holloway, I. and Todres, L. (2003). The status of method: Flexibility, consistency and coherence, *Qualitative Research*, 3, 345–357.

Husserl, E. (1913/1962). *Ideas Pertaining to a Pure Phenomenology and to a Phenomenological Philosophy. Book One: General Introduction to Pure Phenomenology* (Trans. W.R.B. Gibson). New York: Collier Books.

Husserl, E. (1913/1983). *Ideas Pertaining to a Pure Phenomenology and to a Phenomenological Philosophy. Book One: General Introduction to a Pure Phenomenology* (Trans. F. Kersten). Nijhoff: The Hague.

Husserl, E. (1928/1989). *Ideas Pertaining to a Pure Phenomenology and to a Phenomenological Philosophy, Second Book: Studies in the Phenomenology of Constitution* (Trans. R. Rojcewicz and A. Schuwer). Boston, MA: Kluwer. (Original work written in 1928 and published posthumously in 1952.)

Husserl, E. (1936/1970). *The Crisis of European Sciences and Transcendental Phenomenology.* Evanston, IL: Northwestern University Press.

Husserl, E. (1970). *Logical Investigations, Vol. I* (Trans. J.N. Findlay). London: Routledge and Kegan Paul.

Hycner, R.H. (1991). *Between Person and Person: Toward a Dialogical Psychotherapy.* Highland, NY: Gestalt Journal Press.

Hycner, R. and Jacobs, L. (1995). *The Healing Relationship.* New York: Gestalt Journal Press.

Ihde, D. (1993). *Postphenomenology: Essays in the Postmodern Context.* Evanston, IL: Northwestern University Press.

Ihde, D. (2003). Postphenomenology – Again? Accessed October 2008 from: http://sts.imv.au/dk/arbejdspapierer/wp3.pdf.

Jacobson, K. (2009). A developed nature: a phenomenological account of the experience of home, *Continental Philosophy Review, 42,* 355–375. Accessed September 2010 from: http://umaine.academia.edu/KirstenJacobson/Papers/150644/A_Developed_Nature_A_Phenomenological_Account_of_the_Experience_of_Home.

Jager, B. (2010). About 'Doing Science' and 'Contemplating the Human Condition': Address to the International Human Science Research Conference at Molde, Norway, June 2009, *The Humanistic Psychologist, 38,* 67–94.

Junker, B.H. (1960). *Field Work: An Introduction to the Social Sciences* (with an introduction by Everett C. Hughes). Chicago, IL: University of Chicago Press.

Kemp, R. (2009). The lived-body of drug addiction, *Existential Analysis,* January.

Kielhofner, G., Borell, L., Freidheim, L., Goldstein, K., Helfrich, C., Jonsson, H., Josephsson, S., Mallinson, T. and Nygård, L. (2002). Crafting occupational life. In G. Kielhofner (Ed), *Model of Human Occupation: Theory and Application,* 3rd edn. Baltimore, MA: Lippincott Williams and Wilkins.

King, N., Finlay, L., Ashworth, P., Smith, J.A., Langdridge, D. and Butt, T. (2008). 'Can't really trust that, so what can I trust?': A polyvocal, qualitative analysis of the psychology of mistrust, *Qualitative Research in Psychology, 5,* 80–102.

Kiser, S. (2004). An existential case study of madness: Encounters with divine affliction, *Journal of Humanistic Psychology, 44,* 431–454.

Kohut, H. (1984). How does analysis cure? In A. Goldberg & P.E. Stepansky (Eds), *Kohut's Legacy: Contributions to Self Psychology.* Chicago, IL: University of Chicago Press.

Krüger, A. (2007). An introduction to the ethics of gestalt research with informants, *European Journal for Qualitative Research in Psychotherapy, 2,* 17–22.

Kunz, G. (1998). *The Paradox of Power and Weakness: Levinas and an Alternative Paradigm for Psychology.* Albany: State University of New York Press.

Kunz, G. (in press). What's human, what's pathological, and what's therapeutic? In G. Kunz, G. Sayre and K. Krycka (Eds), *Putting Levinas to Work: Levinas and Psychotherapy.* Seattle University.

Kvale, S. (1996). *Interviews: An Introduction to Qualitative Research Interviewing.* London: Sage.

Langdridge, D. (2007). *Phenomenological Psychology: Theory, Research and Method.* Harlow: Pearson Education.

Langdridge, D. (2008). Phenomenology and critical social psychology: Directions and debates in theory and research, *Social and Personality Psychology Compass, 2,* 1126–1142.

Langdridge, D. (2009). Relating through difference: A critical narrative analysis. In L. Finlay and K. Evans (Eds), *Relational-Centred Research for Psychotherapists: Exploring Meanings and Experience.* Chichester, Sussex: Wiley-Blackwell.

Leder, D. (1990). *The Absent Body.* Chicago: University of Chicago Press.

Levin, D.M. (1985). *The Body's Recollection of Being: Phenomenological Psychology and the Deconstruction of Nihilism.* London: Routledge & Kegan Paul.

Levinas, E. (1961/1969). *Totality and Infinity* (Trans. A. Lingis). Pittsburgh, PA: Duquesne University Press.

Levinas, E. (1974/1981). *Otherwise Than Being, or, Beyond Essence* (Trans. A. Lingis). Pittsburgh, PA: Duquesne University Press.

Lincoln, Y.S. and Guba, E.G. (1985). *Naturalistic Inquiry*. Beverley Hills, CA: Sage.

Lincoln, Y.S. and Guba, E.G. (1986). But is it rigorous? Trustworthiness and authenticity in naturalistic evaluation, *New Directions for Program Evaluation, 30*, 73–84.

Lingis, A. (1989). *Deathbound Subjectivity (Studies in Phenomenology and Existential Philosophy)*. Indiana Press.

Lingis, A. (2007). Contact: Tact and caress, *Journal of Phenomenological Psychology, 38*, 1–6.

Madison, G. (2005). *'Existential migration': Voluntary migrant's experiences of not being-at-home in the world*. PhD thesis, London: School of Psychotherapy and Counselling at Regent's College.

Madison, G. (2010). *The End of Belonging: Untold Stories of Leaving Home and the Psychology of Global Relocation*. Createspace Publications.

Martin, C. (2009). Religious existentialism. In H.L. Drefus and M.A. Wrathall (Eds), *A Companion to Phenomenology and Existentialism*. Chichester, Sussex: Wiley-Blackwell.

Maslow, A.H. (1956). Self-actualizing people: A study of psychological health. In C.E. Monstakes (Ed), *The Self: Explorations in Personal Growth* (pp. 160–194). New York: Harper & Row.

Mason, J. (2002). *Qualitative Researching*, 2nd edn. London: Sage.

Mattingly, C. (1998). *Healing Dramas and Clinical Plots: The Narrative Structure of Experience*. Cambridge: Cambridge University Press.

Mattingly, C. & Fleming, M. (1994). *Clinical Reasoning: Forms of Inquiry in a Therapeutic Practice*. Philadelphia, PA: FA Davis.

Mazis, G.A. (2001). Emotion and embodiment within the medical world. In S.K. Toombs (Ed), *Handbook of Phenomenology and Medicine* (pp. 197–214). Dordrecht: Kluwer Academic.

McGreevy, D. (2010). *Overweight nurses' experiences of their interactions with overweight patients*. PhD dissertation, Brighton, Sussex: University of Brighton.

McGuire, A. (1999). Cited in Moodley, R. (2001). (Re)Searching for a client in two different worlds: Mind the research-practice gap, *Counselling and Psychotherapy Research, 1*, 18–23.

McLeod, J. (1999). *Practitioner Research in Counselling*. London: Sage.

McLeod, J. (2001). *Qualitative Research in Counselling and Psychotherapy*. London: Sage. (Reprinted 2006.)

Mellor-Clark, J. and Barkham, M. (2003). Bridging evidence-based practice and practice-based evidence: Developing rigorous and relevant knowledge for thepsychological therapies, *Clinical Psychology and Psychotherapy, 106*, 319–327.

Merleau-Ponty, M. (1945/1962). *Phenomenology of Perception* (Trans. C. Smith). London: Routledge & Kegan Paul.

Merleau-Ponty, M. (1960/1964). *Signs* (Trans. R.C. McCleary). Evanston, IL: Northwestern University Press.

Merleau-Ponty, M. (1964). The film and the new psychology. In M. Merleau-Ponty (Ed), *Sense and Non-Sense*. Evanston, IL: Northwestern University Press.

Merleau-Ponty, M. (1964/1968). *The Visible and the Invisible* (Trans. A. Lingis). Evanston, IL: Northwestern University Press.

Milloy, J. (2005). Gesture of absence: Eros of writing, *Janus Head, 8,* 545–552.

Milloy, J. (2010). *Attending to the somatic fringes of the moment* (panel presentation). Paper given at the International Human Science Research Conference, Seattle University.

Mitchell, S.A. and Aron, L. (Eds) (1999). *Relational Psychoanalysis.* Hillsdale, NJ: Analytic Press.

Moodley, R. (2001). (Re)Searching for a client in two different worlds: Mind the research–practice gap, *Counselling and Psychotherapy Research, 1,* 18–23.

Mook, B. (1999). Metabletics and the family. In The Simon Silverman Phenomenology Center (Ed), *Metabletics: J.H. van den Berg's Historical Phenomenology.* Pittsburgh, PA: Duquesne University.

Mook, B. (2006). The changing nature of childhood: A historical phenomenological study. In C. Thiboutot (Ed), *Essais de Psychologie Phenomenologique-Existentialle* (pp. 183–212). Montreal: Collection du CIRP.

Mook, B. (2008). J.H. van den Berg revisited: Reflections on the changing nature of neurosis, *Janus Head, 10,* 461–475.

Moran, D. (2000). *Introduction to Phenomenology.* London: Routledge.

Moran, D. and Mooney, T. (2002). *The Phenomenology Reader.* London: Routledge.

Morley, J. (2001). Inspiration and expiration: Yoga practice through Merleau-Ponty's Phenomenology of the Body, *Philosophy East and West, 51,* 73–82.

Morrow, S.L. (1992). *Voices: Constructions of survival and coping by women survivors of child sexual abuse.* Unpublished Doctoral Dissertation. Arizona State University, December 1992.

Morrow, S.L. (2006). Honor and respect: Feminist collaborative research with sexually abused women. In C.T. Fischer (Ed), *Qualitative Research Methods for Psychology: Introduction through Empirical Studies.* Amsterdam: Elsevier.

Moustakas, C. (1990). *Heuristic Research: Design, Methodology and Applications.* Newbury Park, CA: Sage.

Moustakas, C. (1994). *Phenomenological Research Methods.* Thousand Oaks, CA: Sage.

Mugerauer, R. (1994). *Interpreting Environments: Tradition, Deconstruction, Hermeneutics.* Austin, TX: University of Texas Press.

Myers, S. (2000). Empathic listening: Reports on the experience of being heard, *Journal of Humanistic Psychology, 40,* 148–173.

Norberg-Schulz, C. (1985). *The Concept of Dwelling.* New York: Rizzoli.

Orange, D.M. (2010). *Thinking for Clinicians: Philosophical Resources for Contemporary Psychoanalysis and Humanistic Psychotherapies.* New York: Routledge.

Osborn, M. and Smith, J.A. (1998). The personal experience of chronic benign lower back pain: An interpretative phenomenological analysis, *British Journal of Health Psychology, 3,* 65–83.

Packer, M. (2011). *The Science of Qualitative Research.* Cambridge: Cambridge University Press.

Padilla, R. (2003). Clara: A phenomenology of disability, *American Journal of Occupational Therapy, 57*, 413–423.

Polkinghorne, D.E. (1983). *Methodology for the Human Sciences.* Albany, NY: State University of New York Press.

Polkinghorne, D.E. (1988). *Narrative Knowing and the Human Sciences.* Albany, New York: State University of New York Press.

Polkinghorne, D.E. (1989) Phenomenological research methods. In R.S. Valle and S. Halling (Eds), *Existential-Phenomenological Perspectives in Psychology: Exploring the Breadth of Human Experience.* New York: Plenum.

Polt, R. (1999). *Heidegger: An Introduction.* London: UCL Press.

Puig, J. (2010). *A Fullfilling Challenge: Psychologists' Experience of Working with Refugees and Asylum Seekers.* City University, London.

Qualls, P.A. (1998). On being with suffering. In R. Valle (Ed), *Phenomenological Inquiry in Psychology: Existential and Transpersonal Dimensions.* New York: Plenum Press.

Raingruber, B. and Kent, M. (2003). Attending to embodied responses: A way to identify practice-based and human meanings associated with secondary trauma, *Qualitative Health Research, 13*, 449–468.

Rao, R. (2006). Wounding to heal: The role of the body in self-cutting, *Qualitative Research in Psychology, 3*, 45–58.

Ratcliffe, M. (2008). *Feelings of Being: Phenomenology, Psychiatry and the Sense of Reality.* Oxford: Oxford University Press.

Reason, P. (1988). *Human Inquiry in Action: Developments in New Paradigm Research.* London: Sage.

Reason, P. and Rowan, J. (Eds) (1981) *Human Inquiry: A Sourcebook of New Paradigm Research.* Chichester: Wiley.

Reissman, C.K. (1993). *Narrative Analysis.* Thousand Oaks, CA: Sage.

Reissman, C.K. (2003). Performing identities in illness narrative: Masculinity and multiple sclerosis, *Qualitative Research, 3*, 5–33.

Relph, E. (1976). *Place and Placelessness.* London: Pion.

Rennie, D.L. (1992). Qualitative analysis of the client's experience of psychotherapy: The unfolding of reflexivity. In S.G. Toukmanian and D.L. Rennie (Eds), *Psychotherapy Process Research: Paradigmatic and Narrative Approaches* (pp. 211–233). Thousand Oaks, CA: Sage.

Reynolds, F. and Lim, K.H. (2007). Contribution of visual art-making to the subjective well-being of women living with cancer: A qualitative study, *Arts in Psychotherapy, 34*, 1–10.

Richardson, L. (1994). Writing: A method of inquiry. In N.K. Denzin and Y.S. Lincoln (Eds), *Handbook of Qualitative Research.* Thousand Oaks, CA: Sage.

Ricoeur, P. (1970). *Freud and Philosophy: An Essay on Interpretation* (Trans. D. Savage). New Haven, CT: Yale University Press.

Ricoeur, P. (1971/1979). The model of the text: Meaningful action considered as a text (Reprinted from *Social Research*, 38). In P. Rabinow and W.M. Sullivan (Eds), *Interpretive Social Science: A Reader* (pp. 73–101). Berkeley, CA: University of California Press.

Ricoeur, P. (1973/1990). Hermeneutics and the critique of ideology. In G.L. Ormiston and A.D. Schrift (Eds), *The Hermeneutic Tradition: From Ast to Ricoeur* (pp. 298–334). Albany, NY: State of University of New York Press.

Ricoeur, P. (1976). *Interpretation Theory: Discourse and the Surplus of Meaning*. Fort Worth, TX: Texas Christian University Press.

Ricoeur, P. (1984). *Time and Narrative*, Vol. 1. (Trans. K. McLaughlin and D. Pellaver). Chicago, IL: University of Chicago Press.

Ricoeur, P. (1985). *Time and Narrative*, Vol. 2. (Trans. K. McLaughlin and D. Pellauer). Chicago, IL: University of Chicago Press.

Ricoeur, P. (1988). *Time and Narrative*, Vol. 3. (Trans. K. McLaughlin and D. Pellauer). Chicago, IL: University of Chicago Press.

Ricoeur, P. (1992). *Oneself as Another* (Trans. K. Blamey). Chicago, IL: University of Chicago Press.

Rilke, R.M. (1904). *Letters to a young poet*, letter 8, August 1904. Accessed October 2010 from: http://www.carrothers.com/rilke8.htm.

Robbins, B. (2006). An empirical, phenomenological study: Being joyful. In C.T. Fischer (Ed), *Qualitative Research Methods for Psychologists: Introduction through Empirical Studies*. Amsterdam: Elsevier.

Robinson, F.A. (1998). Dissociative women's experiences of self-cutting. In R. Valle (Ed), *Phenomenological Inquiry in Psychology: Existential and Transpersonal Dimensions*. New York: Plenum Press.

Rogers, C.R. (1951). *Client-Centred Therapy*. Boston, MA: Houghton Mifflin.

Rogers, C.R. (1969). *Freedom to Learn*. Columbus, OH: Merrill.

Roland-Price, A. and Del Roewenthal, D. (2007). A case of heuristic research: Is counselling/psychotherapy helpful to midwives in relation to breaking bad news to pregnant women? In D. Del Roewenthal (Ed), *Case Studies in Relational Research: Qualitative Research Methods in Counselling and Psychotherapy*. Palgrave Macmillan.

Romanyshyn, R. (2007). *The Wounded Researcher: Research with Soul in Mind*. New Orleans, LA: Spring Journal.

Saakvitne, K.W. and Pearlman, L.A. (1996). *Transforming the Pain: A Workbook on Vicarious Tramatization*. New York: Norton.

Sartre, J-P. (1939/1970). Intentionality: A fundamental idea of Husserl's phenomenology, *Journal of the British Society for Phenomenology*, *1*, 4–5.

Sartre, J.-P. (1943/1969). *Being and Nothingness* (Trans. H. Barnes, 1958.) London: Routledge.

Savin-Baden, M. and Fisher, A. (2002). Negotiating 'honesties' in the research process, *British Journal of Occupational Therapy*, *65*, 191–193.

Sayre, G., Lamb, D. and Navarre, H. (2006). On being a couple: A dialogal inquiry, *Journal of Phenomenological Psychology*, *37*, 197–215.

Schutz, A. (with T. Luckmann) (1973). *The Structures of the Life-World* (Trans. R.M. Zaner and T. Engelhardt). Evanston, IL: Northwestern University Press.

Scott, D. (1997). The researcher's personal responses as a source of insight in the research process, *Nursing Inquiry*, *4*, 130–134.

Seamon, D. (1979). *A Geography of the Lifeworld: Movement, Rest and Encounter*. New York: St Martin's Press.

Seamon, D. (1980). Body-subject, time-space routines, and place ballets. In A. Buttimer and D. Seamon (Eds), *The Human Experience of Space and Place* (pp. 148–165). London: Croom Helm.

Seamon, D. (1993a). Different worlds coming together: A phenomenology of relationship as portrayed in Doris Lessing's Diaries of Jane Somers. In D. Seamon (Ed), *Dwelling, Seeing and Designing: Toward a Phenomenological Ecology* (pp. 219–246). Albany, NY: State University of New York Press.

Seamon, D. (Ed) (1993b). *Dwelling, Seeing, and Designing: Toward a Phenomenological Ecology.* Albany, NY: State University of New York Press.

Seamon, D. (2000). A way of seeing people and place: Phenomenology in environment–behavior research. In S. Wapner, J. Demick, T. Yamamoto and H. Minami (Eds), *Theoretical Perspectives in Environment–Behavior Research* (pp. 157–178). New York: Plenum.

Seamon, D. (2002a). *Phenomenology, place, environment, and architecture: A review of the literature.* Accessed August 2010 from http://www.arch.ksu.edu/seamon/Seamon_reviewEAP.htm

Seamon, D. (2002b). Physical comminglings: Body, habit, and space transformed into place, *Occupational Therapy Journal of Research, 22,* 42S–51S.

Seamon, D. (2010a). A singular impact: Edward Relph's *Place and Placelessness.* Accessed October 2010 from http://www.arch.ksu.edu/seamon/Relph.htm.

Seamon, D. (2010b). Gaston Bachelard's topoanalysis in the 21st century: The lived reciprocity between houses and inhabitants as portrayed by American Writer Louis Bromfield. In L. Embree (Ed), *Phenomenology 2009*, Zeta Books. Accessed September 2010 from: http://ksu.academia.edu/DavidSeamon/Papers/169389/Gaston_Bachelards_Topoanalysis_in_the_21st_Century_The_Lived_Reciprocity_between_Houses_and_Inhabitants_as_Portrayed_by_American_Writer_Louis_Bromfield.

Seamon, D. (2010c). *The place of home and at-homeness in Alan Ball's HBO television series, Six Feet Under*, Paper presented at International Human Science Research Conference, Seattle, WA, August 2010.

Seamon, D. and Mugerauer, R. (Eds) (1985). *Dwelling, Place and Environment: Towards a Phenomenology of Person and World.* New York: Columbia University Press.

Seamon, D. and Sowers, J. (2008). Place and placelessness (1976): Edward Relph. In P. Hubbard, R. Kitchin and G. Valentine (Eds) *Key Texts in Human Geography.* Los Angeles, CA: Sage.

Sela-Smith, S. (2002). Heuristic research: Review and critique of the Moustakas method, *Journal of Humanistic Psychology, 42,* 53–88.

Shields, L. (1998). Integrated, feminist writing. In W. Braud and R. Anderson (Eds), *Transpersonal Research Methods for the Social Sciences: Honoring Human Experience.* Thousand Oaks, CA: Sage.

Silverman, D. (1993). *Interpreting Qualitative Data: Methods for Analysing Talk, Text and Interaction.* London: Sage.

Simms, E.M. (2008a). *The Child in the World: Embodiment, Time, and Language in Early Childhood.* Detroit, MI: Wayne State University Press.

Simms, E.M. (2008b). Children's lived spaces in the inner city: Historical and political aspects of the psychology of place, *The Humanistic Psychologist, 36,* 72–89.

Smith, J.A. (1996) Beyond the divide between cognition and discourse: Using interpretative phenomenological analysis in health psychology, *Psychology and Health, 11,* 261–271.

Smith, J.A. (2007). Hermeneutics, human sciences and health: linking theory and practice, *International Journal of Qualitative Studies on Health and Well-being, 2,* 3–11.

Smith, J.A. (in press). Evaluating the contribution of interpretative phenomenological analysis, *Health Psychology Review.*

Smith, J.A. and Eatough, V. (2007). Interpretative phenomenological analysis. In A. Coyle and E. Lyons (Eds), *Analysing Qualitative Data in Psychology: A Practical and Comparative Guide* (pp. 35–50). London: Sage.

Smith, J.A., Flowers, P. and Larkin, M. (2009). *Interpretative Phenomenological Analysis: Theory, Method and Research.* Los Angeles, CA: Sage.

Smith J.A. and Osborn, M. (2003). Interpretative phenomenological analysis. In J.A. Smith (Ed), *Qualitative Psychology: A Practical Guide to Research Methods.* London: Sage.

Smith, S.J. (2006). Gesture, landscape and embrace: A phenomenological analysis, *Indo-Pacific Journal of Phenomenology, 6,* 1–10. Accessed March 2010 from: http://www.ipjp.org/index.php?option=com_jdownloads&Itemid=25&view=finish&cid=66&catid=12&m=0

Social Research Association (2003). *Advancing the conduct, development and application of social research since 1978: Ethical guidelines.* Accessed November 2008 from: www.the-sra.org.uk/ethical.htm.

Spiegelberg, H. (1982). *The Phenomenological Movement: A Historical Introduction,* 3rd edn. (with the collaboration of Karl Schuhmann). The Hague: Marinus Nijhoff.

Spiegelberg, H. (1984). Three types of the given: The encountered, the search-found and the striking, *Husserl Studies, 1,* 69–78.

Stanley, L. and Wise, S. (1983). *Breaking Out: Feminist Consciousness and Feminist Research.* London: Routledge and Kegan Paul.

Stevens, R. (1996). The reflexive self: an experiential perspective. In R. Stevens (Ed), *Understanding the Self.* London: Sage.

Steward, B. (2006). Strategic choices in research planning. In L. Finlay and C.Ballinger (Eds), *Qualitative Research for Allied Health Professionals: Challenging Choices.* Chichester, West Sussex: John Wiley & Sons.

Stewart, J. (Ed) (1998). *The Debate Between Sartre and Merleau-Ponty.* Evanston, IL: Northwestern University Press.

Stolorow, R.D. and Atwood, G.E. (1992). *Contexts of Being.* Hillsdale, NJ: Analytic Press.

Svenaeus, F. (2001a). The phenomenology of health and illness. In S.K. Toombs (Ed), *Handbook of Phenomenology and Medicine* (pp. 87–108). Dordrecht: Kluwer Academic.

Svenaeus, F. (2001b). *The Hermeneutics of Medicine and the Phenomenology of Health: Steps Towards a Philosophy of Medical Practice*, 2nd edn. Dordrecht: Kluwer Academic Publishers.

Todres, L. (1999). The bodily complexity of truth-telling in qualitative research: Some implications of Gendlin's theory, *The Humanistic Psychologist, 27*, 283–300.

Todres, L. (2007). *Embodied Enquiry: Phenomenological Touchstones for Research, Psychotherapy and Spirituality*. Basingstoke, Hampshire: Palgrave Macmillan.

Todres, L. (2011). Experiential-existential therapy: Embodying freedom and vulnerability. In L. Barnett and G. Madison (Eds), *Existential Psychotherapy: Vibrancy, Legacy and Dialogue*. London: Routledge.

Todres, L. and Galvin, K. (2006). Caring for a partner with Alzheimer's disease: Intimacy, loss and the life that is possible, *International Journal of Qualitative Studies on Health and Well-being, 1*, 50–61.

Todres, L. and Galvin, K.T. (2008). Embodied interpretation: A novel way of evocatively re-presenting meanings in phenomenological research, *Qualitative Research, 8*, 568–583.

Todres, L. and Galvin, K. (2010). 'Dwelling-mobility': An existential theory of well-being, *International Journal of Qualitative Studies in Health and Well-being, 5*, 5444.

Todres, L., Galvin, K.T. and Dahlberg, K. (2007). Lifeworld-led healthcare: Revisiting a humanising philosophy that integrates emerging trends, *Medicine, Health Care and Philosophy, 10*, 53–63.

Toombs, S.K. (1993). *The Meaning of Illness: A Phenomenological Account of the Different Perspectives of Physician and Patient*. Dordrecht: Kluwer Academic.

Toombs, S.K. (2001). Reflections on bodily change: The lived experience of disability. In S.K. Toombs (Ed), *Phenomenology and Medicine*. Dordrecht, Holland: Kluwer Academic.

Usher, K. and Holmes, C. (1997). Ethical aspects of phenomenological research with mentally ill people, *Nursing Ethics, 4*, 49–56.

Valle, R.S. and Halling, S. (Eds.) (1989). *Existential-Phenomenological Perspectives in Psychology: Exploring the Breadth of Human Experience*. New York: Plenum Press.

Valle R., King, M. and Halling, S. (1989). An introduction to existential-phenomenological thought in psychology. In R. Valle and S. Halling (Eds), *Existential-Phenomenological Perspectives in Psychology* (pp. 3–16). New York: Plenum Press.

van den Berg, J.H. (1972). *A Different Existence: Principles of Phenomenological Psychopathology*. Pittsburgh: Duquesne University Press.

Van der Bruggen, H. and Widdershoven, G. (2004). Being a Parkinson's patient: Immobile and unpredicatably whimsical. Literature and existential analysis, *Medicine, Health Care and Philosophy, 7*, 289–301.

van Deurzen-Smith, E. (1997). *Everyday Mysteries: Existential Dimensions of Psychotherapy*. London: Routledge.

van Manen, M. (1990). *Researching Lived Experience: Human Science for an Action Sensitive Pedagogy*. New York: State University of New York Press.

van Manen, M. (2002). *The Heuristic Reduction: Wonder*. Accessed November 2007 from: www.phenomenologyonline.com/inquiry/11.html

van Manen, M. (2007). Phenomenology of practice, *Phenomenology and Practice*, *1*, 11.

von Eckartsberg, R. (1971). On experiential methodology. In A. Giorgi, W.F. Fischer and R. von Eckartsberg (Eds), *Duquesne Studies in Phenomenological Psychology* (Vol. 1, pp. 66–79). Pittsburgh, PA: Duquesne University Press.

von Eckartsberg, R. (1998). Introducing existential-phenomenological psychology. In R. Valle (Ed), *Phenomenological Inquiry in Psychology: Existential and Transpersonal Dimensions* (pp. 3–20). New York: Plenum Press.

Walsh, R. (2004). The methodological implications of Gadamer's distinction between statements and speculative language, *The Humanistic Psychologist*, *32*, 105–119.

Wasserfall, R. (1997). Reflexivity, feminism and difference. In Hertz, R. (Ed), *Reflexivity and Voice*. Thousand Oaks CA: Sage.

Wertz, F. (1983). From everyday to psychological description: Analyzing the moments of a qualitative data analysis, *Journal of Phenomenological Psychology*, *14*, 197–241.

Wertz, F. (2005). Phenomenological research methods for counseling psychology, *Journal of Counseling Psychology*, *52*, 167–177.

Wertz, F.J. (1985). Methods and findings in an empirical analysis of 'being criminally victimized.' in A. Giorgi (Ed), *Phenomenology and Psychological Research* (pp. 155–216). Pittsburgh, PA: Duquesne University Press.

Wertz, F.J. (1986/2000). The rat in modern psychology, *The Humanistic Psychologist: Double Issue Collection of Outstanding Articles*, *28*.

Wertz, F.J. (2010). The method of eidetic analysis for psychology. In T.F. Cloonan (Ed), *The Redirection of Psychology: Essays in Honor of Amedeo P. Giorgi*. Montreal, Quebec: Collection du Cirp.

Wertz, F.J. (in press). A phenomenological psychological approach to trauma and resiliency. In F.J. Wertz, K. Charmaz, L. McMullen, R. Josselson, R. Anderson and E. McSpadden (Eds), *Five Ways of Doing Qualitative Qnalysis: Phenomenological Psychology, Grounded Theory, Discourse Analysis, Narrative Research, and Intuitive Inquiry*. New York: Guilford Press.

Wetherell, M. (1996). Defining social psychology. In R. Sapsford (Ed), *Issues for Social Psychology*. Milton Keynes: Open University.

White, M. & Epston, D. (1990). *Narrative Means to Therapeutic Ends*. New York: W.W. Norton.

Wilkinson, H. (2009). *The Muse as Therapist: A New Poetic Paradigm for Psychotherapy*. London: Karnac.

Willis, P. (2002). Don't call it poetry, *Indo-Pacific Journal of Phenomenology*, *2*, 1–17.

Willis, P. (2008). Getting a feel for the work: Mythopoetic pedagogy for adult educators through phenomenological evocation. In Leonard, T. and Willis, P. (Eds), *Pedagogies of the Imagination*. The Netherlands: Springer.

Willis, P. (2010). Two 'listening reading' and illness stories, *Eremos*, *111*, 23–28.

Wise, S.(1987) A framework for discussing ethical issues in feminist research: a review of the literature. In V. Griffiths, M. Humm, R. O'Rourke, J. Batsleer,

F.Poland and S.Wise (Eds) *Writing Feminist Biography 2: Using Life Histories. Studies in Sexual Politics No. 19*, Manchester: University of Manchester.

Wolcott, H.F. (1990). *Writing Up Qualitative Research.* Newbury Park, CA: Sage.

Yontef, G. (1993). *Awareness, Dialogue and Process. Essays on Gestalt Therapy.* Highland, NY: Gestalt Journal Press.

Yoshida, A. (2010). A phenomenological explication of a master teacher's questioning practices and its implications for the explanation/understanding issue in psychology as a human science. In T.F. Cloonan and C. Thiboutot (Eds), *The Redirection of Psychology: Essays in Honor of Amedeo P. Giorgi* (pp. 279–297). An Edition of the Interdisciplinary Circle of Phenomenological Research, University of Quebec in Montreal and Rimouski.

Young, I.M. (1984). Pregnant embodiment: Subjectivity and alienation, *Journal of Medicine and Philosophy*, 9, 45–62.

Zaner, R.M. (1981). *The Context of Self: A Phenomenological Inquiry Using Medicine as a Clue.* Ohio: Ohio University Press.

Index

Aanstoos, C., 17, 41, 275
ambiguity, 17, 232–3
analysis
  creative, 241–3
  ethics, 222–4
  method, general, 99–100, 111–6,
    187–8, 227–33
  narrative, 237–8
  reflexive, 38, 39, 167, 239–41
  thematic. *See also* findings; themes,
    142, 233–7
anonymity, 191, 218
argument, constructing/evidencing,
    252–4, 260
Ashworth, P., 76, 88, 125, 128, 131–3,
    135, 136, 137, 223, 234, 275–6
audio-recording. *See* recording
authenticity, 50, 60, 213
autobiography. *See* first-person
    research

being-in-the-world, 14, 50, 56
between, 22, 58, 166, 214
body. *See also* embodiment; lived body,
    17, 20, 29–42

bracketing, 23–4, 45, 46–7, 52, 68, 73,
    74–7, 78–9, 81, 83, 96, 128, 161,
    183, 208
breast feeding, experience of, 29–30
bridling. *See also* phenomenological
    attitude, 127
Buber, M., 57–8, 69, 160, 176, 218, 251,
    277

chiasm. *See also* intertwining
    body-world, 56–7
Churchill, S., 40, 78, 84, 109, 113, 121,
    214, 215, 228, 277
cochlear implant research, 10–12, 14,
    24, 205–206, 234, 249, 254
co-creation, 80, 104, 159, 174, 213
Colaizzi, P., 76, 83, 94, 277
collaborative research, 161, 165
confidentiality, 190–91, 218
consciousness, 30, 37, 44, 54, 60, 69, 94
contract. *See* ethics
co-researcher. *See also* participant, 175
creative presentations. *See also* analysis,
    creative; poetry, 164, 171, 187,
    214, 241–3

hermeneutic reflexivity, 79

hermeneutics. *See also* Interpretation;
   phenomenology, hermeneutic
   approach, 52–4, 59, 63–4, 68,76,
   78, 79, 81, 83, 88, 115–6, 126–8,
   129–30 139–41, 165, 239, 261

heuristic research, 7, 162–5, 169–71,
   176

human science, 7, 9, 69, 93, 94, 106,
   109, 111, 115, 175, 248, 260

humanistic, 74, 77–9, 106, 209

Husserl, E., 3, 4, 43, 44–9, 66, 67, 68,
   74, 82, 92, 95, 283

idiographic approach, 128, 135, 136,
   140

imaginative variation, 48, 81, 97–9,
   137, 161

informed consent. *See* ethics

intentionality, 37, 45

interpretation, 27, 52–4, 67, 70, 109,
   111–3, 263

interpretative phenomenological
   analysis (IPA), 79, 83, 90, 121,
   139–48, 196, 261, 263

interpretivism, 67

intersubjectivity. *See also between*;
   subjectivity, 209, 234

intertwining body-world, 21–3, 27, 29,
   30, 35, 36–7, 41, 56–7

interviews, 97, 198–201

intuition, 14, 105, 187, 215 228

I-Thou, 58, 251, 218

Jager, B., 21–2, 122, 284

kindred spirit research, 232

Langdridge, D., 64, 120, 174, 244, 284

language, 19, 52, 53–4, 65, 68, 110,
   132–3, 230

Levinas, E., 41, 61–2, 70

lifeworld, 3, 17, 19, 45, 88, 92, 103,
   125–6, 131–3, 230, 234

lifeworld-led care, 127–8

listening, 52, 209–10

Literary accounts, 206–207, 255–6

literature review, 184–6

lived body
   flesh, 30, 40–41, 56–7
   habitual body, 31, 55
   objective body, 31, 35, 36, 55, 56, 69
   patient's, 20, 25, 33–6, 38, 41,
      130–31, 143–5, 151–2, 153–4, 207
   subjective body, 20, 30, 35, 45, 55
   therapist's, 22, 32–3, 37, 39, 40, 42

lived experience, 10, 15, 16–7, 140, 151

meaning units, 97, 99, 103

meanings, 6, 9, 16, 19, 25, 65, 96, 97,
   102, 109, 144–5

member checking. *See* participant
   validation

mental health, research, 33, 80–81,
   237–8

Merleau-Ponty, M., 21, 23, 27, 33, 36,
   38, 40–43, 54–7, 66, 67, 69, 74,
   76–7, 80, 83, 84, 92, 160, 165,
   210–13, 285–6

metaphor, 20–21, 65, 114, 142, 151,
   195, 235, 256, 257

methodology, 87–92, 186

methods, research. *See also* analysis;
   data collection, 9, 59, 99, 103, 116,
   142, 150–51, 161–4, 186–9

Mitsein, being-with, 50, 208, 250–52

Moustakas, C., 7, 162–3, 174, 176, 181,
   208, 286

multiple sclerosis research, 34–5, 38,
   152, 222–3

narrative, 7, 56, 61, 64, 88, 237–8, 242,
   244

natural attitude, 47, 49, 125

noema/noesis, 45

non-verbal aspects, 32, 38, 40, 65

observation. *See* participant
   observation

occupational therapists experience,
   16–7, 32–3, 203–204

ontology, 27